A Guide to
   Training in
Clinical Pharmacology
   in Europe

A Guide to Training in Clinical Pharmacology in Europe

Edited by
Kim Brøsen
Odense, Denmark

Odense University Press
1999

© Kim Brøsen and Odense University Press 1999
Printed by Special-Trykkeriet Viborg a-s
Cover design by Christen Tofte
ISBN 87-7838-459-1

Odense University Press
Campusvej 55
DK-5230 Odense M
Phone +45 66 15 79 99
Fax +45 66 15 81 26
E-mail: press@forlag.sdu.dk
Internet-bookstore: www.sdu.dk/press

Distribution in the United States and Canada:

International Specialized Book Services
5804 NE Hassalo Street
Portland, OR 97213-3644
USA
Phone +1-800-944-6190

Contents

Preface 7

Editors Note 11

Council 12

Upcoming Congresses 13

Austria 15

Belgium 21

Bulgaria 27

Croatia 29

Czech Republic 35

Denmark 41

Estonia 49

Finland 53

France 59

Germany 117

Greece 175

Hungary 183

Israel 187

Italy 191

Netherlands 209

Norway 217

Poland	*221*
Portugal	*229*
Republic of Ireland	*231*
Romania	*233*
Russia	*237*
Slovakia	*243*
Spain	*251*
Sweden	*263*
Switzerland	*281*
Turkey	*289*
United Kingdom	*299*
Yugoslavia	*339*

Preface to the European Guide

Clinical Pharmacology and Therapeutics (CPT) has been developing as an academic discipline over the last 30 years or so, but its impact on health care services has so far been less impressive than had originally been hoped. In the European region, CPT has developed well in some countries but less well in others. The World Health Organisation (WHO) produced an overall document on CPT in 1970 (1) and some 15 years ago the European Office of WHO started a Europe wide initiative to stimulate the development of CPT. This led to a number of publications (e.g. 2, 3) in relevant fields and to the general idea that there needed to be a Europe-wide organization whose remit was the overall development of CPT in the region.

At the same time as these discussions were taking place, the discipline was making advances in a number of countries. Thus in France, Germany, Denmark, and Spain the subject area was being increasingly recognized by official bodies and the impact of the discipline in the educational field was growing rapidly. In addition, the map of Europe was changing as the former Iron Curtain dissolved and the number of countries in the European Union [initially European Economic Community (EEC)] increased. The desire to help the emerging discipline of CPT in the Eastern European countries was strong and at a meeting in Verona in 1991, it was agreed to create an organization which soon became known as the European Association for Clinical Pharmacology and Therapeutics (EACPT).

The statutes of the Association were agreed at a further meeting in Verona in March 1993 and these were modelled on those of the European Federation of Pharmacological Societies. These statutes have now been given legal credibility in European Union law through legal officers in Germany, where the Assocation's bank is currently located.

Statutes of the Association
As exemplified in these Statutes, the aims of the Association are to develop clinical pharmacology and therapeutics in Europe by:

a. Promoting the utilization of clinical pharmacological services in health care delivery;

b. Improving and harmonizing the teaching of the rational use of drugs at both undergraduate and postgraduate levels;

c. Contributing with clinical pharmacological expertise to policy decisions regarding drug regulation in Europe;

d. Arranging scientific meetings, workshops and courses in clinical pharmacology and therapeutics in Europe;

e. Utilizing the skills of clinical pharmacology and therapeutics in counteracting misuse of prescription drugs and other chemical substances;

f. Promoting problem- and patient-orientated drug information for physicians and other health professionals;

g. Increasing the input of clinical pharmacological skills in the clinical evaluation of drugs;

h. Developing quality control schemes for rational drug prescribing;

i. Enabling individual countries to benefit from the diversification of clinical pharmacology and therapeutics in Europe;

j. Reporting its business and proceedings in a recognized scientific scientific journal.

In addition, the Association determined at an early stage that it would seek to collaborate with other agencies interested in clinical pharmacology and therapeutics in its broadest sense. Thus links with WHO and bodies such as IUPHAR (the International Union of Pharmacology) continue and indeed EACPT is co-sponsoring with the Clinical Division of IUPHAR the next international congress to be held in Florence in July 2000.

Links with other organizations are under active discussion, and these include the European Drug Utilisation Research Group (EURODURG), the European Federation of Pharmaceutical Sciences (EFPS) the European Network of Therapeutic Teachers (ENOTT), and others. A proposal to change the statutes of EACPT (as listed above) will be made at the next meeting of the Council of EACPT in order to formalize these links and to allow for affiliate memberships to occur.

Organization of the Association

The members of EACPT are the national societies of CPT in each country and all members are represented on the Council of EACPT which meets at least every 2 years. Each member has a varying number of delegates on Council depending on the size of the national society. Our statutes only allow for individual members if there is no national society for CPT.

The regular organization of the Association is in the hands of the Executive Committee whose members are elected from the Council delegates and which meets twice each year. In practice, the day-to-day running of matters is dealt with by the Chairman (Professor Folke Sjoqvist, Sweden), the Secretary (Professor Michael Orme, United Kingdom), the Vice-Chairman (Professor Giampaolo Velo, Italy) and the Treasurer (Professor Jochen Kuhlmann, Germany), who communicate regularly with each other.

The aims of the Association are increasingly being met. Thus we have now held two international congresses, in Paris in 1995 and in Berlin in 1997. Both conferences attracted in excess of 1000 delegates to a very full programme of scientific and cultural events. The planning of the third congress to be held in Jerusalem in October 1999 is well underway. The Association reports its business in scientific journals and the abstracts of both congresses were published (in *Therapie* for the Paris Congress and in the *European Journal of Clinical Pharmacology* for the Berlin Congress). The fourth Congress of EACPT will be a major event in Florence in July 2000 in conjunction with the Clinical Division of the International Union of Pharmacology (IUPHAR). The fifth Congress of EACPT will take place in Odense, Denmark in September 2001. The *European Journal of Clinical Pharmacology* is the official journal for EACPT and a regular newsletter concerning the activities of EACPT is published there. EACPT has its own homepage located on the following Internet address: www.sdu.dk/med/homepages/eacpt/

Education and training
The importance of education and training to the Association is obvious from the statutes and a newly formed education sub-committee has been active in bringing forward many of the issues. However, this European Guide is the first outward evidence of the commitment of EACPT to education and training.

One of the products of the WHO involvement in the last decade was a brochure describing the status of clinical pharmacology and therapeutics in the various European Countries (4). This gave a brief description of the discipline in each country and those cities where CPT had an active presence. This brochure was broadly welcomed, but it was recognized that much more detail was required if such a document was to have wide acceptance, along the lines of the Petersen Guide in North America.

This guide is the result of many hours of painstaking work by Professor Kim Brosen and his colleagues from Odense in Denmark in order to provide that necessary detail. It describes the nature and organization of CPT in each country and a map gives the location of the various centres where CPT is undertaken. In addition, each centre of CPT is described in some detail which tells the reader about the main interests of the department concerned, the staff involved, and also gives a short list of relevant research publications. The guide aims to be comprehensive and if it occasionally fails in that aim, the blame should not be attributed to the Danish office. In some cases, it has proved remarkably difficult to persuade senior colleagues to describe their department for the benefit of future generations! The guide is aimed at helping future educational initiatives, particularly as far as training of young scientists and their immediate mentors is concerned. They should find in these pages ample information to guide them as to which centres are best suited for their purpose. There will, we are sure, be additional spin-offs from this work as far as regulatory bodies and research collaboration is concerned. In closing, we would compliment Professor Kim Brosen for his endeavour and we would encourage readers to communicate with him as to how the guide could be improved for the future.

Folke Sjöqvist (Chairman)   *Michael Orme (Secretary)*

References

1. WHO Technical Report Series. No 446 (1970) Clinical Pharmacology, Scope, Organisation and Training: Report of a WHO Study Group.
2. Dukes G, Lunde PKM, Melander A, Orme M, Sjoqvist F, Tognoni G, Wesseling H (1990) Clinical pharmacology and primary health care in Europe: a gap to bridge. Eur J Clin Pharmacol 38: 315-318.
3. Orme M, Sjoqvist F, Bircher J, Bogaert M, Dukes MNG, Eichelbaum M, Gram LF, Huller H, Lunde I, Tognoni G (1990) The teaching and organisation of clinical pharmacology in European medical schools. Eur J Clin Pharmacol 38: 101-105.
4. Anonymous. Clinical Pharmacology: The European Challenge. WHO Regional Publications. European Series. No 39, 84pp.

Editor's Note

This document is available on the following website address:
www.sdu.dk/med/homepages/eacpt/guide.html

Any change, amendment or new texts from centres not already in the printed version of the Guide should be submitted to the editor, and will subsequently be incorporated in the Internet version.

Editor
Professor Kim Brøsen
Institute of Public Health
Clinical Pharmacology
University of Southern Denmark
Main Campus: Odense University
Winsløwparken 18
DK-5000 Odense, Denmark
Phone: +45 65 50 37 51
Fax: +45 65 91 60 89
E-mail: k-brosen@cekfo.sdu.dk
Homep: www.sdu.dk/med/homepages/eacpt/eacpt5.html

European Association for Clinical Pharmacology and Therapeutics

Council

Chairman:	F Sjöqvist, Sweden
Vice-chairman:	GP Velo, Italy
Secretary:	M Orme, United Kingdom
Treasurer:	J Kuhlmann, Germany
Councillors:	M Bogaert, Belgium
	K Brøsen, Denmark
	P Dayer, Switzerland
	P Jaillon, France
	JR Laporte, Spain
	I Roots, Germany
	B Vrhovac, Croatia
Honorary Presidents:	G Cheymol, France
	M Rietbrock, Germany

National Delegates:

Austria:	D Magometschnigg
Belgium:	M Bogaert
Bulgaria:	V Vlahov
Croatia:	B Vrhovac
Czech Republic:	T Sechser
Denmark:	K Brøsen
Estonia:	R Kiivet
Finland:	P Neuvonen
France:	P Jaillon
	P Lechat
Germany:	J Kuhlmann
	I Roots
Greece:	A Iliopoulou
Hungary:	B Gachalyi
Israel:	M Levy
Italy:	G Velo
Netherlands:	JMH Schellens
Norway:	H Olsen
Poland:	A Mrozikiecz
Portugal:	F Teixeira
Romania:	V Voicu
Russia:	V Kukes
	L Olbinskay
Slovakia:	M Kriska
Spain:	JR Laporte
Sweden:	F Sjöqvist
Switzerland:	P Dayer
Turkey:	SO Kayaalp
United Kingdom:	M Orme
	D Barnett
Youguslavia:	T Kazic

Upcoming Congresses under the Auspices of the European Association for Clinical Pharmacology

1999
3rd Congress
Jerusalem, Israel
October 3-8.
Scientific Secretariat:
Professor Micha Levy
Clinical Pharmacology Unit
Division of Internal Medicine
Hadassah University Hospital
P.o.b. 12000
91120 Jerusalem, Israel
Phone: + 972 264 27 427
Fax: +972 2 64 22 384

Organizing Secretariat:
PO Box 50006
Tel Aviv 61500, Israel
Phone: +972 3 514 0000
Fax: +972 3 514 0077/517 5674
E-mail: eacpt3.jc4@kenes.com
Homep: www.kenes.com/eacpt3/

2000
4th Congress of EACPT – VII World Congress in CPT
June 15-20, Florence, Italy
Organizing Secretariat:
CMO
Via San Donato 20
50127 Florence, Italy
Phone: +39 055 33 611
Fax: +39 055 336 125 0/350
E-mail: CPT2000@Mail.Newtours-CMO.it
Homep:www.Newtours-CMO.it/CPT2000

Scientific Secretariat:
Professor Giampaolo Velo
CPT 2000
C/o Institute of Pharmacology
Policlinico Borgo Roma
37134 Verona, Italy
Phone: +39 0455 00 408/807 4899
Fax: +39 0455 81111
E-mail: gpvelo@farma.univr.it

2001
5th Congress of EACPT
12-15 September, Odense, Denmark
Organizing Secretariat:
Odense Congress Center
Ørbækvej 350
5220 Odense, Denmark
Phone: +45 66 15 55 35
Fax: +45 66 15 50 70
E-mail: adm@occ.dk
Homep:www.occ.dk

Scientific Secretariat:
Professor Kim Brøsen
Institute of Public Health
Clinical Pharmacology
University of Southern Denmark
Main Campus: Odense University
Winsløwparken 18
DK-5000 Odense, Denmark
Phone: +45 65 50 37 51
Fax: +45 65 91 60 89
E-mail: k-brosen@cekfo.sdu.dk
Homep:www.sdu.dk/med/homepages/eacpt/eacpt5.html

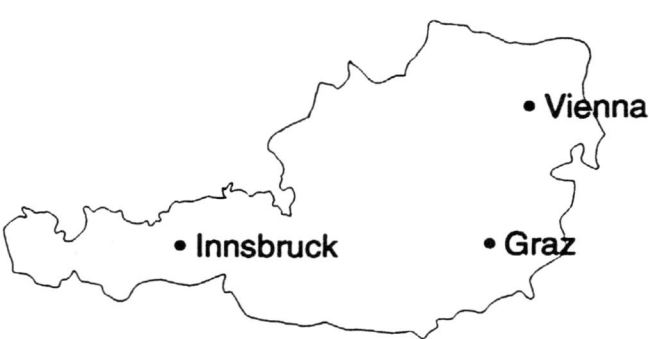

Austria

Clinical pharmacology is an official medical speciality in Austria, but only as a supplement to another medical speciality such as general internal medicine, neurology, psychiatry or pharmacology. For specialists in general internal medicine, neurology or psychiatry, additional training for 18 months at a department or a division of clinical pharmacology and 18 months at an institute of basic pharmacology is required. Specialists in pharmacology need a further 18 months of training in clinical pharmacology as outlined above, and also 18 months at a department of general internal medicine. A more detailed description of the training programme is available at the Ministry of Labour, Health and Social Affairs (Bundesministerium für Arbeit, Gesundheit und Soziales, Radetzkystrasse 2, A-1030 Vienna, Tel: +43 1 71172-0 and Fax: +43 1 71172 4150).

The Austrian Working Group for Clinical Pharmacology was established in 1971. In 1995, the Working Group had 165 members. In order to become a member, an individual must have a scientific interest in clinical pharmacology and must be able to demonstrate specific knowledge in relation to the aims of the Working Group. Private companies and institutions with a scientific interest in clinical pharmacology can also become members. The Working Group has committed itself to support and further develop clinical pharmacology in Austria as a non-profit organization. The Working Group organizes lectures and symposia in clinical pharmacology. So far, 19 symposia have been organized and the proceedings have always been published in the form of a book. The Working Group organizes joint meetings with foreign societies or sections of clinical pharmacology, in particular with the German Society of Clinical Pharmacology and Therapeutics. Joint meetings have also been organized in collaboration with other Austrian institutions or societies with aims that are in agreement with that of the Working Group. Another activity has been to assess, give advice, monitor and document clinical trials. Since 1993, the Working Group has trained investigators. Ad hoc working groups have been established, forming an ethics committee, and another group develops computer software supporting decision-making in individual treatment of hypertension.

The first chair in clinical pharmacology was established in 1971 at the Division of Clinical Pharmacology at the 1st Medical Clinic of the University of Vienna Medical School. The first professor appointed was Dr. Gerhart Hitzenberger (1971-1992).

The Minister for Labour, Health and Social Affairs is politically responsible for clinical pharmacology in Austria. Clinical pharmacologists in Austria provide expert support to the Austrian Drug Regulation Agency. In addition, the Drug Council of the Ministry of Health and Consumers Protection has a clinical pharmacologist as a full time member.

Addresses

Graz
Professor BA Peskar
University of Graz
Institut für Experimentelle und Klinische Pharmakologie
Universitätsplatz 4
A-8010 Graz
Phone: +43 316 380 4305
Fax: +43 316 380 9645

Innsbruck
Professor H Winkler
University of Innsbruck
Institute of Pharmacology
Peter Mayr-Strasse 1A
A-6020 Innsbruck
Phone: +43 512 507 3700
Fax: +43 512 507 2868

Vienna
Professor J Bonelli
Hospital St. Elisabeth
Interne Abteilung
Abteilung für Klinische Pharmakologie
Landstrasser Hauptstrasse 4 a
A-1030 Vienna

Phone: +43 1 71126
Fax: +43 1 7112 612

Professor H-G Eichler
University of Vienna Medical School
Klinische Pharmakologie
Allgemeines Krankenhaus
Währinger Gürtel 18-20
A-1090 Vienna
Phone: +43 1 4040 02980
Fax: +43 1 4040 02998
E-mail: Klin-Pharmakologie@univie.AC.AT

Professor G Hitzenberger
Society for Clinical Pharmacology
Kinderspitalgasse 10/15
A-1090 Vienna
Phone: +43 1 408 451116
Fax: +43 1 408 451117

Professor D Magometschnigg
Society for Clinical Pharmacology
Kinderspitalgasse 10/15
A-1090 Vienna
Phone: +43 1 408 451116
Fax: +43 1 408 451117

Training Centres in Austria

Vienna

Research and training programme: the clinical pharmacology programme in its present form was established in 1992; it is conducted through the Department of Clinical Pharmacology. Major activities are directed to clinical and experimental research as well as teaching of therapeutics and clinical trial methodology.

Clinical and research facilities: The Department is located in the newly constructed 200 bed 'Allgemeines Krankenhaus', Austria's largest teaching hospital, and comprises a modern clinical research centre plus fully equipped laboratory space.

The University: Vienna University, established in 1365, is owned by the Federal Government. The School of Medicine is affiliated with the community-based Allgemeines Krankenhaus.

Current full time staff comprises 10 research physicians, seven trained research nurses plus pharmacists and laboratory technicians. The total number of staff including graduate students is approximately 30.

Application procedures: informal inquiries are always welcomed.

References

Jansen B, Schlagbauer-Wadl H, Eichler HG, Wolff K, van Elsas A, Schrier PI, Pehamberger H (1997) Activated N-Ras contributes to the chemoresistance of human melanoma in severe combined immunodeficiency (SCID) mice by blocking apoptosis. Cancer Res 57: 362-365

Schmetterer L, Findl O, Fasching P, Gerber W, Strenn K, Breiteneder H, Adam H, Eichler HG, Wolzt M (1997) Nitric oxide and ocular blood flow in patients with IDDM. Diabetes 46/4: 653-658

Wolzt M, Schmetterer L, Ferber W, Artner E, Mensik C, Wichler HG, Krejcy K (1997) Effect of nitric oxide synthase inhibition on renal hemodynamics in humans: reversal by L-arginine. Am J Physiol 272 (Renal Physiol 41): F178-182

Müller M, Mader RM, Steiner B, Steger GG, Gnant M, Helbich T, Jakesz R, Eichler HG, Blöchl-Daum B (1997) 5-Fluorouracil kinetics in the extracellular tumour space and clinical response in breast cancer patients. Cancer Research (in press)

Wolzt M, Eder M, Weltermann A, Entlicher S, Eichler HG, Kyrle PA (1997) Comparison of the effects of different low molecular weight heparins on the hemostatic system activation in vivo in man. Thromb Haemost (in press)

Innsbruck

The department is an officially recognized institution for training in clinical pharmacology. It provides training in basic methods. As far as clinical pharmacology is concerned, main interests of the department concern drug evaluation (risk/benefit ratio), drug safety (pharmacovigilance) and rational use of drugs.

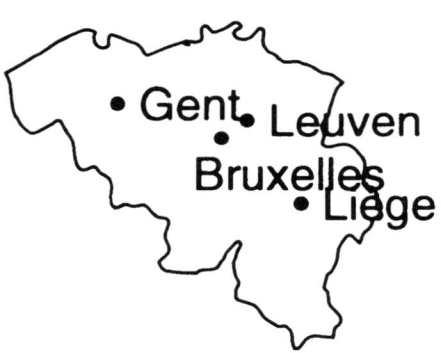

Belgium

There are 25 different medical specialities in Belgium; however, clinical pharmacology is not among them, and is not even considered by the authorities. Accordingly, there are no formal national requirements or a training programme. One is usually considered a specialist in clinical pharmacology if one has a training in basic pharmacology and at the same time is a specialist in a relevant clinical subject, typically general internal medicine, but sometimes also in other fields.

A Section of Clinical Pharmacology has been established within the Belgian Society for Fundamental and Clinical Physiology and Pharmacology. There is an ongoing process trying to identify those members of the National Society who are also members of the Section. It is estimated that about 50 members can be recognized as clinical pharmacologists.

There are no chairs in clinical pharmacology, but in several universities the subject has developed within departments of pharmacology. Clinical pharmacologists in Belgium are active in the National Drug Regulatory Agency. MDs working in the pharmaceutical industry are usually considered as clinical pharmacologists, although they often have no formal training in either basic or clinical pharmacology. One of the medical schools organizes a post-graduate programme in pharmacology and pharmaceutical medicine called 'Pharmed'.

Addresses

Bruxelles
Professor A Dupont
Department of Pharmacology
Vrije Universiteit Brussels
Laarbeeklaan 103
B-1090 Brussels
Phone: +32 2 477 4111
Fax: +32 2 477 5800

Professor A Herchuelz
Université Libre de Bruxelles
Faculté de Medecine
Laboratoire de Pharmacodynamie
et de Thérapeutique (CP 617)
Route de Lennik 808
B-1070 Bruxelles
Phone: +32 2 555 6202

Fax: +32 2 555 6370
E-mail: herchu@ulb.ac.be

Professor JM Maloteaux
Université de Louvain
Dept. of Pharmacology (5410)
Avenue Hippocrate 10
B-1200 Bruxelles
Phone: +32 2 764 1080 or
+32 2 754 5437
Fax: +32 2 764 9336
E-mail: maloteaux@nchm.ucl.ac.be

Gent
Professor M Bogaert
Heymans Institute of Pharmacology
University of Gent
De Pintelaan 185
B-9000 Gent
Phone: +32 9 240 3336
Fax: +32 9 240 4988
E-mail: marc.bogaert@rug.ac.be

Leuven
Professor B Tjandra-Maga
Afdeling Farmacologie
Campus Gasthuisberg
Gebouw Onderwijs en Navorsing
KUL
Herestraat 49
B-3000 Leuven
Phone: +32 16 345806/+32 16 345801
Fax: +32 16 345699

Liège
Professor A Dresse
Université de Liège
Institut de Pathologie
Laboratoire de Pharmacologie
B-4000 Sart-Tilman par Liège
Phone: +32 41 562525
Fax: +32 41 662977

Training Centres in Belgium

Bruxelles
Université libre de Bruxelles
The laboratory is mainly involved in basic pharmacological research, and the staff comprises about 20 persons. The main research interests are Ca^{2+} extrusion mechanisms and ATP-sensitive K^+ channels.

There is a Clinical Pharmacology Unit combined with a sleep laboratory located in a hospital where the unit has six beds and a staff of about six persons. Work is mainly done on demand, and the research programme concerns sleep and drug-drug interactions. The sleep expert is M. Kerkhofs, who is the president of the 'Belgian Association for the Study of Sleep' and Vice-President of the 'European Sleep Research Unit.

The university is also organizing a postgraduate programme in pharmacology and pharmaceutical medicine called Pharmed. It comprises eight seminars of 1 week (one seminar a month) of about 40 hours. The teaching is aimed at providing a specific training for the various functions held in drug companies by physicians, pharmacists, masters and PhDs.

Gent
University of Gent

The unit of clinical pharmacology is mainly involved in teaching of clinical pharmacology and pharmacotherapy, and in research. There is no formal training programme. The research is focused on human kinetics and drug disposition on one hand, and on drug use evaluation and pharmacoepidemiology in general on the other hand. Clinical studies are carried out in collaboration with clinical departments of the University Hospital or other hospitals.

The unit of clinical pharmacology functions within the Heymans Institute of Pharmacology which is the pharmacology department of the Gent University Medical School, and which is in charge of teaching pharmacology and pharmacotherapy for students in medicine, pharmacy and dentistry.

There are no positions specifically aimed at clinical pharmacology, but at any moment one full professorship and several research positions are used for research and service in clinical pharmacology.
There are no formal application procedures as there is no formal training programme. Inquiries can be addressed to Professor Dr M. Bogaert.

References

Belpaire FM, Wijnant P, Van Trappen P, Dhont M, Verstraete A, Bogaert MG (1995) Protein binding of propranolol and verapamil enantiomers in maternal and foetal serum. Br J Clin Pharmacol 39:190-193

De Muynck C, Lefebvre RA, Remon JP (1994) Study of the bioavailability of four indomethacin suppository formulations in healthy volunteers. Int J Pharm 104: 87-91

Fauville J-P, Hantson P, Honore P, Belpaire F, Rosseel MT, Mahieu P (1995) Severe diltiazem poisoning with intestinal pseudo-obstruction: case report and toxicological data. Clin Toxicol 33: 273-277

Lefebvre RA, Van Peer A, Woestenborghs R (1997) Influence of itraconazole on the pharmacokinetics and electrocardiographic effects of astemizole. Brit J Clin Pharmacol 43: 319-322

Rosseel MT, Peleman R, Van Hoorebeke H, Pauwels RA (1997) Measurement of cefuroxime in human bronchoalveolar lavage fluid by high-performance liquid chromatography after solid phase extraction. J Chromatogr-Biomed Appl 689: 438-441

Vander Stichele RH, Bogaert MG (1995) European legislation and research projects regarding patient education for medication. Drug Information J 29: 285-290

Vander Stichele RH, Dezeure EM, Bogaert MG (1995) Systematic review of clinical efficacy of topical treatments for head lice. Br Med J 311: 604-608

Vander Stichele RH, De Potter B, Vyncke P, Bogaert MG (1996) Attitude of physicians toward patient package inserts for medication information in Belgium. Patient Education and Counseling 28: 5-13

Vanscheeuwyck P, Buylaert WA, Vogelaers D, Colardyn F (1993) Cholinesterase reactivation in organophosphorus poisoned patients depends on the plasma concentrations of the oxime pralidoxime methylsulphate and of the organophosphate. Arch Toxicol 67: 79-84

Willems JL, De Bisschop HC, Verstraete AG, Declerck C, Christiaens Y, Laethem ME, Lefebvre RA, Belpaire FM, Vanhoe HL, Bogaert MG (1995) Stereoselective pharmacokinetics of oxprenolol and its glucuronides in humans. Clin Pharmacol Ther 57: 419-424

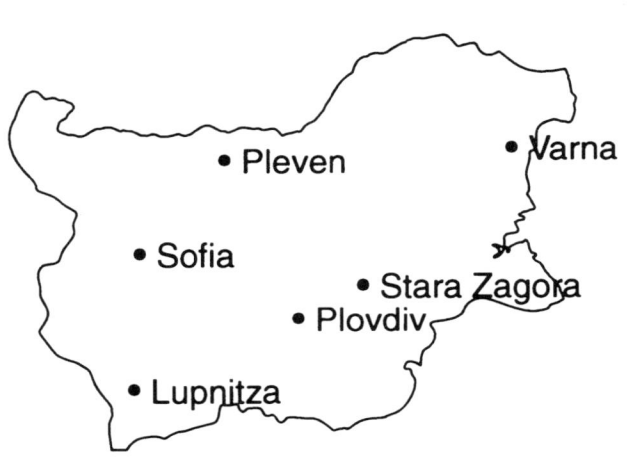

Bulgaria

Clinical pharmacology is not an independent medical speciality in Bulgaria, but part of pharmacology which has this status. A Section of Clinical Pharmacology was established within the Bulgarian Pharmacological Society in 1983. In 1997, the section was transformed into an independent scientific society, namely the Bulgarian Society for Clinical Pharmacology and Therapeutics. The present number of members in the society is 40. 1983 was also the year where the first, and so far only chair in clinical pharmacology was established at the Medical Faculty of the Medical University in Sofia. Teaching in clinical pharmacology during the medical studies takes place during the 5th year at the 9th semester. The course includes 30 lectures and 30 hours of practical exercises.

Clinical pharmacology teaching is also included in the postgraduate training of interns in general internal medicine, neurology, chemotherapy and others. The departments of pharmacology at the medical faculties in Varna, Plovdiv, Pleven and Stara Zagora are authorized to teach clinical pharmacology to medical students.

Clinical pharmacology units are established at the pharmaceutical firms Sopharma Ltd, Sofia, and Pharmacia Ltd, Dupnitza. According to the Bulgarian Drug Law, GCP is an obligatory requirement when performing clinical trials of drugs in the country.

Addresses

Sofia
Professor Dr V Vlahov
Department of Clinical Pharmacology
Queen Giovanna Hospital
8, Belo more St.
1040 Sofia – Bulgaria
Phone: +359 2 946 1646
Fax: +359 2 946 1646

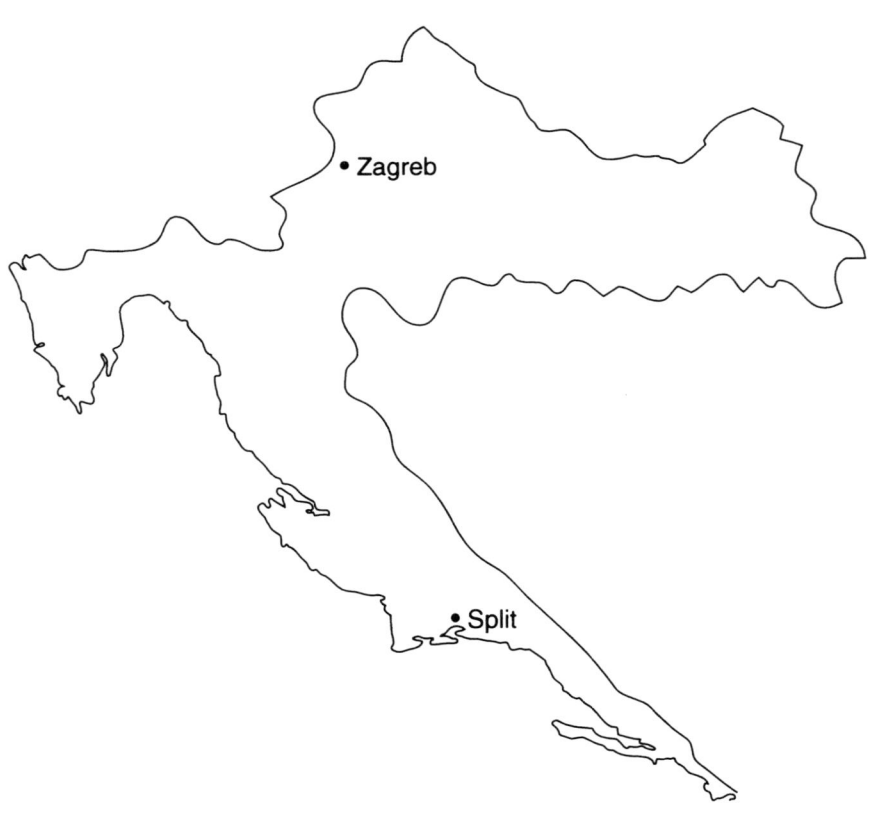

Croatia

Clinical pharmacology has been a separate medical speciality in Croatia since 1974. There was a change in 1994, so that the discipline is now termed 'clinical pharmacology and toxicology'. The national requirement to become a specialist in clinical pharmacology consist of 4 years as a trainee, followed by an examination in clinical pharmacology and toxicology. The 4 years of training in clinical pharmacology consist of the following periods: 1) 6 months at an institute of basic pharmacology or 6 months in a pharmacological laboratory in a pharmaceutical company, 2) 12 months at the Section of Clinical Pharmacology in Zagreb or partly in Zagreb and the rest of the period at the corresponding unit in Split and finally 3) 12 months (actually only 5 months), the contents of the remainder 7 months is chosen by the trainee in a clinical or laboratory institution such as the Institute for Drug Control) of formal education in the form of lectures, seminars and practical work in Zagreb. In fact, this postgraduate course is available to all MDs and not just trainees in clinical pharmacology. During 300 hours of teaching, the following disciplines are taught: the scientific basis of rational drug use, clinical trial methodology, analytical toxicology and toxicokinetics, pharmacodynamics, pharmacokinetics and drug biotransformation, planning of pharmacological and toxicological investigations and drug information (statistics, information technology). During the last 18 months, the trainee works in a clinical department chosen according to the future clinical speciality. In the Section of Clinical Pharmacology in Zagreb, there are subsections for patient care, counselling service, outpatients, clinical trials in particular in healthy volunteers, drug information, hospital drug committee, ADR monitoring centre and pharmacokinetics. After the first 12 months of the training programme, the trainee can add an extra 12 months in order to write a thesis to obtain a so-called magisterium in clinical pharmacology. This is a prerequisite for obtaining a regular PhD thesis.

The Pharmacotherapeutic Section of the Croatian Medical Association was established in the beginning of the 1980s. In 1992, the Section changed name to that of 'Croatian Society of Clinical Pharmacology and Therapeutics'. It has about 150 members, all of whom (chemists, pharmacists and physicians) work in some area of clinical pharmacology. The commitments of the Society are to promote the development of clinical pharmacology in Croatia, to promote the rational prescription of drugs and to provide adequate information on drugs.

Croatia has no chair in clinical pharmacology. Teaching of clinical pharmacology to medical students takes place in connection with the course in drug treatment in general internal medicine and again during the 6th and final year in a new course called 'mother, child and drugs'. In addition to its own separate courses, teaching in clinical pharmacology forms an integrated part of postdoctoral courses for general practitioners and other clinical specialists.

The Ministry of Health is responsible for clinical pharmacology. However, the Science and Technology Ministry is responsible for the academic activities of the discipline. Clinical pharmacology has a very good relationship with the Drug Regulation Agency, the Public Health Assurance and the pharmaceutical industry. Each of these three institutions depends very much on the Sections of Clinical Pharmacology, especially that in Zagreb. One staff member from the Section of Clinical Pharmacology in Zagreb is a member of the Croatian Drug Registration Committee, another is a member of the Committee for Preparation of Drug Regulation and also a member of the very influential Committee for Drug Reimbursement. It is deemed that the pharmaceutical industry is very much dependent on the expert support by Croatian clinical pharmacologists, both in performing clinical trials and in conducting studies with healthy volunteers.

Addresses

Split
Associate professor J Bagatin
KBC Split
Spinciceva 1
21000 Split
Croatia
Phone: +385 21 515055
Fax: +385 21 365738

Zagreb
Professor B Vrhovac
Section of Clinical Pharmacology
Department of Medicine
University Hospital Rebro
Kispaticeva 12
10000 Zagreb
Croatia
Phone: +385 1 213 861
Fax: +385 1 213 861
E-mail: vrhovac@rebro.mef.hr

Training Centres in Croatia

Zagreb

Research and training programme: in healthy volunteers, about 10 bioequivalence studies each with an average of 24 probands are undertaken per year. The studies are sponsored by the domestic and the foreign pharmaceutical industry. In patients, several mainly kinetic studies are performed. Sponsor: Croatian Ministry of Science and Technology and the pharmaceutical industry.

Training programme: the section offers training in all activities important for a clinical pharmacology service listed in the Croatia description, especially practical pharmacotherapeutic care for the patient hospitalized or seen in the outpatient clinic. Dealing with ADR (as a National centre the Unit receives all the documents from WHO Geneva and Uppsala) analysis and feedback to reporters. Performing actively participation in the above mentioned clinical studies (trials). Preparing articles for two drug editions: Bulletin (10/year), since 1976 and Pharmaca (4/year), since 1963, planning of drug information. Hospital drug committee activities. The evaluation of cost/benefit ratio (for Croatian Institute for Health Insurance) of drugs not approved (yet) in Croatia but prescribed by doctors.

Clinical and research facilities: the section has a 10-bed ward for general internal medicine patients according to the research interest or with a pharmacotherapeutic problem (resistance to therapy, ADR, interaction). Outpatient clinic examination of patients, pregnant women who have taken a drug in early pregnancy, advice on teratogenicity, examination of documentation concerning a therapeutic problem. ADR monitoring centre. Headquarters of the Hospital drug committee, editorial office of the two mentioned drug publications. A clinical pharmacology laboratory with good collaboration with the chemical side of drug measurements.

The University: three members of the staff are professors of the Medical School of Zagreb University. The section of Clinical Pharmacology is part of the Department of Medicine which is part of the University Hospital with regular teaching activities on the undergraduate and postgraduate level.

Staff: three professors of internal medicine and clinical pharmacology, two residents in clinical pharmacology plus a number of in-

ternists, or residents in clinical pharmacology who are taken as collaborators when needed. Close collaboration with the Centre for Biomedical Research where drug assays can be and are performed.
Application procedure: a curriculum vitae and a letter stating wishes and a description of working place after obtaining full or partial expertise, specialization in Zagreb.

References
Baudoin Z, Vrhovac B (1996) Dukes MNG, ed. Meyler's side effects of drugs. 13th ed. Amsterdam: Elsevier 265-284
Huic M, Macoli V, Vrhovac B, Francetic I, Bakran I (1994) Adverse drug reactions resulting in hospital admission. Int J Clin Pharmacol Ther 32: 675-682
Huic M, Vrhovac B, Macolic-Sarini V, Francetic I, Bakran I, Giljanovic S (1996) How safe are bioequivalence studies in healthy volunteers? Therapie 51: 410-413
Vrhovac B (1996) Access to information on drug regulation in the countries of Central and Eastern Europe. Int J Risk Safety Med 9: 173-178
Vrhovac B, Sarapa N, Bakran I, Hui M, Macoli-Sarini V, Franceti I, Wolf-Coporda A, Plavsic F (1995) Pharmacokinetic changes in patients with oedema. Clin Pharmacokinet 28: 405-418
Vrhovac B (editor in chief) et al. (1996) Interna medicina (Internal medicine), 2nd edn. Zagreb: Naprijed (1800 pp, 170 coauthors, Croatian language, special section CP, first edn 1991)

Split
In Split, up to March 1997, School of Medicine was a part of the Medical School from Zagreb. Clinical pharmacologists have been giving lessons on rational drug use as a part of internal medicine. From March 1997, the School of Medicine in Split has been completely independent and clinical pharmacology lecturing is a part of basic pharmacology, internal medicine and present also in the sixth and final year in a course called 'Public Health'.

With regard to the organization of a Section of Clinical Pharmacology and Toxicology in Split, there are two parts: clinical and preclinical (outpatient department). The first included 25 beds for patients from the area of general internal medicine and, if the circumstances require, there are patients who are included in research. The other part of the Section is the Outpatient Department for hypertension (24-hour blood pressure monitoring and plethysmography are included).

Our research is predominantly clinical; we investigate antihypertensive drugs, diuretics, antibiotics, and at the moment a low molecular weight heparin in unstable angina pectoris and deep phlebothrombosis. We are also taking part in Syst-Eur and lacidipine versus amlodipine studies in hypertensive patients. For the year to come we have planned to perform some venoconstrictive tests in hypertensives with glaucoma. This trial has been planned in connection with a School of Medicine in Trieste.

Concerning the staff, the Section of Clinical Pharmacology has one doctor, an associate professor, a specialist of clinical pharmacology and internal medicine, two doctors-specialists of internal medicine with master's thesis in the field of cardiovascular pharmacology. If needed, there is a professor of internal medicine and clinical pharmacology who has two functions: chief of the medical clinic and Dean of Split School of Medicine.

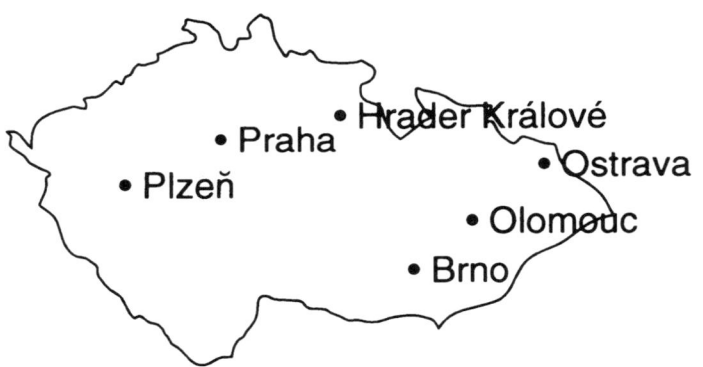

Czech Republic

Clinical pharmacology in the Czech Republic has been recognized as an independent branch of internal medicine since 1981. In 1982, a specialization in clinical pharmacology was introduced. Very briefly, the history of clinical pharmacology in the Czech Republic can be traced to the 1980s, when the vision of Clinical Pharmacology Units in each of 10 regions was adopted by the Ministry of Health. In fact, due to a reorganization of the health care system, especially during the last 7 years, the development of a network of Clinical Pharmacology Units is till now far from complete (see map). The most recent survey to describe clinical pharmacology in the Czech Republic is based on questionnaires mailed to all chairs of departments of pharmacology which were also quoted in lectures in Berlin 1997.
- The national requirements to become a specialist in clinical pharmacology are: a basic licence (attestation) in internal medicine, paediatrics or psychiatry, then 2 years of training in clinical pharmacology in the Department of Clinical Pharmacology. Experimental pharmacologists can be trained in 6-month courses
- The training programme in clinical pharmacology is similar to that of the leading clinical pharmacology departments (e.g. Sweden).

The Society of Clinical Pharmacology (Section of Clinical Pharmacology) has existed since 1992 and is part of the Czech Society for Experimental and Clinical Pharmacology and Toxicology. There are 99 members co-operating on the recent tasks of clinical pharmacology: clinical pharmacological service (when operating in hospital), teaching in clinical pharmacology (not sufficient in both pregraduate and postgraduate education), research (pharmacoepidemiology – in co-operation with the clinical pharmacy, pharmacoeconomics – hospital formularies, clinical outcomes research in hospitals).

Only in a minority of medical schools in the Czech Republic is there an undergraduate training in clinical pharmacology available, which is represented by lectures read by clinical pharmacologists. In the Czech Republic, the accreditation of clinical pharmacology has been achieved by approximately 30 physicians.

Responsible Ministries are the Ministry of Health Care and Ministry of Education.

For many years the chairmen of the Committee of New Drugs of the Ministry of Health were clinical pharmacologists (Professor Elis, Professor Svihovec, Associate Professor Sechser). As far as the pharmaceutical industry is concerned, there are Czech pharmaceutical manufacturers (sharing a majority of the pharmaceutical market) with only genetic products. The R&D Departments of the Czech pharmaceutical companies are a part of this progress with a different impact on the pharmaceutical production.

Conclusion: The field of clinical pharmacology in the Czech Republic is currently facing serious questions that will determine its future.

Addresses

Brno
Professor Alexandra Sulcová
Department of Pharmacology, Masaryk University
Jostova 10
662 43 Brno
Phone: +42 54 2126377
Fax: +42 54 2126377
E-mail: sulcova@med.mun1.cz

Hradec Králové
Professor Jirina Martínková
Department of Pharmacology
Simkova 870
500 01 Hradec Králové
Phone: +42 49 25347
E-mail: farmaks@lfhk.cuni.cz

Jirí Vortel
Department of Clinical Pharmacology
Teaching Hospital
500 05 Hradec Králové

Phone: +42 49 583 3720
Fax: +42 49 583 2003
E-mail: vortel@lfhk.cuni.cz

Olomouc
Professor Jaroslav Jezdínsky
Institute of Pharmacology
Faculty of Medicine, Palacky University
Hnevotínská 3
775 15 Olomouc
Phone: +42 68 414101
Fax:: +42 68 5413541

Ostrava
Associate Professor Milan Grundmann
Department of Clinical Pharmacology
Teaching Hospital Ostrava
17. listopadu 1790
708 52 Ostrava
Phone: +42 69 6912516
Fax: +42 69 436680
E-mail: milan.grundmann@kfa.fnspo.cz

Pilzen
Associate Professor Otto Mayer
Department of Clinical Pharmacology
Teaching Hospital Plzen (Pilsen)
ul. E.Benese 13
300 00 Plzen
Fax:: +42 19 277661

Prague
Associate Professor Frantisek Perlík
Department of Clinical Pharmacology
General Teaching Hospital
1st Medical Faculty, Charles University
U nemocnice 2
128 08 Prague 2
Phone: +42 22 4963118(5)
Fax: +42 22 97932

Olga Votroubková
Department of Clinical Pharmacology
Teaching Hospital Motol
V úvalu 85
150 00 Prague 5
Phone: +42 22 4435652

Associate Professor Tomás Sechser
Department of Clinical Pharmacology
Diabetes Centre
Institute for Clinical and Experimental Medicine
Videnska 800
14000 Prague
Phone: +42 2610 83225
Fax:: +42 2472 1982
E-mail: tomas.sechser@medicon.cz

Professor Hassan Farghali
Institute of Pharmacology
1st Faculty of Medicine
Charles University
Albertov 4
128 00 Prague 4
Phone: +42 22 93254
Fax: +42 22 93254

Professor Jan Svihovec
Department of Pharmacology
2nd Medical Faculty, Charles University
Albertov 4
128 00 Prague 2
Phone: +42 22 90772
Fax:: +42 22 90772
E-mail: Jan.svihovec@lfmotol.cuni.cz

Professor Milos Krsiak
Department of Pharmacology
3rd Medical Faculty, Charles University
Ruská 87
100 00 Prague 10
Phone: +42 267102487(05)
Fax:: +42 26 7102461 or 67311812
E-mail: Miloslav.krsiak@lf3.cuni.cz

Training Centres in the Czech Republic

Prague
Dept of Clinical Pharmacology, Institute for Clinical and Experimental Medicine (IKEM)

Clinical pharmacology was formally constituted in the Czech Republic in 1982. According to the 'Conception of Clinical Pharmacology' published by the Ministry of Health of the Czech Republic in 1982, 'Clinical pharmacology is the horizontal scientific branch that integrates experimental pharmacology with clinical and paraclinical branches with the aim to study and objectively evaluate the efficiency of drugs in healthy people and in patients.' It has its own scientific society, which is a member of the European Society of Clinical Pharmacology. For postgraduate education, the Subdivision of Clinical Pharmacology, IPVZ, was created. The Department of Clinical Pharmacology IKEM has the following activities.

Health care service
- it provides complex information and consultation for efficient and safe utilization of drugs not only in diabetology, but also in all other medical branches in IKEM.
- the clinico-pharmacological service provides analysis and monitoring of drug concentrations in body fluids, pharmacokinetic analysis and the interpretation of its results
- co-operation in pharmacotherapeutically complicated cases.
- consultations in choice of drugs and their combinations, prevention of drug interactions
- analysis of drug consumption in IKEM, providing the optimization of drug prescription regulation.

Research
- research in all four phases of clinical evaluation of new drugs (in healthy volunteers and in patients)
- introduction of good clinical practice principles to the realization of clinical studies in all departments in IKEM.
- methodological help in formation of standard operating procedures.
- research supported by grants from the Ministry of Health.

Teaching
- pre- and postgraduate courses in collaboration with Subdivision of Clinical Pharmacology IPVZ.
- courses of pharmacotherapy in diabetology and other medical specializations in IKEM.

Organization of the department: head of the department and the secretariat - management and coordination of all activities in health care service, research, teaching and expertise (for Ministry of Health).

Laboratories

Pharmacodynamical laboratory: clinical studies in healthy volunteers and in patients, samplings of biological materials for pharmacokinetic studies and pharmacodynamic studies in humans using non-invasive methods.

Laboratory of microbiological titrations: detection of drug concentrations with microbiological and fluoroimmunological methods for clinico-pharmacological service and research.

Laboratory of physico-chemical analyses: detection of drug concentrations with physico-chemical methods.

Laboratory of pharmacokinetical analysis: complex analysis of pharmacokinetic data, information on drugs and consultations of individualization and optimization of pharmaco-therapy.

Collaboration with clinical departments: clinical evaluation of new drugs both in inpatients and outpatients.

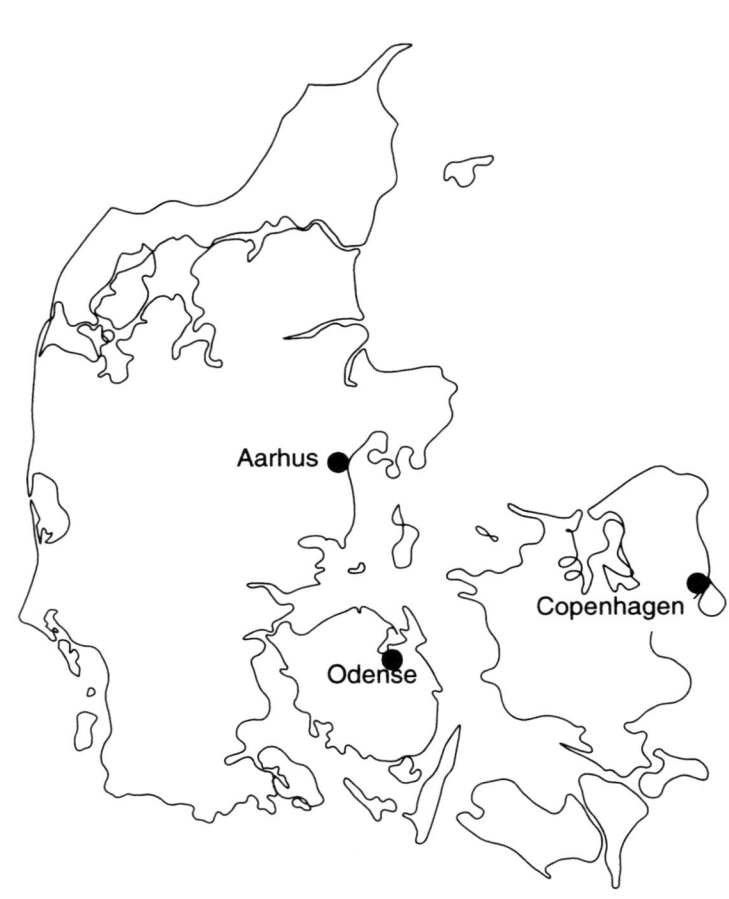

Denmark

Clinical pharmacology became a separate medical speciality in Denmark, June 1996. An MD degree followed by 18 months of internship (6 months of surgery, 6 months of internal medicine and 6 months of general practice) is mandatory before the specialist training can begin. The specialist training lasts 72 months and consists of a clinical part (36 months) and a clinical pharmacology part (36 months). At least 12 months must take place at any department of internal medicine. The remainder 24 months can take place in internal medicine, including subspecialities (cardiology, endocrinology, gastroenterology etc.), anaesthesiology, neurology, psychiatry, oncology, paediatrics or general practice. Only 12 months can take place at any of the three last mentioned specialities. As for the clinical pharmacology part, 24 months usually take place at any of the three university departments in either Copenhagen (National University Hospital), Odense or Århus. The remainder 12 months can take place at an institute of pharmacology, a department of clinical chemistry with TDM responsibility or at the National Board of Drugs or in the pharmaceutical industry (only 6 months for the two latter). Besides, all trainees should follow a series of eight courses in the different areas of clinical pharmacology. The titles are:

1. Pharmacokinetics
2. Drug metabolism and excretion
3. Pharmacodynamics and dose-effect relationships
4. Analytical methods including TDM and clinical toxicology
5. Development of drugs
6. Pharmacoepidemiology and pharmacoeconomy
7. Administrative pharmacology
8. Rational pharmacotherapy

The Danish Society of Clinical Pharmacology was founded in 1976 and it presently has 150 members (all MD). The Society organizes two to four meetings every year either on specific topics with invited speakers or meetings with free communications. The Society is also responsible for the theoretical courses in clinical pharmacology. The Society has tight bonds to its two sister societies, the Danish Society of Pharmacology and Toxicology and the Danish Society of Clinical Chemical Pharmacology.

In 1973, the Medical Research Council established a research unit in clinical pharmacology and in 1977/78 chairs in clinical pharmacology were established at the universities in Copenhagen, Odense and Århus. Pharmacology is a separate course at the three medical faculties, and teaching is provided mainly in the form of about 100 lectures. The research fellows, assistant professors and full professors in clinical pharmacology provide the teaching, along with their colleagues in basic pharmacology. In some of the faculties, there are separate lectures in clinical pharmacology and pharmacotherapeutics during the last year of the medical study. Some senior clinical pharmacologists also teach pharmacology and clinical pharmacy at the Royal School of Pharmacy in Copenhagen. Most of the senior clinical pharmacologists are also very active in postgraduate teaching. The Danish Board of Health offers a 5-day course in clinical pharmacology 3 times a year to all interns. Courses in the research methodology of clinical pharmacology are offered to PhD students at the three Danish faculties.

The pharmaceutical industry in Denmark is very important for the country in terms of export trade and jobs. The industry has had difficulties in recruiting doctors with a basic training in clinical pharmacology. This hampers the development of new drugs in Denmark and might lead to the Danish pharmaceutical industry becoming less competitive. These arguments were taken to the Government, with the result that significant funds were agreed for the development of the discipline. Thus, the Danish Government has provided 70 million DDK over the years 1996-2000, distributed to the centre of Clinical Pharmacology in Odense, the centre of Clinical Pharmacology in Århus and to the Clinical Pharmacology Network in Copenhagen. At the moment, 20-25 MDs undergo training at the three centres to become specialists in clinical pharmacology. In Copenhagen, five of the positions are financed by 50% from industry (Novo Nordisk, Leo Pharmaceuticals and H. Lundbeck). The trainees are involved in drug information, drug rounds, drug evaluation committees and teaching. Many but not all are preparing a PhD thesis while becoming specialists in clinical pharmacology. In the future, the specialists in clinical pharmacology will find jobs in industry, the National Board of Drugs, in hospitals, in the primary health care system and at universities.

The Ministry of Health, the Ministry of Education, the Ministry of Research and the Ministry of Industry are all responsible for clinical pharmacology in Denmark.

Addresses

Copenhagen
Dr P Buch Andreasen
Unit of Clinical Pharmacology
Gentofte Hospital
Niels Andersens Vej 65
DK-2900 Hellerup
Phone: +45 3977 3468
Fax: +45 3965 4156
E-mail: PBA@nethotel.dk

Dr H Rolighed Christensen
Unit of Clinical Pharmacology
Bispebjerg Hospital
Bispebjerg Bakke
2400 Copenhagen NV
Phone: +45 3531 2332
Fax: +45 3531 3711
E-mail: HRCO1@bbh.hosp.dk

Dr JP Kampmann
Unit of Clinical Pharmacology
Bispebjerg Hospital
Bispebjerg Bakke
DK-2400 Copenhagen NV
Phone: +45 3531 2740
Fax: +45 3531 3556

Dr S Loft
Unit of Clinical Pharmacology and Toxicology
Institute of Pharmacology
Copenhagen University

Panum Institute
Blegdamsvej 3
DK-2200 Copenhagen NV
Phone: +45 3532 7649
Fax: +45 3532 7610
E-mail: steffen.loft@farmakol.ku.dk

Professor H Enghusen Poulsen
Department of Clinical Pharmacology Q 7642
National University Hospital (Rigshospitalet)
Tagensvej 20
DK-2200 Copenhagen NV
Phone: +45 3545 7671
Fax: +45 3545 2745
E-mail: henrikep@rh.dk

Dr J Sonne
Unit of Clinical Pharmacology
Gentofte Hospital
Niels Andersens Vej 65
DK-2900 Hellerup
Phone: +45 3977 3997
Fax: +45 3977 7656
E-mail: jsonne@nethotel.dk

Odense
Professor K Brøsen
Institute of Public Health
Clinical Pharmacology
University of Southern Denmark

Main Campus: Odense University
Winsløwparken 18
DK-5000 Odense C
Phone: +45 6550 3751
Fax: +45 6591 6089
E-mail: k-brosen@cekfo.sdu.dk
Homep: www.sdu.dk/med/homepages/
eacpt/ eacpt5.html

Professor LF Gram
Institute of Public Health
Clinical Pharmacology
University of Southern Denmark
Main Campus: Odense University
Winsløwparken 18
DK-5000 Odense C
Phone: +45 6550 3750

Fax: +45 6591 6089
E-mail: lf-gram@cekfo.sdu.dk

Aarhus
Professor F Andreasen
Department of Clinical Pharmacology
Institute of Pharmacology
Århus University
Bartholin Building
Universitetsparken
DK-8000 Århus
Phone: +45 8942 1712
Fax: +45 8612 8804
E-mail: fa@farm.aau.dk
Homep: www.pharmacology.aau.
dk/staff/Frederik Andreasen.html

Training Centres in Denmark

Aarhus

Centre for Clinical Pharmacology, University of Aarhus and Aarhus University Hospital
The activities of the Centre for Clinical Pharmacology are aimed at initiating and supporting research and education within clinical pharmacology. A board with representatives for clinical departments, the university and the pharmaceutical industry is responsible for the achievement of an optimal balance between science, economy and education. The professor of clinical pharmacology is chairman of the board. The centre offers postgraduate training programmes in clinical pharmacology at three levels.

Level (1): combined educational and research positions leading to the recognition as a Danish specialist in clinical pharmacology. The training programme is established in close collaboration with the programmes offered by the two other Danish centres of clinical pharmacology. As special fields of interest, the centre offers clinical pharmacological training programmes for 2-1 year at clinical research units in A) psychiatry, B) oncology or C) circulatory pharmacology. According to the plan, the trainee in clinical pharmacology should spend half of the time on a research project and half the time performing education related tasks.

Level (2): the centre encourages and supports the initiation and performance of research projects within clinical pharmacology. Present research fields concern individual variation in metabolic responses to drug therapy of endocrinological diseases, heart diseases and diseases of the CNS.

Level (3): the centre offers two open PhD courses of 4-5 days duration: 'Research in Pharmacotherapy' and 'The patient in Clinical Pharmacological Research'.

Inquiries: The Centre for Clinical Pharmacology. Department of Clinical Pharmacology, The Bartholin Building, University of Aarhus.

Copenhagen
Clinical Pharmacology Network Copenhagen (CPNC)
Clinical Pharmacology in Copenhagen consists of four subcentres: three at University Hospitals: Rigshospitalet, Bispebjerg Hospital and Gentofte Hospital and one subcenter at the Clinical Pharmacology Department at the University of Copenhagen. Each of these subcentres are responsible for the education of clinical pharmacologists.

Several of the senior clinical pharmacologists have additional specialist degrees (internal medicine, pulmonary medicine, gastroenterology) and have strong affiliations with daily contact with departments of internal medicine.

The subcentres are involved in
- Basic clinical pharmacological scientific work.
- National counselling in toxicology affairs.
- Therapeutic drug monitoring in close relationship with the clinicians, including ward rounds.
- Quality assurance covering the whole domain of drug usage in the primary and secondary health sectors.
- Preparation of evidence based standard operation procedures for different diseases.
- A general counselling in all medical and therapeutic affairs for the hospital staff including administrators and health authorities.
- Education of all physicians in rational pharmacotherapy.
- Chairs in Drug Committees.

Odense

The Department of Clinical Pharmacology at Odense University was established on 1 August 1978 by professor Lars F. Gram. The research mainly falls into three categories: 1) clinical research [controlled trials of antidepressants and pain research (diabetic neuropathy and experimental pain models)], 2) pharmacoepidemiology (prescription database) and 3) pharmacokinetics (drug metabolism, pharmacogenetics and drug-drug interactions). The department serves as a 2-year training centre for residents in clinical pharmacology. All of our residents write a Ph.D. in clinical pharmacology while they receive their specialist training. Therefore, training usually lasts 3 years. The department provides drug information to the island of Funen and the southern part of Jutland comprising a population of about 1 million inhabitants. The department has no beds and no direct clinical responsibility for patients. In order to support the pharmaceutical industry in Denmark, the Danish Government has funded the Centre of Clinical Pharmacology in Odense with 6 million DKK (0.5 million , or 1.6 million DM) each year. The funding is part of a larger national programme with a total budget of 70 million DKK for research and research based training in clinical pharmacology. Training posts approved for 1 year in the specialist training are offered at the Section of Clinical Pharmacology at the Clinical Chemistry Department of Odense University Hospital. Formally the section will be responsible for a Unit for Good Clinical Practice and a Clinical Trial Unit. The residents at the section are involved in Therapeutic Drug Monitoring and also in drug information. The total staff at the Centre (department and section) consists of two full professors, one guest professor, one assistant professor, eight part time associate professors in pharmacotherapy, one part-time associate professor in clinical chemical pharmacology, 10-12 residents, three clinical pharmacists, one computer ingeneer, one or two research nurses, one analytical chemist, three laboratory technicians, and two or three secretaries. Odense University was established in 1966, and it has 4 faculties: Humanities, Natural Sciences, School of Business and Economics and Health Sciences. The total number of students is about 11,000 and the staff consists of about 1,000 people. An amalgamation between Odense University, the Business Highschool/Engineer Highschool of Southern Jutland and the University Centre of Southern Jutland took place during 1998. By the year 2001, the amalgamated university named University of Southern Denmark is expected to have about 17,000 students in Odense, Kolding, Sønderborg and Esbjerg, and thus it will be the second or third largest university in Denmark.

Positions at the Centre are announced in Ugeskrift for Læger (The weekly magazine of the Danish Medical Association). Applications should be sent to either Professor Lars F. Gram or Professor Kim Brøsen. The Centre will host the 5th EACPT Congress in 2001.

References

Gaist D, Hallas J, Sindrup SH, Gram LF (1996) Is overuse of sumatriptan a problem? Eur J Clin Pharmacol 50: 161-166

Gaist D, Sørensen HT, Hallas J (1997) The Danish prescription registries. Dan Med Bull 44: 444-448

Gram LF (1994) Fluoxetine (review). N Engl J Med 331:1354-1361

Hallas J (1996) Evidence of depression provoked by cardiovascular medication: a prescription sequence symmetry analysis. Epidemiology 7: 478-484

Jeppesen U, Loft S, Poulsen HE, Brøsen K (1996) A fluvoxamine-caffeine interaction study. Pharmacogenetics 6: 213-222

Madsen H, Hansen TS, Brøsen K (1996) Imipramine metabolism in relation to the sparteine oxidation polymorphism - a family study. Pharmacogenetics 6: 513-519

Poulsen L, Arendt-Nielsen L, Brøsen K, Sindrup SH (1996) The hypoalgesic effect of tramadol in relation to CYP2D6. Clin Pharmacol Ther 60: 636-644

Rasmussen BB, Mäenpää J, Pelkonen O, Loft S, Poulsen HE, Lykkesfeldt J, Brøsen K (1995) Selective serotonin reuptake inhibitors and theophylline metabolism in human liver microsomes: potent inhibition by fluvoxamine. Br J Clin Pharmacol 39: 433-439

Rosholm JU, Gram LF, Isacsson G, Hallas J, Bergmann U (1997) Changes in the pattern of antidepressant use upon the introduction of new antidepressants. A prescription database study. Eur J Clin Pharmacol 52: 205-209

Sindrup SH, Brøsen K (1995) The pharmacogenetics of codeine hypoalgesia (review). Pharmacogenetics 5: 335-346

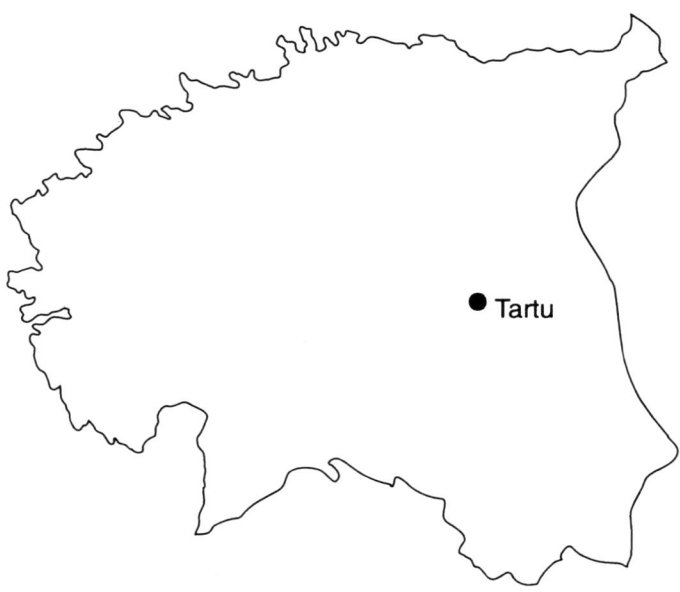

Estonia

Clinical pharmacology is not yet a separate medical speciality in Estonia, but is likely to become one in the near future, due to the fact that an increasing number of physicians receive training in the discipline. The training takes place at the Department of Clinical Pharmacology in Tartu. In order to enter training, the candidates must have obtained their MD degree. The training programme is formally linked to a PhD programme in pharmacology or a similar research project in a relevant area of clinical medicine. As an alternative, a continuing medical education programme in clinical pharmacology is available from 1997. It is called residentship in clinical pharmacology and should entail 2-4 years training depending on the previous clinical experience of the applicant.

The Estonian Society of Pharmacology has a Section of Clinical Pharmacology. The contact address for the Section is the Department of Pharmacology in Tartu (see below). The members of the Section are the teachers of clinical pharmacology and also clinical pharmacologists at the National Drug Regulatory Authority, but also clinicians in general internal medicine who perform clinical trials. Clinical pharmacology is not very strong in the domestic pharmaceutical industry, and this is mainly due to the fact that industry in Estonia is not research-oriented.

The only medical faculty in Estonia is situated in Tartu. Clinical pharmacology has been an integrated part of the undergraduate teaching of medical students since the beginning of the 1980s. A chair in clinical pharmacology was established in 1992 at the Department of Pharmacology, which is responsible for the teaching. The curriculum consists of a 20-hours lecture and a 60-hours (2 weeks) seminar programme in clinical pharmacology during the final year of the undergraduate medical study. Pharmacotherapy makes up a substantial part of the postgraduate programme which is compulsory for practising physicians.

At present, there are no routine clinical pharmacological services in

Estonia, but they are under way in several of the major hospitals. The main priority is given to drug information. The clinical pharmacologists have been involved in creating a National Formulary type handbook for physicians and editing in co-operation with the National Drug Regulatory Authority bimonthly Drug Information Bulletin. Workshops for physicians and pharmacists on selected topics of pharmacotherapy are held. Experts in the relevant clinical disciplines or clinical pharmacologists have been responsible for the teaching. By far the majority of research in clinical pharmacology is performed at the University in Tartu. The research is focused on pharmacokinetics, pharmacogenetics and pharmacoepidemiology.

The experts both in basic and clinical pharmacology among the academic staff at the University of Tartu provide assistance to the national drug regulatory authority at the Ministry of Social Affairs, the so-called State Agency of Medicines in Tartu. The expert assistance is given both for registration purposes and for post-marketing surveillance. The postgraduate training programme in clinical pharmacology also includes work at the Agency.

Addresses

Tartu
Professor L Raego
Department of Pharmacology
University of Tartu
18 Ülikooli Str.
EE 2400 Tartu
Estonia
Phone: +372 7 441219
Fax: +372 7 441 549
E-mail: lembit@sam.ee

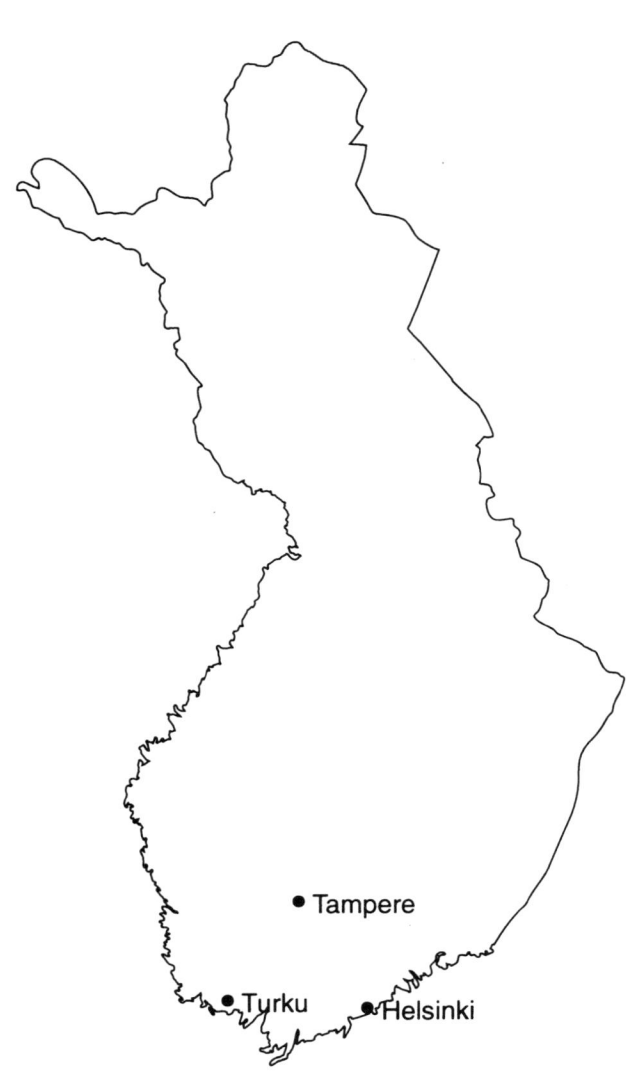

Finland

Clinical pharmacology has been an official medical speciality in Finland since 1966. The national requirements for the speciality in clinical pharmacology are: 1) a general training as a physician for 2 years, 2) a special training in clinical pharmacology for 4 (2) years, 3) a written speciality board examination and 4) theoretical courses for 80 hours (at least 60 hours clinical pharmacology). The requirements may be changed in the near future.

The general training consists of at least 6 months in general practice at a 'health centre' and 6 months in anaesthaesiology, internal medicine, psychiatry or paediatrics. The remainder of the 2 years can consist of two different clinical areas but can also include research for up to 6 months.

The special training (either according to A or B): A) 4 years in clinical pharmacology; this may include 1 year of basic pharmacology, clinical chemistry, clinical physiology, pharmaceutical medicine (industry) or work at the National Agency for Medicines, or B) 2 years in clinical pharmacology if the trainee has a previous speciality either in internal medicine, paediatrics, anaesthesiology neurology or psychiatry.

For the written speciality board examination, the following books are used: 1) Neuvonen, Himberg, Iisalo, Mattila & Ylitalo: *Kliininen Farmakologia (Clinical Pharmacology)* 2) Speight & Holford: *Avery's Drug Treatment*, 3) Pocock: *Clinical Trials, A Practical Approach*, 4) Rowland & Tozer: *Clinical Pharmacokinetics, Concepts and Applications* and 5) *Guideline for Good Clinical Practice*. In addition, three latest annual volumes of the following journals: *Drugs, Clinical Pharmacology & Therapeutics, Lancet, New England Journal of Medicine, British Medical Journal, Duodecim, Finnish Medical Journal,* and publications of the Finnish National Agency for Medicines.

Each of the three departments of clinical pharmacology in Finland has its own training programme. It will be tailored according to the background of the trainee and contains, e.g. clinical pharmacokinetics, TDM, GCP, biostatistics, drug evaluation and registration, treatment of various diseases and intoxications. During the specialist training, the trainee performs TDM, consultations in drug-related problems at hospital wards and out-patient clinics, clinical drug trials, works at the Poison Information Centre, etc. There are six or seven training posts in clinical pharmacology. The graduate school 'Clinical Drug Trials' gives eight additional posts.

The Finnish Society of Clinical Pharmacology was founded in 1994. Before that, there was a Section of Clinical Pharmacology within the Finnish Pharmacological Society. The number of members is 86 (August 1997). The Society arranges two scientific meetings annually and post-graduate courses, e.g. »Clinical Drug Trial«. The society has good relationships with sister societies, e.g. to pharmacology, internal medicine, anaesthesiology, etc.

The first chair in clinical pharmacology was established in 1968 at the University of Helsinki, i.e. the chair is one of the oldest in Europe. At present, there are three chairs [Helsinki, Turku (1983) and Tampere (1989)]. The professors are also chief physicians in clinical pharmacology at the respective university hospital. Clinical pharmacology is an obligatory discipline (30-60 hours) with examinations of medical students, and it is important to postgraduates within many clinical fields. A problem-oriented Finnish textbook of clinical pharmacology was published in 1994.

The minister responsible for clinical pharmacology is the Minister of Education. There is a good co-operation between clinical pharmacologists working in academia and hospitals and the pharmaceutical industry and the National Agency for Medicines.

Addresses

Helsinki
Professor PJ Neuvonen
Department of Clinical Pharmacology
University of Helsinki & Helsinki University Central Hospital
Haartmanink. 4
FIN-00290 Helsinki
Finland
Phone: +358 9 4713315
Fax: +358 9 4714039
Email: pertti.neuvonen@huch.fi

Tampere
Professor Pauli Ylitalo
Department of Pharmacology
Clinical Pharmacology and Toxicology
University of Tampere
Box 607
FIN-33101 Tampere
Finland
Phone: +358 3 2156731
Fax: +358 3 2156170
E-mail: klpayl@uta.fi

Turku
Professor Mika Scheinin
Department of Pharmacology and Clinical Pharmacology
University of Turku
Kiinamyllynk. 10
FIN-20520 Turku
Finland
Phone: +358 2 3337502
Fax: +358 2 3337216
E-mail: m.schein@utu.fi

Training Centres in Finland

Helsinki
University of Helsinki and Helsinki University Central Hospital
The research includes:
- drug interactions (absorption/metabolism/elimination)
- pharmacokinetic principles (activated charcoal etc.) for the treatment of acute intoxications
- pharmacokinetic characterization of drugs
- paediatric clinical pharmacology
- drug efficacy studies
- effect of diseases on pharmacokinetics

The training includes
- methods in clinical pharmacology
- clinical pharmacokinetics
- clinical trials

- clinical toxicology
- drug therapy

Three universities and university hospitals, industry and The National Agency for Medicines are participating in the graduate-school "Clinical Drug Trial - Planning, Performance and Critical Evaluation". Annually, about 40,000 drug analyses (60 items) are performed in TDM and 30,000 phone consultations are received in the National Poison Information centre (around-the-clock).

The department consists of 700 m2 laboratory and office rooms, facilities for human studies but no hospital beds. The department belongs to the University of Helsinki and Helsinki University Central Hospital.

The staff includes one professor, one assistant professor, one senior physician, three research associates/registrars, four MDs in graduate school, one chemist, several pharmacists, laboratory nurses, etc., in total 40 persons.

Applications should be addressed to the head (Professor Pertti Neuvonen).

References

Ahonen J, Olkkola KT, Neuvonen PJ (1997) Effect of route of administration of fluconazole on the interaction between fluconazole and midazolam. Eur J Clin Pharmacol 51: 415-419

Backman JT, Olkkola KT, Neuvonen PJ (1996a) Rifampin drastically reduces plasma concentrations and effects of oral midazolam. Clin Pharmacol Ther 59: 7-13

Backman JT, Olkkola KT, Ojala M, Laaksovirta H, Neuvonen PJ (1996b) Concentrations and effects of oral midazolam are greatly reduced in patients treated with carbamazepine or phenytoin. Epilepsia 37: 253-257

Jalava K-M, Olkkola KT, Neuvonen PJ (1997) Itraconazole greatly increases plasma concentrations and effects of felodipine. Clin Pharmacol Ther 61: 410-415

Neuvonen PJ, Jalava M (1996) Itraconazole drastically increases plasma concentrations of lovastatin and lovastatin acid. Clin Pharmacol Ther 60: 54-61

Neuvonen PJ, Varhe A, Olkkola KT (1996) The effect of ingestion time interval on the interaction between itraconazole and triazolam. Clin Pharmacol Ther 60: 326-331

Olkkola KT, Aranko K, Luurila H, Hiller A, Saarnivaara L, Himberg J-J, Neuvonen PJ (1993) A potentially hazardous interaction between erythromycin and midazolam. Clin Pharmacol Ther 53: 298-305

Olkkola KT, Backman JT, Neuvonen PJ (1994) Midazolam should be avoided in patients receiving systemic antimycotics ketoconazole or itraconazole. Clin Pharm Ther 55: 481-485

Varhe A, Olkkola KT, Neuvonen PJ (1994) Oral triazolam potentially hazardous to patients receiving systemic antimycotics ketoconazole or itraconazole. Clin Pharmacol Ther 56: 601-607

Villikka K, Kivistö KT, Backman J, Olkkola KT, Neuvonen PJ (1997) Triazolam is ineffective in patients taking rifampin. Clin Pharmacol Ther 61: 8-14

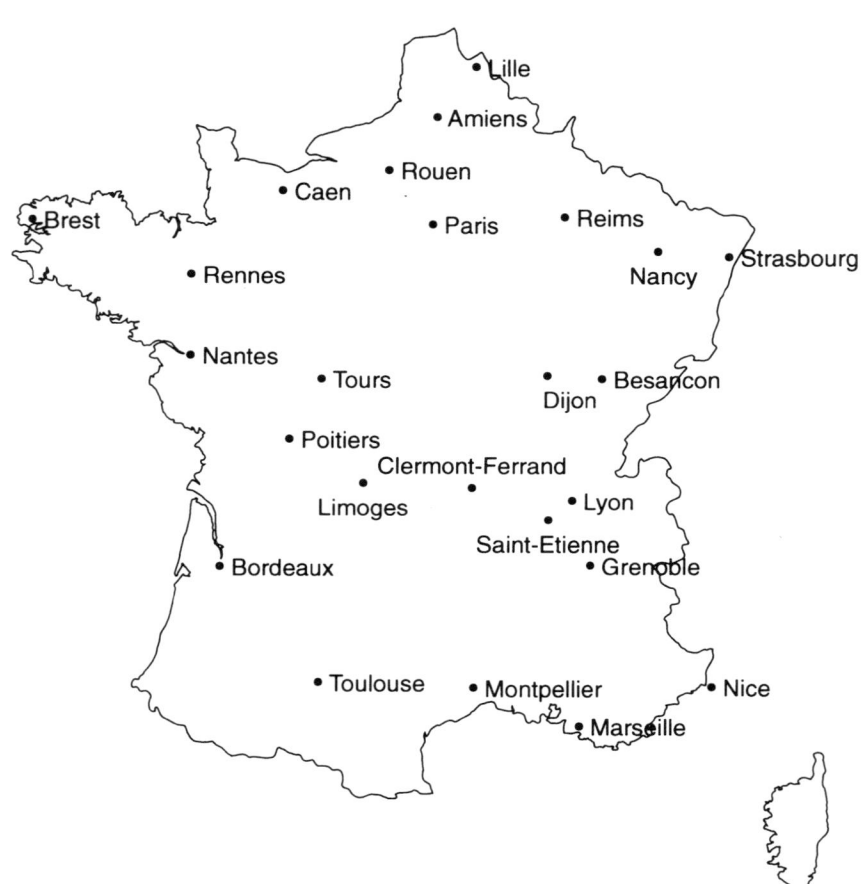

France

Clinical pharmacology is an official speciality in the medical faculties of the universities in France. The university departments of pharmacology have distinct units for basic pharmacology and clinical pharmacology. The head of the department can either be a basic pharmacologist or a clinical pharmacologist. Specialists in clinical pharmacology must have an MD degree followed by 4 years of clinical training as residents at university hospitals. In addition, a PhD thesis in pharmacology is required, after which employment as assistant professor in clinical pharmacology becomes possible. There are no uniform rules concerning the training programme in clinical pharmacology. It depends on the actual medical department of pharmacology. However, it is common practice to work for 4 years as an assistant in a unit of clinical pharmacology prior to the position as assistant professor.

In 1997, the French pharmacologists decided to join forces by unifying in one Societé Francaise de Pharmacologie (SFP), four societies which had been created at different times: the Association of Pharmacologists (which included a section of Clinical Pharmacology), the French Society of Clinical Pharmacology and Therapeutics, The Association of Experimental Pharmacology and The French Association of Pharmacovigilance Centres. This new society is organized to have an official section of Clinical Pharmacology, Pharmacovigilance and Therapeutics. This section has about 700 members. The new society will organize one national meeting and one 2-day seminar in basic and clinical pharmacology each year. It will continue to publish two journals, *Fundamental and Clinical Pharmacology* (in English) and *Therapie* (in French). It will support EACPT, EPHAR, IUPHAR and IUPHAR-CPT activities. The society will promote the participation of young pharmacologists at national and international meetings through the distribution of educational grants. Through its members, the society has a widespread network to most of the clinical societies (cardiology, gastroenterology, neurology, etc.).

The first chair in clinical pharmacology was established in 1981 in Paris at the University Hospital Henri Mondor – Créteil. Since then, a total of 30 professors of clinical pharmacology have been nominated. The professors teach clinical pharmacology to medical students, to MDs (specialized certificates and diplomas) and to physicians during their continued medical training.

The Minister of Health and Social Affairs and the Minister of Education both are responsible for clinical pharmacology. The French Drug Agency supports an official network of 30 centres for clinical pharmacology and therapeutics through annual research grants. An Orientation Committee of Clinical Pharmacology headed by Professor Patrice Jaillon is in charge of the network. Most of the clinical pharmacologists are experts for one or more of the four commissions at the agency: drug authorization (AMM), transparence, pharmacovigilance and control of drug advertising. Three of these commissions are directed by a professor of clinical pharmacology or a professor of therapeutics. Most of the centres of clinical pharmacology are affiliated with the drug industry through research contracts, and besides, many clinical pharmacologists serve as consultants for drug development in industry.

Addresses

Amiens
Professor M Andrejak
Service de Pharmacologie
Hôpital Sud
C.H.R.U. d'Amiens
80054 Amiens Cedex
Phone: +33 322 455 788
Fax: +33 322 455 660

Besançon
Professor P Bechtel
Service de Pharmacologie Clinique
Hôpital Jean Minjoz
25030 Besancon Cedex
Phone: +33 381 668 300
Fax: +33 381 669 499

Bobigny
Professor G Perret
Laboratoire de Pharmacologie
Faculté de Médicine
74 rue Marcel Cachin
93012 Bobigny
Phone: +33 148 387 704
Fax: +33 148 387 777

Bordeaux
Professor B Bégaud
Department of Pharmacology
Université Victor-Segalen – Bordeaux 2
CHU Bordeaux Pellegrin
33076 Bordeaux Cedex
Phone: +33 557 571 561
Fax: +33 556 981 291
E-mail: bernard.begaud@pharmaco.u-bordeaux2.fr

Professor J Dangoumau
Department of Pharmacology
Université Victor-Segalen – Bordeaux 2
CHU Bordeaux Pellegrin
33076 Bordeaux Cedex
Phone: +33 557 571 560
Fax: +33 556 245 889

Professor B Bannwarth
Départment de Thérapeutique
Université Victor-Segalen – Bordeaux 2
CHU Bordeaux Pellegrin
33076 Bordeaux Cedex
Phone: +33 557 571 560
Fax: +33 556 245 889

Professor N Moore
Department of Clinical Pharmacology
Université Victor-Segalen – Bordeaux 2
CHU Bordeaux Pellegrin
33076 Bordeaux Cedex
Phone: +33 557 571 560
Fax: +33 556 245 889
E-mail: nicholas.moore@pharmacc.u-bordeaux2.fr

Brest
Professor C Riche
C.H.U.
5 avenue Foch
29285 Brest Cedex
Phone: +33 298 223 310
Fax: +33 298 016 466

Caen
Professor P Bustany
Laboratoire de Pharmacologie
U.E.R. de Médicine
Avenue de la Côte de Nacre
14033 Caen Cedex
Phone: +33 231 064 669
Fax: +33 231 064 673
E-mail: bustany-p@chu.caen.fr

Professor M Moulin
Laboratoire de Pharmacologie
U.E.R. de Médicine
Avenue de la Côte de Nacre
14032 Caen Cedex
Phone: +33 231 068 213
Fax: +33 231 064 673

Clermont Ferrand
Professor A Eschalier
Laboratoire de Pharmacologie
Faculté de Médicine
28 place Henri Dunant – B.P. 38
63001 Clermont Ferrand Cedex
Phone: +33 473 608 033
Fax: +33 473 277 162

Professor C. Dubray
Laboratoire de Pharmacologie
Faculté de Médicine
28 place Henri Dunant – B.P. 38
63001 Clermont Ferrand Cedex
Phone: +33 473 608 033
Fax: +33 473 277 162

Creteil
Professor I Macquin-Mavier
Service de Pharmacologie Clinique
Hôpital Henri Mondor
51 Avenue du Maréchal de Lattre de Tassigny
94010 Créteil
Phone: +33 149 812 761
Fax: +33 149 812 765
E-mail: isabelle.macquin-mavier@hmr.ap-hop-paris.fr

Professor JP Tillement
Laboratoire de Pharmacologie
Centre Hospitalier Intercommunal
40 Avenue de Verdun
94000 Creteil
Phone: +33 145 175 380
Fax: +33 142 175 389
E-mail: tillement@univ-paris12.fr

Dijon
Professor M Dumas
Laboratoire de Pharmacologie Médicale
U.F.R de Médicine
7 boulevard Jeanne d'Arc
21033 Dijon Cedex
Phone: +33 380 393 356
Fax: +33 380 393 300

Professor A Escousse
Service Pharmacologie Cliniqùe
Centre Régional de Pharmacocigilance
Hôpital Général
3, rue du Faubourg Raines
21033 Dijon Cedex
Phone: +33 380 293 742
Fax: +33 380 293 723
Grenoble

Professor G Bessard
Laboratoire de Pharmacologie
Hôpital Michallon
BP 217
F-38043 Grenoble Cedex 9
Phone: +33 476 765 492
Fax: +33 476 765 655

Lille
Professor B Dupuis
Laboratoire de Pharmacologie
Faculté de Médecine
1 place de Verdun
59 045 Lille Cedex
Phone: +33 320 445 449
Fax: +33 320 539 223
E-mail: ciclille@chru-lille.fr

Professor Ch Libersa
Laboratoire de Pharmacologie
C.H.U. de Lille
1 place de Verdun
59045 Lille Cedex
Phone: +33 320 445 449
Fax: +33 320 626 992
E-mail: ciclille@chru-lille.fr

Limoges
Professor L Merle
Centre Régional de Pharmacovigilance
Hôpital Universitaire Dupuytren
2 avenue Martin Luther King
87042 Limoges Cedex
Phone: +33 555 056 123
Fax: +33 555 056 667

Lyon
Professor J-P Boissel
Claude Bernard University
Faculty Hospital Lyon
DRED EA Mo 643
Service de Pharmacologie Clinique
B.P. 3041
69394 Lyon Cedex3
Phone: +33 472 115 232
Fax: +33 478 531 030

Professor J Descotes
Department of Pharmacologie, Medical Toxicology
and Environmental Medicine
INSERM U 80
Faculté de Médecine Lyon-R.t.H. Laënnec
69372 Lyon cedex 08
Phone: +33 478 778 664
Fax: +33 476 329 249
E-mail:
descotes@laennec1.univ.lyon1.fr

Professor JC Evreux
Centre Antipoison – Centre de Pharmacovigilance
Hôpital E. Herriot – Pavillon N
5 place d'Arsonval
69003 Lyon
Phone: +33 472 116 987
Fax: +33 472 116 985

Marseille
Professor O Blin
Laboratoire de Pharmacologie Clinique

Timone Hospital
27 bld Jean Moulin
13385 Marseille Cedex 5
Phone: +33 491 387 563
Fax: +33 491 472 140
E-mail: oblin@ap-hm.fr

Professor G Bouvenot
Laboratoire de Méthodologie des Essais
Faculté de Médicine
27 bld Jean Moulin
13385 Marseille Cedex 5
Phone: +33 491 834 488

Professor B Bruguerolle
Laboratoire de Pharmacologie Clinique
Hôpital La Timone
27 bld Jean Moulin
13385 Marseille Cedex 5
Phone: +33 491 387 024
Fax: +33 491 256 526

Montpellier
Professor P Petit
Centre Hospitalier Universitaire de Montpellier
Hopital la Colomiere
Polyclinique de Psychiatrie
39, avenue Charles Flahault
F-34295 Montpellier Cedex 5
Phone: +33 467 336 690
Fax: +33 467 336 670
E-mail: ppetit@sc.univ-montpl.fr

Nancy
Professor P Gillet
Laboratoire de Pharmacologie
Faculté de Médecine de Nancy
Av de la Fôret de Haye, B.P. 184
54505 Vandoevre Les Nancy
Phone: +33 383 592622
Fax: +33 383 592622
E-mail: pharmaco@pharmaco-med.u.nancy.fr

Professor P Netter
Laboratoire de Pharmacologie
Faculté de Médecine de Nancy
Université Henri Poincaré, Nancy I
Av de la Fôret de Haye, B.P. 184
54505 Vandoevre Les Nancy
Phone: +33 383 592622
Fax: +33 383 592622
E-mail: pharmaco@pharmaco-med.u.nancy.fr

Professor RJ Royer
Laboratoire de Pharmacologie
Faculté de Médecine de Nancy
Av de la Fôret de Haye, B.P. 184
54505 Vandoevre Les Nancy
Phone: +33 383 592622
Fax: +33 383 592622
E-mail: pharmaco@pharmaco-med.u.nancy.fr

Dr F Zannad
Pharmacologie Clinique
Centre d'Investigation Clinique INSERM-CHU
Hôpital Jeanne d'Arc
F-54200 Dommartin les Toul
Phone: +33 383 656 625
Fax: +33 383 656 619
E-mail: cic@chu-nancy.fr

Nantes:
Professor M Bourin
Unité de Psychopharmacologie
Hôpital St.-Jacques
U.F.R. de Médicine
1 rue Gaston Veil
44035 Nantes Cedex
Phone: +33 240 846 432
Fax: +33 240 846 433

Nice:
Dr MD Drici
Service de Pharmacologie
Faculté de Médicine

Avenue de Vallombrose
06107 Nice Cedex
Phone: +33 493 377 749
Fax: +33 493 536 121

Paris:
Professor M Alexandre
Service de Pharmacologie Clinique
Hôpital Broussais
96 rue Didot
75674 Paris Cedex 14
Phone: +33 143 959 100
Fax: +33 143 958 100

Professor J-F Bergmann
Service Médecine Interne A
Therapeutics and Research Unit
Hôpital Lariboisière
2 rue Ambroise Paré
75475 Paris Cedex 10
Phone: +33 149 956 341
Fax: +33 149 958 446

Professor F Calvo
Centre for Clinical Investigation
Hôpital Saint-Louis
1, Avenue Claude Vellefaux
75475 Paris Cedex 10
Phone: +33 142 499 494
Fax: +33 142 499 397
E-mail: fabien.calvo@chu-StLouis.fr

Professor C Caulin
Service Médecine Interne A
Hôpital Lariboisère
2 rue Ambroise Paré
75475 Paris Cedex 10
Phone: +33 149 958 126
Fax: +33 149 958 446

Professor J-L Elghozi
Laboratoire de Pharmacologie
Faculté de Médecine Necker CNRS
URA 1482
156 rue de Vaugirard
75015 Paris
Phone: +33 145 665 585
Fax: +33 140 615 584

Professor C Funck-Brentano
Unité de Pharmacologie Clinique
Hôpital St Antoine
184 rue du Fg St Antoine
75012 Paris
Phone: +33 149 282 200
Fax: +33 143 413 884

Professor JP Giroud
Labo. de Pharmacologie Clinique
CHU Cochin-Port Royal, Pav. G. Roussy
27 rue du Fg St Jacque
75674 Paris Cedex
Phone: +33 142 341 995
Fax: +33 144 412 557

Professor E Jacqz-Aigrain
Perinatal and Paediatric Clinical Pharmacology
Hôpital Robert Debré
48 Boulevard Séruier
75019 Paris
Phone: +33 140 032 150
Fax: +33 140 034 759

Professor P Jaillon
Universié Pierre et Marie Curie – Paris IV
Unité de Pharmacologie Clinique
Hôpital St. Antoine
184 rue du Fg St. Antoine
75012 Paris
Phone: +33 140 011 393
Fax: +33 140 011 404

Professor G Lagier
Service de Pharmacologie
Hôpital Fernand Widal
200 rue du Fg Saint Denis
75010 Paris

Phone: +33 140 054 338
Fax: +33 140 054 856

Professor S Laurent
Service de Pharmacologie Clinique
Hôital Broussais
96 rue Didot
75674 Paris Cedex 14
Phone: +33 143 959 100
Fax: +33 143 958 100

Professor P Lechat
Département de Pharmacologie Clinique
Hôpital Pitié-Salpétrière
47 bd de l'Hôpital
75013 Paris
Phone: +33 142 161 661
Fax: +33 142 161 688

Professor F Lhoste
Pharmacologie
Faculté de Médecine
Necker
156 rue de Vangirard
75015 Paris
Phone: +33 140 615 339
Fax: +33 140 615 584

Professor G Pons
Service de Pharmacologie Périnatale et Pèdiatrique
Hôpital Saint Vincint de Paul
82 Avenue Denfert Rochereau
75674 Paris 14
Phone: +33 140 488 211
Fax: +33 140 488 328
E-mail: gerard.pons@svp.ap-hop-paris.fr

Professor A Puech
Service de Pharmacologie
Hôpital Pitié-Salpétrière
47 Bd de l'hôpital
75651 Paris Cedex 13

Phone: +33 142 161 661
Fax: +33 142 161 688

Professor M Safar
Service de Médecine Interne 1 et 7
Hôpital Broussais
96 rue Didot
75074 Paris Cedex 14
Phone: +33 143 959 122
Fax: +33 145 433 894

Poitiers
Professor B Vandel
Service de Pharmacologie Clinique
Pavillon Le Blaye
Cité Hospitalière de la Milétrie B.P. 557
86021 Poitiers Cedex F
Phone: +33 549 444 453
Fax: +33 549 443 845

Reims
Professor Ph Devillier
Laboratoire de Pharmacologie – Toxicologie
Centre Régional de Pharmacovigilance
Hopital Maison Blanche
45 rue Cognacq-Jay
51092 Reims Cedex
Phone: +33 326 787 531
Fax: +33 326 788 456
E-mail: denis-lamiable
@email.msn.com

Professor H Millard
Laboratoire de Pharmacologie – Toxicologie
Centre Régional de Pharmacovigilance
Hopital Maison Blanche
54 rue Cognacq-Jay
51092 Reims Cedex
Phone: +33 326 787 531
Fax: +33 326 788 456
E-mail: denis-lamiable
@email.msn.com

Rennes
Professor H Allain
Laboratoire de Pharmacologie
C.H.U. Pontchaillou/Faculté de
Médecine
Université Rennes I
2 avenue Pr Léon-Bernard
35043 Rennes cedex
Phone: +33 299 336872
Fax: +33 299 336890
E-mail: Herve.Allain@univ-rennesl.fr
Homep: www.med.univ.rennesl.fr/galesne/pharmaco

Professor E Belissant
Laboratoire de Pharmacologie
C.H.U. Pontchaillou/Faculté de
Médecine
Université Rennes I
2 avenue Pr Léon-Bernard
35043 Rennes cedex
Phone: +33 299 336 872
Fax: +33 299 336 890
E-mail: Herve.Allain@univ-rennesl.fr
Each site: http://www.each.be
Wfdc site: http://www.sfdc.corn/h_allain

Rouen
Professor C Thuillez
Service de Pharmacologie Clinique
CHU de Rouen
Hôpital de Boisguillaume
76031 Rouen Cedex
Phone: +33 232 889 030
Fax: +33 235 889 049
E-mail: Pharmacologie @chu-rouen.fr

Saint Etienne
Professor H Decousus
Unité de Pharmacologie Clinique
Service de Médecine Interne et Thérapeutique
Pavillon 5 Hôpital Bellevue
42055 Saint Etienne Cedex
Phone: +33 477 427 788
Fax: +33 477 427 820

Professor M Ollagnier
Laboratoire de Pharmacologie
Centre de Pharmacovigilance
Hôpital de Bellevue
Boulevard Pasteur
42055 Saint Etienne Cedex 2
Phone: +33 477 427 737
Fax: +33 477 427 774

Professor P Queneau
President of APNET
Hôpital Bellevue
Boulevard Pasteur
42055 Saint-Etienne Cedex 2
Phone: +33 477 427 773
Fax: +33 477 420 482
Strasbourg

Professor P Bousquet
Professeur de Pharmacologie Expérimentale
Institut de Pharmacologie et de
Médecine Expérimentale
11 rue Humann
67085 Strasbourg Cedex
Phone: +33 388 358 754
Fax: +33 388 360 715

Professor J-L Imbs
Professeur de Pharmacologie et de
Médecine Expérimentale
Service d'Hypertension, maladies vasculaires et pharmacologie Clinique
Faculté de Médecine
11 rue Humann
67085 Strasbourg Cedex
Phone: +33 388 358 754
Fax: +33 388 360 715
E-mail: Jean-Louis.Imbs@pharmaco-ulp.u.strasbg.fr

Professor D Stephan
Institut de Pharmacologie et de
Médecine Expérimentale
Service d'Hypertension, maladies vasculaires et Pharmacologie Clinique
Hôpitaux Universitaires
Faculté de Médecine
11 rue Humann
67085 Strasbourg Cedex
Phone: +33 388 358 755
Fax: +33 388 360 715
E-mail: Stephan@mailserver.u.strasbg.fr

Toulouse
Professor Jean-Louis Montastruc
Service de Pharmacologie Clinique
Centre Hospitalier Universitaire
Faculté de Médecine
37 allées Jules Guesde
31073 Toulouse Cedex
Phone: +33 561 145 960
Fax: +33 561 255 116
E-mail: montastruc@cict.fr

Professor O Rascol
Laboratoire de Pharmacologie Medicale et Clinique
Faculté de Médecine
37 allées Jules Guesde
31073 Toulouse Cedex
Phone: +33 561 145 962
Fax: +33 561 255 116
E-mail: rascol@cict.fr

Professor JM Senard
Service de Pharmacologie Clinique
Centre Hospitalier Universitaire
Faculté de Médecine
37 allées Jules Guesde
31073 Toulouse Cedex
Phone: +33 561 145 961
Fax: +33 561 255 116
E-mail: senard@cict.fr

Tours
Professor E Autret-Leca
Sce de Pharmacologie Clinique
et Centre Régional de Pharmacovigilance
Hôpital Bretonneau
2 Boulevard Tonnellé
37044 Tours Cedex 01
Phone: +33 247 478 029
Fax: +33 247 473 826

Training Centres in France

Amiens

Research programme
- Antihypertensive drugs evaluation with a special reference to the use of ambulatory blood pressure measurement and to the assessment of arterial compliance.
- Clinical Pharmacokinetics
- Drug Safety Evaluation after post-marketing of drugs (pharmacovigilance).

Training programme
- Teaching of basic and clinical pharmacology during the universitary course in the medical faculty.
- Postgraduate training of general practioners.

Clinical and research facilities
Clinical Pharmacology Unit (cardiovascular pharmacology: assessment of drugs on blood pressure, heart rate and blood pressure variability (spectral analysis), arterial compliance (pulse wave velocity). Clinical pharmacokinetics: HPLC measurements of drugs. Blood samples for kinetic studies in humans and drug monitoring. Kinetics analysis. Drug safety: (Regional Centre of Pharmacovigilance): Adverse effects spontaneous reporting. Surveys with the French network of pharmacovigilance and local epidemiologic studies concerning drug safety and utilization.

Staff: one professor and an additional five academic positions in Clinical Pharmacokinetics and Drug Monitoring, clinical investigations in cardiovascular pharmacology and pharmacovigilance.

Application procedures: according to the French and to the Huriet Law 'Lieu de Recherches san bénéfice thérapeutique'.

References

Andréjak M (1996) Aims of ambulatory blood pressure monitoring during phase II and III clinical trials. Blood Pressure Monitoring 1: 309-311

Andréjak M, Gersberg M, Sgro C, Decocq G, Hamel J-D, Morin M, Gras V (1998a) French pharmacovigilance survey evaluating the hepatic toxicity of coumarin. Submitted to Pharmaco Epidemiol Drug Safety

Andréjak M, Genes N, Vaur L, Poncelet P, Clerson P, Carré A (1998b) Electronic pill-boxes in the evaluation of antihypertensive treatment compliance: comparison of once daily versus twice daily regimen. Submitted to J Cardiovasc Pharmacol

Chetaille E, de Cagny B, Chatelain-Trouvé B, Hellmuth D, Hary L, Fournier A, Andréjak M (1996) Pharmacokinetic parameters of meprobamate during continous veno-venous haemofiltration (CVVHF) after a severe intoxication. Nephro Pharmacology. Berlin 28-29.

Chetaille E, Redeker S, Picard C, Hary L, Schmit JL, Andréjak M (1997) Study in HIV-seropositive patients and healthy volunteers of correlations between the sulphamethoxazole and metabolism after 5 days of treatment and their acetylation and oxidative status. EACPT Congress, Berlin 17-20 September

Daelman F, Andréjak M, Rajaonarivony D, Bryselbout E, Jezraoul P, Ossart M (1994) Phenylephrine eyedrops, systemic atropine and cardiovascular adverse events. Thérapie 49: 467

de Cagny B, Chetaille E, Sechet A, Decocq G, Hary L, Fournier A, Andréjak M (1996) Acute renal failure induced by vancomycin overdose: usefulness of continuous haemofiltration. Nephrol Pharmacology. Berlin 28-29 juin

Decocq G, Brazier M, Hary L, Hubau C, Fortaine MR, Gondry J, Andréjak M (1997) Serum bupivacaine concentrations and transplacental transfer following repeated epidural administrations in term parturients during labour. Fundam Clin Pharmacol 11: 365-370

Makdassi M, de Cagny B, Lobjoie E, Andréjak M, Fournier A (1996) Convulsions, hypertension crisis and acute renal failure in postpartum: role of bromocriptine? Nephron 72: 732-733

Muir JF, Peiffer G, Richard MO, Benhamou D, Andréjak M, Hary L and Moore N (1993) Lack of effect of magnesium-aluminium hydroxide on the absorption of theophyline given as a pH-dependent sustained release preparation. Eur J Clin Pharmacol 44: 85-88

Besançon

Research programme: drug metabolism in psychiatry and allo- and xenotransplantation.

Training programme: clinical pharmacology in organ transplantation.

Research facilities: chromatographic technics, mass spectrometry, P.C.R.

Staff: one professor, one maitre de conference, one docent praticien hospitalier, two praticiens hospitalier-pharmacists, six technicians, three doctorants.

References

Bendriss A, Bechtel Y, Paintaud G, Bendriss EK, Joanne C, Bresson-Hadni S, Magnette J, Becker MC, Gillet M, Mantion G, Miguet JP, Bechtel PR (1995) Stability of debrisoquine CYP2D6 phenotype in liver transplant patients. Ther Drug Monit 17: 113-119

Catteau A, Bechtel YC, Poisson N, Bechtel PR, Bonaiti-Pellie C (1995) A population and family study of CYP1A2 using caffeine urinary metabolites. Eur J Clin Pharmacol 47: 423-430

Bechtel PR (1995) Relevance and limits of Pharmacogenetics to detect patients at risk of adverse drug reactions. Pharmacoepidemiology and Drug Safety 4: 31-36

Bechtel PR, Bechtel YC (1995) Interethnic differences in arylamine N-acetyltransferase activity, clinical consequences. In Advances in drug metabolism in man. 137-149 Ed. GM Pacifici and GN Fracchia. EUR 14539-EN

Bendriss EK, Bechtel Y, Bendriss A, Humbert PH, Paintaud G, Magnette J, Agache P, Bechtel PR (1996) Inhibition of caffeine metabolism by 5 methoxypsoralen in patients with psoriasis. Br J Clin Pharmacol 41: 421-424

Bendriss EK, Bechtel YC, Paintaud G, Brientini MP, Mantion G, Miguet JP, Bennani A, Bechtel PR (1997) Acetylation polymorphism expression in patients before and after liver transplantation. Influence of host-/graft genotypes. Pharmacogenetics, accepted 26-11-97

Maboundou CW, Paintaud G, Bresson-Hadni S, Mantion G, Miguet JP, Bechtel PR (1996a) Effect of the transition from intravenous to oral dosing on cyclosporin A through concentrations in liver transplant patients. Ther Drug Monit 18 (3): 310-314

Maboundou CW, Paintaud G, Vanlemmens C, Magnette J, Bresson-Hadni S, Mantion G, Miguet JP, Bechtel PR (1996b) A single dose of ursodiol does not affect cyclosporine absorption in liver transplant patients. Eur J Clin Pharmacol 50: 335-337

Monek O, Paintaud G, Bechtel Y, Miguet JP, Mantion G, Bechtel PR (1997) Influence of donor and recipient genotypes on CYP2D6 phenotype after liver transplantation: a study of mutations CYP2D6* and CYP2D6*4. Eur J Clin Pharmacol, accepted 1-09-97

Paintaud G, Bechtel P, Brientini MP, Miguet JP, Bechtel PR (1996) Effects of liver diseases on drug metabolism. Therapie 51 (4): 384-390

Bordeaux

University Victor Segalen

The Department of Clinical Pharmacology

Research programmes

- Pharmacokinetics: drug lipophilicity and tissue penetration (fundamental and clinical), plasma protein and tissue binding, bioavailability.
- Clinical pharmacology: cardiovascular pharmacology, effects of drugs on reactivity to stress; effects of physical training on drug metabolism and effects; cardiotoxicity of anticancer drugs. Effects of drugs, autacoids, and cytokines on human bronchi in vivo and in vitro.
- Pharmacoepidemiology: drug utilization studies, methodology of spontaneous reporting of adverse drug reactions, cohort studies (elderly, tacrine and Alzheimer's disease, clozapine, case control studies; pharmacodependencies).
- Pharmacoeconomics: prevalence, incidence and cost of adverse drug reactions and suicide attempts.

Training/teaching programmes: diplomas for investigators in clinical trials, pharmacoepide-miology, pharmacochemistry, fundamental and applied pharmacology.

Clinical and research facilities:
- Fundamental pharmacology lab: human bronchi in vitro.
- Pharmacokinetics lab for plasma drug assays, pharmacokinetic studies.
- Clinical pharmacology unit (healthy volunteers).
- Links with clinical departments in oncology, cardiology, respiratory medicine.
- Pharmacoepidemiology unit.

Staff: three Professors [Bernard Begaud (head of department, pharmacoepidemiology], Jacques Dangoumau (pharmacoeconomics), Nicholas Moore (clinical pharmacology, cardiovascular pharmacology), two associate professors (Fabienne Pehourcq (pharmacokinetics), Mathieu Molimard (respiratory pharmacology), one hospital practitioner [Françoise Haramburu (Pharmacovigilance, Pharmacodependence)], three assistants, research assistants, technicians. More than 40 persons overall.

Application procedures: contact any of the professors for initial contact.

References

Abenhaim L, Moride Y, Brenot F, Rich S, Benichou J, Kurz X, Higenbottam T, Oakley C, Wouters E, Aubier M, Simonneau G, Begaud B (1996) Appetite-suppressant drugs and the risk of primary pulmonary hypertension. International Primary Pulmonary Hypertension Study Group. N Engl J Med 335 (9): 609-616

Auzou P, Ozsancak C, Hannequin D, Moore N, Augustin P (1996) Clozapine for the treatment of psychosis in Parkinson's disease: a review. Acta Neurol Scand 94 (5): 329-336

Compagnon P, Thiberville L, Moore N, Thuillez C, Lacroix C (1996) Simple high-performance liquid chromatographic method for the quantitation of 5-fluorouracil in human plasma. J Chromatogr B Biomed Appl 677 (2): 380-383

Fourrier A, Letenneur L, Begaud B, Dartigues JF (1996) Nonsteroidal antiinflammatory drug use and cognitive function in the elderly: inconclusive results from a population-based cohort study. J Clin Epidemiol 49 (10): 1201

Mercie P, Rue-Fenouche C, Fournier A, Constans J, Begaud B, Conri C (1996) Prevalence of adverse effects of peripheral vasodilator agents in the elderly over the age of 65 years Therapie 51 (5): 602-603

Molimard M, Advenier C (1996) The human bronchus model in vitro. Pharmacological approach of various components involved in the functional response. Cell Biol Toxicol 12 (4-6): 233-237

Moore N, Breemeersch C, Noblet C (1996) Renal failure with fluoroquinolones.Therapie 51 (4): 421-423

Moride Y, Haramburu F, Requejo AA, Begaud B (1997) Under-reporting of adverse drug reactions in general practice. Br J Clin Pharmacol 43 (2): 177-181

Naline E, Molimard M, Regoli D, Emonds-Alt X, Bellamy JF, Advenier C (1996) Evidence for functional tachykinin NK1 receptors on human isolated small bronchi. Am J Physiol 271 (5 Pt 1): L763-L767

Rosenberg L, Begaud B, Bergman U, Brown B, Buist AS, Cramer D, Daling J, Grimes D, Kemper F, Mills A (1996) What are the risks of third-generation oral contraceptives? Are third-generation oral contraceptives safe? Hum Reprod 11 (4): 687-688

Brest

Research Programme

Phase one and phase two metabolism and drug interactions in vitro in human cells and in vivo in relation to hepatotoxicity observed in post-marketing survey.

Training and teaching programme: in charge of clinical pharmacology for medical students.

Clinical and research facilities: human hepatocytes in culture and other species, human hepatic microsomes. Liquid chromatography for metabolism or pharmakokinetic studies. Pharmacokinetic analysis. Meta-analysis. Possibility of clinical trial in cancer patients and in healthy volunteers in cardiology.

Staff: five researchers

References

Becquemont L, Le Bot MA, Riché C, Beaune P (1996) Influence of fluvoxamine on tacrine metabolism in vitro: potential implication for the hepatotoxicity in vivo. Fundam Clin Pharmacol 10: 156-157

Becquemont L, Ragueneau I, Le Bot MA, Riché C, Funck-Bretano C, Jaillon P (1997) Influence of the CYP1A2 inhibitor fluvoxamine on tacrine pharmacokinetics in humans. Clin Pharmacol Ther (in press)

Berson A, Renault S, Leitéron P, Robin MA, Fromenty B, Fau D, Le Bot MA, Riché C, Durant-Schneider AM, Feldmann G, Pessayre D (1996) Uncoupling of rat and human mitochondria: a possible explanation for tacrine-induce liver dysfunction. Gastroenterology 110: 1878-1890

Haaz MC, Rivory LP, Riché C, Robert J (1997a) The transformation of irinotecan (CPT-II) to its active metabolite SN-38 by human liver microsomes. Differential hydrolysis for the lactone and carboxylate forms. Naunyn-Schmiedeberg's Arch Pharmacol 356: 257-262

Haaz MC, Rivory L, Jantet S, Ratanasavanh D, Robert J (1997b) Glucuronidation of of SN-38, the active metabolite of irinotecan, by human hepatic microsomes. Pharmacol Toxicol 80: 91-96

Haaz MC, Rovory L, Riché L, Vernillet L, Robert J (1997c) Metabolism of CPT-II by human hepatic microsomes: participation of cytochrome P-450 3A and drug interactions. Cancer Res (in press)

Iribarne Ch, Berthou F, Carlhant D, Dréano Y, Picart D, Lohézic F, Riché C (1997) Inhibition of methadone and buprenorphine N-dealkylations by three HIV-1 protease inhibition. Drug Metab Dispos (in press)

Lagadic-Gossmann D, Rissel M, Le Bot MA, Gunlouzo A (1997) Toxic effects of tacrine on primary hepatocytes and liver epithelial cells in culture. Soumis à Cell Biology and Toxicology

Le Bot MA, Kernaleguen D, Simon I, Berlion M, Riché C (1996) Effet du S9788, de la ciclosporine A et du vérapamil sur l'accumulation intracellulaire de la doxorubicine, de la daunorubicine, de la daunorubicine et du daunorubicinol dans les hépatocytes de rat en culture primaire. Ann Biol Clin 54: 21-24

Ratanasavanh D, Lamiarne E, Biour M, Guédès Y, Gersbero M, Leutenegger E, Riché C (1996) Metabolism and toxicity of coumarin on cultured human, rat, mouse and rabbit hepatocytes. Fundam Clin Pharmacol 10: 504-510

Caen

Research Programme

Pharmacokinetic of psychotropic drugs and others (>40 molecules). Modelling for PET of new ligands metabolisms by animal studies. Protein Synthesis modelling in vivo (PET or QAR). Pharmacogenetic of DA receptor and behaviour, binding on receptors, quantitative autoradiography, tissue pharmacokinetics, toxicology and illegal drugs (detection and dosages).

Training and teaching programme

Medical pharmacology (second and third levels in medical and pharmaceutical courses). Important participations in fundamental science certificates. Midwifery and nursing teaching.

Clinical and research facilities

Numerous clinical departments and medical laboratories in the same site (1700 beds), IRM, Spectro IRM, PET and cyclotron, DNA analysis and sequencing in the hospital. Regional centre for Drug Adverse Effects and Pharmacodependence Study centre in the lab.

Staff: two professors, one MD, two pharmacists and one PhD

References

Barre L, Debruyne D, Lasne MC, Gourand F, Bonvento G, Camsonne R, Moulin M, Baron JC (1992) Synthesis and regional rat brain distribution of [11C]MDL 72222: a 5HT3 receptor antagonist. Int J Appl Radiat Isotopes 43 (4): 509-516

Besret L, Debruyne D, Rioux P, Bonvalot T, Moulin M (1996) A comprehensive investigation of plasma and brain regional pharmacokinetics of imipramine and its metabolites during and after chronic administration in the rat. J Pharm Sci 85(3): 291-295

Bustany P, Trenque T, Crambes O, Moulin M (1995) Restoration of brain protein synthesis in mature and aged rats by a DA agonist, piribedil. Fundam Clin Pharmacol 9 (5): 458-468

Camsonne R, Bustany P, Bigot MC, Pottier D, Moulin M (1994) Persistent low plasma levels of HIV-1 in patients on AZT Therapy and its implications. Thérapie 49 (2): 146-147

Debruyne D, Ryckelynck JP, Moulin M, Hurault De Ligny B, Levaltier B, Bigot MC (1990) Pharmacokinetics of fluconazole in patients undergoing continous ambulatory peritoneal dialysis. Clin Pharmacokinet 18 (6): 491-498

Debruyne D, Moulin M, Tartiere J, Bigot MC, Gerard JL, Bricard H (1990) Clinical pharmacokinetics after repeated intrapleural bupivacaine administration. Clin Pharmacokinet 18 (3): 240-244

Debruyne D, Abadie P, Barre L, Albessard F, Moulin M (1991) Plasma pharmacokinetics and metabolism of the benzodiazepine antagonist [11C]Ro 15-1788 (flumazenil) in baboon and human during position emission tomography studies. Eur J Drug Metab Pharmacokinet 16(2): 141-152

Debruyne D, Tartiere J, Albessard F, Samba D, Deshayes JP, Moulin M (1995) Clinical pharmacokinetics of propofol in postoperative sedation after orthotopic liver transplantation. Clin Drug Invest 9 (1): 8-15

Trenque T, Bustany P, Lamiable D, Legros S, Choisy H (1994) Pharmacokinetics and brain distribution of zolpidem in the rat after acute and chronic administratioin. J Pharm Pharmacol 46 (7): 611-613

Trenque T, Bustany P, Lamiable D, Vistelle R, Moreau F, Millart H, Choisy H (1997) Effects of acute and chronic treatment by zolpidem on serotoninergic and dopaminergic brain levels. Pharm Sci 3 (2): 153-155

Creteil

Centre Hospitalier Intercommunal
Research programme
Relationship between plasma protein binding and drug distribution. Preservation of kidney function in cyclospirin treated patients.

Training programme
Training in general pharmacology and in advanced pharmacology. Clinical pharmacology of organ transplantation.

Clinical and research facilities
- Statistical unit
- Chromatographic assays
- Use of radiopharmaceuticals
- Spectroscopic and fluorometric assays

Staff: seven full time researchers, three practicien hospitaliers, eight students and technicians

References

Doit C, Barre J, Cohen R, Bonacorsi S, Bourrillon A, Bingen EH (1997) Bactericidal activity against intermediately cephalosporin-resistant streptococcus pneumoniae in cerebrospinal fluid of children with bacterial meningitis treated with high doses of cefotaxime and vancomycin. Antimicrob Agents Chemother 41 (9): 2050-2052

Elimadi A, Morin D, Albengres E, Chauvet-Monges AM, Allain V, Crevat A, Tillement JP (1997) Differential effects of zidovudine and zidovudine triphosphate on mitochondrial permeability transition and oxidative phosphorylation. Br J Pharmacol 121: 1295-1300

Hauet T, Bauza G, Mothes D, Le Moyec L, Goujon JM, Dore B, Caritez JC, Carretier M, Eugene M, Tillement JP (1997) Beneficial effects on rat kidney preservation of the antiischemic agent trimetazidine during cold storage and reperfusion/assessment by 31P nuclear magnetic resonance spectroscopy. Transplant Proc 29: 2343-2344

Hauet T, Mothes D, Goujon JM, Caritez JC, Carretier M, Le Moyec L, Eugene M, Tillement JP (1997) Trimetazidine prevents renal injury in the isolated perfused pig kidney exposed to prolonged cold ischemia. Transplantation 64 (7): 1082-1086

Hervé F, Duche JC, D'Athis P, Marche C, Barre J, Tillement JP (1996) Binding of disopyramide, methadone, dipyridamole, chlorpromazine, lidocaine and progesterone to the two main genetic variants of human alpha1-acid glycoprotein: evidence for drug-binding differences between the variants and for the presence of two separate drug binding sites on alpa1-acid glycoprotein. Pharmacogenetics 6 (5): 403-415

Lebargy F, Benhammou K, Morin D, Zini R, Urien S, Bree F, Bignon J, Branellec A, Lagrue G (1996) Tobacco smoking induces expression of very-high-affinity nicotine binding sites on blood polymorphonuclear cells. Am J Respir Crit Care Med 153: 1056-1063

Russo H, Urien S, Duboin MP, Bres J, Bressolle F (1997a) Pharmacokinetics of high-dosage thopental sodium in patients with cerebral injuries. Influential factors on kinetic model and on parameter variability. Clin Drug Invest 13 (5): 255-269

Russo H, Simon N, Duboin MP, Urien S (1997b) Population pharmacokinetics of high-dose thiopental in patients with cerebral injuries. Clin Pharmacol Ther 62 (1): 15-20

Simon N, Zini R, Morin C, Bree F, Tillement JP (1997a) Prednisolone and azathioprine worsen the cyclosporine A-induced oxidative phosphorylation decrease of kidney mitochondria. Life Sci 61 (6): 659-666

Simon N, Brunet P, Roumenov D, Dussol B, Barre J, Duche JC, Albengres E, D'Athis P, Chauvet-Monges AM, Berland Y, Tillement JP (1997b) Trimetazidine does not modify blood levels and immunosuppressant effects of cyclosporine A in renal allograft recipients. Br J Clin Pharmacol 44 (6): 591-594

Henri Mondor Hospital
Research programme
– Angiogenesis in cardiovascular diseases (in collaboration with INSERM)
– Heart rate and blood pressure variability in heart failure patients
– Baroreflex function in cardiovascular diseases
– Respiratory pharmacology

Training/teaching programme
– Experimental and clinical pharmacology for medical students
– Host laboratory for clinical research assistant
– Participation to inter-University PhD teaching programme on clinical pharmacology

Clinical and research facilities
– Pharmacodynamic explorations in the cardiovascular field (orthostatic hypotension, vaso-vagal syncope, dysautonomia, ambulatory blood pressure monitoring)
– Clinical trials with cardiovascular drugs with the cardiologists of the institution.
– Collaboration with clinicians for clinical trials with methdological and logistic support in various fields (dermatology, hepatology, neurology)

Staff: one professor of clinical pharmacology, one full-time assistant, two part-time MDs. One full-time clinical research nurse and one secretary.

Application procedures: by fax or by mail.

References

Calvet JH, Coste A, Levame M, Harf A, Macquin-Mavier I, Escudier E (1996) Airway epithelial damage induced by sulphur mustard in guinea pigs. Effects of glucocorticoids. Hum Exp Toxicol 15: 964-971

Carvalhaes-Neto N, Lorino H, Gallinari C, Escolano C, Mallet A, Zerah F, Harf A, Macquin-Mavier I (1995) Cognitive function and assessment of lung function in institutionalized elderly patients. Am J Respir Crit Care Med 152: 1611-1615

Cloarec-Blanchard L, Funk-Bretano C, Lipski M, Jaillon P, Macquin-Mavier I (1997) Repeatablilty of spectral components of short-term blood pressure and heart rate variatiliby during acute symathetic activation in healthy young male subjects. Clin Sci 93: 21-28

Delacourt C, D'Ortho M-P, Macquin-Mavier I, Pezet S, Harf A, Lafuma C (1995) Increased 92-kDa gelatinase activity from alveolar macrophages in newborn rats. Am J Respir Crit Care Med 151: 1939-1945

Delacourt C, d'Ortho M-P, Macquin-Mavier I, Pezet S, Housset B, Lafuma C, Harf A (1996) Oxidant-antioxidant balance in alveolar macrophages from newborn rats. Eur Respir J 9: 2517-2524

D'Ortho MP, Jarreau Ph, Delacourt C. Pezet S, Lafuma C, Harf A. Macquin-Mavier I (1995) Tachykinins induce gelatinase production from guinea pig alveolar macrophages. Involvement of NK2 receptors. Am J Physiol (Lung Cell Mol Physiol) 269: L631-L636

Jarreau Ph, Harf A, Boyer V, Macquin-Mavier I (1996) Aerosolized non peptide NK1 and NK2 tachykinin receptor antagonists inhibit pentamidine-induced bronchoconstriction in the guinea pig. Fundam Clin Pharmacol 10: 518-523

Partovian C, Jacqz E, Keundjian A, Jaillon P, Funck-Bretano C (1995) Comparison of chloroguanide and mephenytoin for the in vivo assessment of genetically determined CYP2C19 activity in humans. Clin Pharmacol Ther 58: 257-63

Partovian C, Benetons A, Pommies JP. Safar ME (1998) Effects of high salt diet associated with bradykinin receptor blockade on arterial structure. Am J Physiol (in press)

Zerah F, Lorino AM, Lorino H, Brochard P, Harf A, Macquin-Mavier I (1995) Forced oscillation technique vs spirometry to assess bronchodilatation in patients with chronic obstructive diseases. Chest 108: 41-47

Dijon

Research programme
Clinical pharmacology of immunosuppresive drugs; pharmacogenetics of thiopurine methyl transferase; gene regulation of glucuronosyl transferase; pharmacoepidemiology of drug induced hepatitis.

Training and teaching programmes
Medical students: clinical pharmacology and pharmacokinetics; pharmacovigilance and pharmacoepidemiology.

PhD: clinical pharmacology of immunosuppresive drugs

Staff: one professor (MD), two PhDs (pharmacists) and one pharmacist

References
Bernard P, Hamdoune M, Mounie J, Goudonnet H, Magdalou J, Santona L, Escousse A. Effect of dietary vitamin A and thyroidal status on the binding characteristics of

the T3 nuclear receptors and glucuronidation of flurbiprofen. Actualités en Pharmacie et Biologie Clinique. Garnier JP, Le Moel G, Bousquet B, Dreux C, Eds. VARIA Publ., Paris, 7ème série, pp. 230-234

Charmollaux M, Goudonnet H, Mounie J, Magdalou J, Escousse A, Truchot RC (1991) Comparative and simultaneous effects of simvastatin and ciprofibrate on plasma lipids parameters and upon drug metabolising and peroxisome proliferation markers. Cell Mol Biol 37 (8): 765-771

Escousse A (1995) Clinical pharmacology of azathioprine in transplant recipients. In Organ transplantation and tissue grafting, Hervé P, Rifle G, Vuitton D, Dureau G, Bechtel P, Justrubo E. INSERM/John Libbey & Company Ltd: 29-40

Escousse A, Mousson C, Sanrona L, Zanetta G, Mounie J, Tanter Y, Duperray D, Rifle G, Chevet D (1995a) Azathrioprine induced pancytopenia in homozygous thiopurine methyl transferase deficient renal transplant recipient. Family study. Transplant Proc, 27 (2): 1739-1742

Escousse A, Rifle G, Sgro C, Mousson C, Zanetta G, Chevet D (1995b) Azathioprine toxicity, 6-mercaptopurine bioavaibility, and the 'poor' 6thiopurine methylator phenotype. Eur J Clin Pharmacol 48: 309-310

Hamdoune M, Mounie J, Magdalou J, Masmoudi T, Goudonnet H, Escousse A (1995) Characterization of the in vitro glucuronidation of flurbiprofen enantiomers. Drug Metab Dispos 23 (3): 343-348

Grenoble

Research programme: pharmacokinetics of narcotics opoid analgesics pharmakinetics, psychoactive drugs, therapeutic monitoring of eicosanoids and cardio-vascular system.

Staff: one professor and five pharmacists.

References

Amalfitano G, Bessard J, Vincent F, Eysseric H, Bessard G (1996) Gas chromatographic quantitation of dextropropoxyphene and norpropoxyphene in urine after solid-phase extraction. J Anal Toxicol 20: 547-554

Bessard G, Alibeu JP, Cartal M, Nicolle E, Serre Debeauvais F, Devillier P (1997) Pharmacokinetics of intrarectal nalbuphine in children undergoing general anaesthesia. Fundam Clin Pharmacol 11: 133-137

Bois F, Desfougeres A, Boumendjel A, Mariotte A, Bessard G, Caron F, Devillier P (1997) Genistein and fluorinated analogs suppress agonist-induced airway smooth muscle contraction. Bioorg Med Chem Lett 7: 1323-1326

Corompt E, Bessard G, Lantuejoul S, Naline E, Advenier C, Devillier P (in press) Inhibitory effects of large Ca2+-activated K+-channel blockers on b-adrenergic- and NO-donor-mediated relaxations of human and guinea-pig airway smooth muscles. Naunyn-Schmiedebergs's Arch Pharmacol

Devillier P, Bessard G, Advenier C (1995) Benzodiacepines and GABA-induced effects. In 'Airway Smooth Muscle: Neurotransmitters, Amines and Signal Transduction'; Eds Reaburn D, Giernbyez M, Birkhauser Verlag AG, London, Vol IV; ch. 9: 309-324

Devillier P, Bessard G, Thromboxane A (1996) Antagonists and thromboxane synthase inhibitors. In 'Antiasthmatic Drugs' in 'Progress in Basic and Clinical Pharmacology' by Pauwels R, Advenier C, O'Byrne P; Karger Publishers AG, Basel Switzerland

Nicolle E, Michaut S, Serre Debeauvais F, Bessard G (1995) Rapid and sensitive high-performance liquid chromatographic assay for nalbuphine in plasma. J Chromatogr B 603: 111-117

Nicolle E, Devillier P, Delanoy B, Durand C, Bessard G (1996) Therapeutic monitoring of nalbuphine: transplacental transfer and estimated pharmacokinetic in the neonate. Eur J Clin Pharmacol 49: 485-489

Stanke F, Jourdil N, Bessard J, Bessard G (1996) Simultaneous determination of zolpidem and zopiclone in human plasma by gas chromatography-nitrogen-phosphorus detection. J Chromatogr, 675: 43-51

Stanke F, Cracowski JL, Chavanon O, Magne JL, Blin D, Bessard G, Devillier P (in press) Glibenclamide inhibits thromboxane A2-induced contraction in human internal mammary artery and saphenous vein. Eur J Pharmacol

Limoges

Research programme
- Development of sensitive and specific methods for the assay of drugs and toxic compounds (HPLC, GC, LC-MS, LC-ES, GC-MS).
- Population pharmacokinetics applied to anticancer drugs and to patients in intensive care units or in geriatric units.
- Addiction to, pharmacokinetics of methadone, buprenorphine.
- Effect of environmental and industrial toxics in humans.
- Mechanism of anti-thyroid effect of tricyclic antidepressants and phenothiazines.
- Paraoxonase and atherosclerosis in ageing.
- Population pharmacovigilance in geriatrics

Training and teaching programmes
- Medical students: general principles of pharmacology in 3rd year, clinical pharmacology in 6th year.
- Pharmacy students: pharmacovigilance in 6th year
- Continuous medical education

Clinical and research facilities
Premises both in the faculty and in the hospital shared between the bi-

ological and clinical (pharmacovigilance) activities. The department also includes the sampling centre of the hospital together with two beds for out patient-explorations.

Staff: supervisory staff: six permanent staff (four MD, two Pharm D), one chemical engineer, four part-time staff (two MD, two pharm D). Other staff: 17 technicians, three secretaries.

References

Debord J, Pessis C, Voultoury JC, Marquet P, Lotfi H, Merle L, Lachâtre G (1995) Population pharmacokinetics of amikacin in intensive care unit patients studied by NPEM algorithm. Fundam Clin Pharmacol 9: 57-61

Debord J, Charmes JP, Marquet P, Merle L, Lachâtre G (1997) Population pharmacokinetics of amikacin in geriatric patients studied with the NPEN-2 algorithm. Int J Clin Pharmacol Ther 35: 24-27

Lotfi H, Dreyfuss MF, Marquet P, Debord J, Merle L, Lachâtre G (1996) Screening procedure for determination of thirteen oral anticoagulants and rodenticides. J Anal Toxicol 20: 93-100

Marquet P, François B, Vignon P, Lachâtre G (1996) A soldier who had seizures after drinking quarter of litre of wine. Lancet 348: 1070

Marquet P, Chevret J, Lavignasse P, Merle L, Lachâtre G (1997) Buprenorphine withdrawal syndrome in a newborn. Clin Pharmacol Ther 62: 569-571

Merle L, Reidenberg MM, Camacho MT, Drayer DE (1980) Renal injury in patients with rheumatoid arthritis treated with gold. Clin Pharmacol Ther 28: 216-222

Merle L, Charmes JP, Valette JP, Tronchet J, Lachâtre G, Nicot G (1981) Enzymuria and low molecular weight proteinuria as markers of aminoglycoside nephrotoxicity. Organ directed toxicity. Chemical indices and mechanisms. Brown SS, Davies DS (Eds), Pergamon Publ. 85-90

Nicot G, Merle L, Valette JP, Charmes JP, Lachâtre G (1982) Gentamicin and sisomicin induced renal toxicity. Eur J Clin Pharmacol 83: 161-166

Nicot G, Valette JP, dupuy JL, Merle L, Lachâtre G, Nouaille Y (1984a) Characterization of the esterases of the mitochondrial fraction of guinea pig cortical renal cells. Proc soc Exp Biol Med 176: 467-471

Nicot G, Merle L, Charmes JP, Valette JP, Nouaille Y, Lachâtre G, Leroux-Robert C (1984b) Transient glomerular proteinuria, enzymuria and nephrotoxic reaction induced by radiocontrast media. JAMA 252: 2432-2434

Lyon

Claude Bernard University

Field of interest and main topics
– regression of left ventricular hypertrophy
– treatment of prevention and regression of atheroclerosis
– antithrombotic drugs and prevention of thrombosis

- post-menopausal replacement therapy
- treatment of peripheral arterial disease
- clinical trial logistic and computer network
- safety and efficacy monitoring
- biostatistics applied to therapy target population definition
- cardiovascular drug pharmacodynamics
- PK-PD modelling
- evidence based medicine
- mathematical modelling and computer simulation
- methods in meta-analysis
- multiple sclerosis
- quality of life in clinical trials
- cardiovascular effect of steroids hormon
- therapeutic information: concepts and methodology

The department is responsible for teaching clinical and fundamental pharmacology to medical students in one of the four medical schools in Lyon, and for teaching clinical pharmacology and methodology of clinical trials to post graduates all over France, with two courses: one for research fellows, the other for professionals of the pharmaceutical industry.

Main research approaches
- investigations in healthy volunteers of pharmacodynamic of cardiovascular drugs
- clinical trials, especially multicentre, multinational trials, mainly in cardiovascular domains also in oncology, neurology and paediatric.

Staff
About 50 persons are working in the department: one professor, two assistant professors, eight researchers, 10 post graduate fellows, three engineers, 12 technicians, secretaries, CRAs (12). Some are payed by the university, others by INSERM and by a non profit organization.

References
Acar J, Iung B, Boissel JP, Samama MM, Michel PL, Teppe JP, Pony JC, Le Breton H, Thomas D, Isnard R, de Gevigney G, Viguier E, Sfihi A, Hanania G, Ghannem M, Mirode A, Nemoz C and the AREVA Group (1996) AREVA: multicenter ran-

domized comparison of low-dose vs standard dose anticoagulation in patients with mechanical prosthetic heart valves. Circulation 94: 2107-2112

Boissel JP, Collet JP, Lion L, Ducruet T, Moleur P, Luciani J, Milon H, Madonna O, Gillet J, Gerini P, Dazord A, Haugh MC and the OCAPI Study Group (1995) A randomized comparison of the effect of four antihypertensive monotherapies on the subjective quality of life in previously untreated asymptomatic patients: field trial in general practice. J Hypertension 13: 1059-1067

Cornu C, Cochat P, Collet JP, Delair S, Haugh MC, Rolland C, the GEP (1994) Survey of the attitudes to management of acute pyelonephritis in children. Pediatr Nephrol 8: 275-277

European Study of Prevention of Infarct with Molsidomine (ESPRIM) Group (1994) The ESPRIM Trial: short-term treatment of acute myocardial infarction with molsidomine. Lancet 344: 91-97

Girard P, Laporte-Simitsidis S, Mismetti P, Decousus H, Boissel JP (1995) Influence of confounding factors on designs for dose-effect relationship estimates. Stat Med 14: 987-1005

Girard P, Sheiner LB, Kastrissios H, Blaschke TF (1996) Do we need full compliance data for population pharmacokinetic analysis? J Pharmacokinet Biopharm 24 (2): 265-282

Leizorovicz A, Simonneau G, Decousus H, Boissel JP (1994) Comparison of efficacy and safety of low molecular weight heparins and unfractionated heparin in initial treatment of deep venous thrombosis: a meta-analysis. Br Med J 309: 299-304

Lièvre M, Guéret P, Gayet Ch, Roudaut R, Haugh MC, Delair S, Boissel JP on behalf of the HYCAR Study Group (1995) Ramipril-induced regression of left ventricular hypertrophy independent of changes in blood pressure in hypertensive patients: The HYCAR (HYpertrophie CArdiaque et Ramipril) Study. Hypertension 25: 92-97

The Multicenter Acute Stroke Trial - Europe Study Group (1996) Thrombolytic therapy with streptokinase in acute ischemic stroke. N Engl J Med 335: 145-150

Uzzan B, Campos J, Cucherat M, Nony P, Boissel JP, Perret GY (1996) Effects on bone mass of long term treatment with thyroid hormones: a meta-analysis. J Clin Endocrinol Metab 81: 4278-89

Lyon Poison Centre

The Department of Pharmacology, Toxicology and Environmental Medicine, headed by Professor J Descotes, is mainly interested in methods of immunotoxicity evaluation, mechanisms of immunotoxic effects, fundamental immunopharmacology and diseases of medicinal and environmental origin (mainly hypersensitivities and autoimmunity). The clinical facilities are located in Lyon Poison Centre.

Training programmes include Postdoctoral Degree in Medical Toxicology, Postdoctoral Degree for Study Directors in Regulatory Toxicology, Continuing Education in Immunotoxicology, PreDoctoral and

PhD Training in Immunology and Toxicology.

The staff consists of 12 members in the research team and 25 in Poison Centre.

Applications can be sent to Head of Department.

References

Descotes J (1996) Human Toxicology. Elsevier Science, Amsterdam

Krasteva M, Garrigue JL, Horrand F, Tchou I, Descotes J, Nicolas JF (1996) Suboptimal non-inflammatory concentrations of haptens may elicit a contact sensitivity reaction when used as a mix. Contact Dermatitis 35: 279-282

Pham E, Nicolas B, Vial T, Descotes J (1995) Modelization of warning procedures to detect the toxic effects of drugs and chemicals to man: application to a sentinel disease programme in immunotoxicology. Toxicology Modelling 1: 207-218

Testud F, Granclaude JM, Descotes J (1996) Acute hexogen poisoning after occupational exposure. Clin Toxicol 34: 109-111

Verdier F, Aujoulas M, Condevaux F, Descotes J (1995) Determination of lymphocyte subsets and cytokine levels in nonhuman primates: cross-reactivity of human reagents. Toxicology 105: 81-90

Verdier F, Patriarca C, Descotes J (1997) Autoantibodies in conventional toxicity testing. Toxicology 119: 51-58

Vial T, Descotes J (1994) Contact sensitization assays. Do they predict the risk for hyper-sensitivity? Toxicology 93: 63-75

Vial T, Descotes J (1996) Drugs acting on the immune system. In: Meyler's Side Effetcs of Drugs, 13th ed., MNG Dukes (ed.), Elsevier Sciences, Amsterdam, p.1090-1165

Vial T, Tedone R, Patriarca C, Descotes J (1995) Effect of serotonin on the chemiluminescence response of rat peripheral blood leucocytes. Int J Immunopharmacol 17 : 813-819

Vial T, Nicolas B, Descotes J (1997) Drug-induced autoimmunity. Experience of the French Pharmacovigilance system. Toxicology 119: 23-27

Marseilles

Aix-Marseille II University

Research programme: clinical trials methodology.

Training and teaching programme
- Pharmaco-therapeutics for medical students
- Participation in French inter-university programmes on pharmacology, clinical trials methodology, pharmacoepidemiology, clinical research assistants formation and biostatistics applied to biology and medicine

Clinical and research facilities
In the Laboratory of Clinical Trials methodology: methodological support in clinical trials and medical evaluation for clinical reseachers and pharmaceutical industry. In the Clinical Investigation Centre of Sainte-Marguerite University Hospital, a five-bed facility opened to clinicians, researchers and pharmaceutical industry methodological support.
Staff: two professors of therapeutics, one assistant professor and one assistant.
Application procedure: by mail.

References
Bouvenot G (1994a) Réflexions sur la méthodologie de l'évaluation des traitements de l'arthrose. Rev Rheum 61(2): 74-79. Considerations on the methodology of studies evaluation treatment for osteo arthritis. Engl Ed 61 (2) 74-76
Bouvenot G (1994b) Critéres substitution. Rev Rhum 61 (11): 801-803 Surrogate end-points. Engl. Ed 61 (11): 711-713
Bouvenot G (1996a) La Médecine Factuelle. Thérapie 51: 209-211
Bouvenot G (1996b) Justification des pratiques thérapeutiques. Rev Rhum. 63 (6): 461-462 What should our treatment decisions be based on? Engl Ed 63 (6) 383-384
Bouvenot G (1996c) Le placebo des essais cliniques: mise en examen. Rev Rhum (Ed Fr) 63 (9): 663-666 Placebo-controlled clinical trials: a reappraisal (Engl Ed) 63 (9): 565-568
Bouvenot G, Vray M (1994) Validité interne et portée des résultats des essais cliniques. Rev Méd Int 15: 9-12
Bouvenot G, Teule-Espie M (1994) Analyse des stratégies du traitement médicamenteux de la douleur et de leur évaluation. Thérapie 50: 235-238
Compston J, Audran M, Avouac B, Bouvenot G, Devogelaer JP et al. (Group for the Respect of Ethics and Excellence in Science) (1996) Recommendations for the registration of agents used in the prevention and treatment of glucocorticoid-induced osteoporosis. Calcif Tissue Int 59: 323-327
Dougados M, Devogelaer JP, Annefeldt M, Avouac B, Bouvenot G et al (Group for the Respect of Ethics and Excellence in Science) (1996) Recommendations for the registration of drugs used in the treatment of osteoarthritis. Am Rheum Disease 55: 552-557
Eschwege E, Bouvenot G (1994) Essais clinique explicatifs ou pragmatiques: le dualisme. Rev Méd Interne 15: 357-361
Reginster JY, Compston JE, Jones EA, Kaufman JM, Audran M, Bouvenot G, Prati L, Mazzuoli G, Lemmel EM, Ringe JD, Sebert JL, Avouac B (1995) Recommendations for the registration of new chemical entities used in the prevention and treatment of osteoporosis. Calcif Tissue Int 57: 247-250

The Department of Clinical Pharmacology of the Timone Hospital
Research and training programme: CNS drugs: pharmacokinetics and pharmacodynamics on healthy volunteers, clinical trials in schizophrenia, Parkinson's Disease.

Clinical and Research facilities: Hospital Phase I Unit (the CPCET): 1000 m^2, eight beds, four rooms for pharmacodynamics (vigilance, performances and memory; ophthalmology and infrared oculomotor recording; choice reaction time and electromyography; emotion induction).

The University: formal University Research Unit (UPRES 2199)
Staff:15 medical doctors, pharmacists, CRNs, CRAs, biostatistician, QA
Application procedures: letter and interview
Inquiries: Professor O Blin

References
Azorin JM et al. (1994) Aspects cliniques de la dépression chez le psychotique. Encéphale 20 SP 4: 663-666
Blin O et al. (1996) Antipsychotic and anxiolytic properties of risperidone, haloperidol and methotrimeprazine in schizophrenic patients. J Clin Psychopharmacol 1: 38-44
Masson G et al. (1993) Dopaminergic modulation of visual perception in man. Fundam Clin Pharmacol 7: 449-463
Paut O et al. (1995) Evaluation of saccadic eye movements as an objective test during recovery from anaesthesia. Acta Anaesth Scand 39: 1117-1124

Montpellier
University Montpellier I, France
Research and training programme: pharmacology of the central nervous system, particularly psychopharmacology, pharmacology of glucose homeostasis, insulin secretion and feeding behaviour, in patients and healthy volunteers.

Clinical and research facilities: Psychopharmacology Unit, comprising two beds devoted to pharmacological investigations, with five additional beds functionally localized in the surrounding psychiatric departments. Standardized evaluations of psychopathology, cognitive and executive functions as well as subjective drug effects.

Biomedical Research centre, comprising two beds devoted to biomedical investigations, particularly drugs, physiology and pathophysiology, with hospital environment of internal medicine, intensive care and various medical departments including endocrinology and metabolism. Technical facilities for the handling and storage of biological samples and for standard medical evaluations and monitoring.

Staff: Professor Pierre Petit, MD, PhD, in charge of the Psychopharmacology Unit and the Biomedical Research centre. Coworkers: one Senior Lecturer (Doctor in Pharmaceutical Sciences), one Medical Assistant (Medical Doctor), one Resident in Industrial Pharmacy, one part-time Secretary. Medical and nursing staff according to clinical protocols in progress.

Application procedure: medical doctors, licenced to practice medicine in their home country and justifying a background in general pharmacology may apply for a training period (at least 6 months). Applicants must also be proficient in speaking and writing French and English languages.

Inquiries: Professor P Petit

References
Botta T, Cartault F, Pouget R, Blayac JP, Petit P (1995a) An imidazopyridine anxiolytic alters glucose tolerance in patients: a pilot investigation. Clin Neuropharmacol 18: 79-82

Botta T, Hüe B, Hillaire-Buys D, Barbe A, Alric R, Pouget R, Petit P (1995b) Clonazepam in acute mania: time-blind evaluation of clinical response and concentrations in plasma. J Affect Disord 36: 21-27

Giacardi-Paty M, Botta T, Pujelte D, Lainey E, Petit P (1993) Neuroleptic rechallenge after neuroleptic malignant syndrome. Br J Psychiatry 163: 121-122

Humbert T, Pujelte D, Bottai T, Hüe B, Pouget R, Petit P (1997) Pilot investigation of TRHinduced TSH and prolactin release in anxious patients treated with diazepam. Clin Neuropharmacol, in press

Loubatieres-Mariani MM, Petit P, Chapal J, Hillaire-Buys D, Bertrand G, Ribes G (1994) Effects of purinoceptor agonists on insulin secretion. In: Adenosine and Adenine Nucleotides: From Molecular Biology to Integrative Physiology. Balardinelli L, Pelleg A, eds. Martinus Nijhoff Publishers, Boston 337-345

Petit P, Lonjon R, Cociglio M, Slazewska A, Blayac JP, Hüe B, Alric R, Pouget R (1991) Carbamazepine and its 10,11-epoxide metabolite in acute mania: clinical and pharmacokinetic correlates. Eur J Clin Pharmacol 41: 541-546

Petit P, Manteghetti M, Berdeu D, Ribes G, Loubatieres-Mariani MM (1992) Effects of a peripheral-type benzodiazepine on glucose-induced insulin secretion. Eur J Pharmacol 221: 359-363

Petit P, Sauvaire Y, Hillaire-Buys D, Leconte O, Baissac Y, Ponsin G, Ribes G (1995) Steroid saponins from fenugreek seeds: extraction, purification and pharmacologi-

cal investigation on feeding behaviour and plasma cholesterol. Steroids 60: 674-680
Petit P, Loubatieres-Mariani MM, Keppens S, Sheehan MJ (1996) Purinergic receptors and metabolic function. Drug Dev Res 39: 413-425
Pujalte D, Bottai T, Hüe B, Alric R, Pouget R, Blayac JP, Petit P (1994) A double-blind comparison of clonazepam and placebo in the treatment of neuroleptic-induced akathisia. Clin Neuropharmaco. 17: 236-242

Nancy
University Henri Poincaré

Research and training programme: cardiovascular pharmacology; time-effect profile of drugs; clinical trials; methodology; drugs for heart failure and hypertension.

Clinical and research facilities: Centre de dépistage et de prévention cardiovasculaire. Out- patients and in-patients (36 beds): clinical and research programme in atherosclerotic risk factors and drug prevention. Centre d'Investigation Clinique INSERM-CHU. A clinical research facility with full time clinical research staff + four beds + cardiovascular, autonomic nervous system, respiratory and metabolic non-invasive investigations. Funded by the University Hospital and INSERM.

The University: University Henri Poincar: Science + Pharmacy + Medicine University. Equipe d'Accueil 'Insuffisance Cardiaque'
Staff: Medical doctors, pharmacist, clinical research assistants and research nurses + secretary, biostatistician and computer specialist.

Application procedures: Contact Dr F. Zannad

References

Chati Z, Zannad F, Robin-Lherbier B, Escanye JM, Jeandel C, Robert J, Aliot E (1994) Contribution of specific abnormalities to limitation of exercise capacity in patients with chronic heart failure: a phosphorus 31 nuclear magnetic resonance study. Am Heart J 128: 781-792
Chati Z, Mertes PM, Aliot A, Zannad F (1996) Plasma levels of atrial natriuretic peptide and of other vasoconstricting hormones in patients with chronic heart failure: relationship to exercise capacity. Int J Cardiol 135-142
Khder Y, El Ghawi R, Bray Des Boscs L, Aliot E, Zannad F (1996) Investigations of the peripheral vascular mechanisms implicated in congestive heart failure by the non invasive evaluation of the radial artery compliance and reactivity. Int J Cardiol 56: 149-158
Zannad F (1995a) Clinical pharmacology of Nisoldipine coat core. Am J Cardiol 75: 41E-45E

Zannad F (1995b) Practical pharmacology of the 24-hour trough: peak ratio of antihypertensive drugs. J Hypertens 13 (suppl 2): S109-S112

Zannad F, Chati Z (1994) Skeletal muscle metabolic, morphohistological and biochemical abnormalities in congestive heart failure. Heart Failure 10: 58-66

Zannad F, Bray des Boscs L, El Ghawi R, Donner M, Thibout E, Stoltz JF (1993) Effects of lisinopril and hydrochlorotiazide on platelet function and function rheology in essential hypertension: a randomly allocated double-blind study. J Hypertens 11: 559-564

Zannad F, Vaur L, Dutrey-Dupagne C, Genes N, Clerson P (1996a) Antihypertensive effects of trandolapril and nitrendipine in the elderly: a controlled trial with special emphasis on time effect profiles. J Hum Hypertens 10: 51-55

Zannad F, Matzinger A, Larche J (1996b) Trough/peak ratios of once daily angiotensin converting enzyme inhibitors and calcium antagonists. Am J Hypertens 9: 633-643

Nantes

Research programme
Mainly psychometric studies with healthy volunteers in the field of neurobiology of anxiety, i.e. introduction of panicogenic agents; study of action of small dosages of benzodiazepines; refractory depression.

Training programme
The training programme is the formation of investigators in the field of clinical trials and teaching of residents in the field of psychopharmacology.

Clinical and research facilities
The clinical facilities consist of 150 m^2 with eight beds in the Academic Service of Psychiatry. These eight beds are dedicated to research mainly in the field of refractory depression.

Staff: There are two psychiatrists, two residents and two research clinical assistants and four nurses.

References

Bourin M, Malinge M (1995a) Controlled comparison of the effects and abrupt discontinuation of buspirone and lorazepam. Prog Neuro-Psychopharmacol Biol Psychiatr 19: 567-575

Bourin M, Malinge M (1995b) A new design of trial for hypnotics comparison: a double-blind cross-over trial with patient's preference assessment and continuation of preferred treatment. Prog Neuro Psychopharmacol Biol Psychiat 20: 373-385

Bourin M, Couëtoux du Tertre A, Colombel MC, Auget JL (1994) Effects of low dos-

es of lorazepam on psychometric tests in healthy volunteers. Int Clin Psychopharmacol 9: 83-88
Bourin M, Colombel MC, Malinge M (1995) Lorazepam 0.25 mg twice a day improves aspects of psychometric performance in healthy volunteers. J Psychopharmacol 9: 251-257
Bourin M, Bougerol T, Guitton B, Broutin E (1997) A combination of plant extracts in the treatment of outpatients with adjustment disorder with anxious mood: controlled study versus placebo. Fundam Clin Pharmacol 11: 127-132
Bradwejn J, Koszycki D, Bourin M (1991) Dose ranging study of the effects of cholecystokinin in healthy volunteers. J Psychiatr Neurosci 16: 91-95
Bradwejn J, Koszycki D, Payeur R, Bourin M, Borthwick H (1992) Replication of action of cholecystokinin tetrapeptide in panic disorder: clinical and behavioural findings. Am J Psychiatry 149: 962-964
Bradwejn J, Koszycki D, Couëtoux du Tertre A, Paradis M, Bourin M (1994) Effects of flumazenil on cholecystokinin-tetrapeptide-induced panic symptoms in healthy volunteers. Psychopharmacology 114: 257-261
Koszycki D, Bradwejn J, Bourin M (1991) Comparison of the effects of cholecystokinin-tetrapeptide and carbon dioxide in healthy volunteers. Eur Neuropsychopharmacol 1: 137-141
Lecrubier Y, Bourin M, Moon CA, Schifano F, Blanchard C, Danjou P, Hackett D (1997) Efficacy of venlafaxine in depressive illness in general practice. Acta Psychiatr Scand 95: 485-493

Paris
Hôpital Broussais - Service de Pharmacologie Clinique
Our research and training programme concerns mainly cardiovascular pharmacology, focusing on arterial remodelling in various diseases, and during antihypertensive treatment.

The department is connected to an INSERM (French N.I.H.) unit (U337: about 30 physicians and technicians), and therefore to the fundamental part of this research.

The staff consists of three senior physicians: Professor Stéfane Laurent, Dr Pierre Boutouyrie, Dr Carmen Kreft-Jais, one senior biologist: Dr Eliane Billaud

References
Azizi M, Veyssier-Belot C, Alhenc-Gelas M, Chatellier G, Billaud-Mesguish E, Fiessinger JN, Aiach M (1995) Comparison of biological activities of two low molecular weight heparins in 10 healthy volunteers. Br J Clin Pharmacol 40: 577-584
Bonithon-Khopp C, Ducimeiere P, Touboul PJ, Feve JM, Billaud E, Courbon Heraud

V (1994) Plasma angiotensin-converting enzyme activity and carotid wall thickening. Circulation 89: 952-954

Boutouyrie P, Laurent S, Girerd X, Beck L, Abergel E, Safar M (1995) Common carotid artery distensibility and patterns of left ventricular hypertrophy in hypertensive patients. Hypertension 25 [part 1]: 651-659

Heron D, Chatellier G, Billaud E, Plouin JF (1996) The urinary metanephrine-to-creatinine ratio for the diagnosis of pheochromocytoma. Ann Int Med 125: 300-310

Kreft-Jais C, Laforest L, Bonnardeau A, Dumont C, Plouin PF, Jeunemaire X (1994a) ACE inhibitors, cough and genetics. Lancet 343: 740

Kreft-Jais C, Caviezel B, Beck L, Girerd X, Billaud E, Boutouyrie P, Hoeks A, Safar M (1994b) Carotid artery distensibility and distending pressure in hypertensive humans. Hypertension 23 [part 2]: 878-883

Laurent S (1995) Arterial wall hypertrophy and stiffness in essential hypertensive patients. Hypertension 26: 355-362

Laurent S, Girerd X, Mourad JJ, Boutouyrie P, Safar M (1994) Elastic modulus of the redial artery wall is not increased in patients with essential hypertension. Arteriosclerosis and Thrombosis 1223-1231

Laurent S, Vanhoutte P, Cavero I, Chabrier PE, Dupuis B, Elghozi JL, Hamon G, Janiak P, Juillet Y, Kher A, Koen R, Madonna O, Maffrand JP, Pruneau D, Thuilliez C (1996) The arterial wall: a new pharmacological and therapeutic target. Fundam Clin Pharmacol 10: 243-257

Safar M, Laurent S (1996) Large arteries and veins in hypertension. In: Handbook of hypertension; pathophysiology and hypertension. Ed A. Zanchetti, G. Mancia, Elsevier, Amsterdam, Lausanne, New York, pp 334-383

Hôpital Cochin
Research programme
- Phase I and phase II antibiotic and antiviral drug clinical trials
- Pathogenesis and therapy of sepsis
- Pharmacokinetic-pharmacodynamic relationship of anti-infectives
- Clinical pharmacology of cytokines
- New strategies of vaccine development

Study types: first administration to man; safety and tolerability; bioavailability, bioequivalence; drug interactions; development of pharmacodynamic models and measurement of pharmacodynamic parameters in healthy volunteers; dose finding response;
comparative studies; long term studies; drug metabolism studies; PK-PK studies.

Traning/teaching programme: teaching clinical pharmacology for medical students as well as post graduate lectures for investigators

Clinical and research facilities
Clinical facilities: clinic with a floor area of 500 m² and two beds, intensive care unit available, blood sampling room, sample work-up room and -80°C freezer for sample storage, examination room.

Research facilities: enzyme-immunoassay (EIA), high performance liquid chromatography (HPLC), two flow cytometers (FacSCAN), enzyme linked immunoabsorbent assay (ELISA), spectrofluorometer

Staff: five scientific staff (physicians and biologists), two nurses, two medical laboratory technicians.

Hôpital Lariboisière
Unité de Recherches Thérapeutiques

– Inpatients: prophylaxis of deep vein thrombosis in medical patients; pharmacokinetics of antiviral therapies in AIDS patients; deep vein thrombosis management; anticoagulant therapy in patients in atrial fibrillation; thrombogenesis in patients with hypertension
– In healthy volunteers: pharmacodynamics in gastroenterology (pH-metry, digestive transit time, fibroscopy, transgastric potential diference); liver metabolism of drugs (CYP450 3A4: erythromycin C14 breath test); pharmacokinetics in healthy volunteers; veinous and arterial thrombogenesis and effect of antithrombotic drugs
– Various: methodology of clinical trials; registration procedures; quality of life in clinical trials

Training programme: (1) PhD in clinical pharmacclogy (DEA), (2) University diploma in methodology of clinical trials. (3) Formations for the monitoring of clinical trials.

Clinical and research facilities
Internal medicine unit: internal medicine hospitalization (20 beds), gastroenterology hospitalization (10 beds), cardiology hospitalization (15 beds), infectious disease and AIDS hospitalization (12 beds), outpatients clinics for internal medicine, infectious disease and AIDS.

Research Centre: phase II centre with healthy volunteers trials authorization. Facilities for pharmacokinetics. Centre for phase III therapeutic trials.

Staff: two professors and six MDs.

Further information can be requested from Professor JF Bergmann.

References

Bergmann JF (1997) Prévention de la thrombose veineuse e milieu médical. La Recue du prat 47: 1399-1401

Blondon H, Bergmann JF (1996) Hépatite chronique C: les incertitudes thérapeutiques. Gastroenterol Clin Biol 20: 1043-1046

Chassany O, Bergmann JF, Simoneau G, Elouaer-Blanc L, Segrestaa JM, Caulin C (1996) The comparative effets of single intravenous doses of cimetidine, ranitidine, famotidine and omeprazole on intragastric pH. Current Therapeutic Research 57 (3): 159-167

Chassany O, Bergmann JF, Marquis P, Scherrer B, Genève B, Sapede C. XXXVIe congrès de la Société Nationale Française de Médecine Interne, Nîmes Juin (1997) Etude européenne de validation psychométrique d'une échelle de qualité de vie spécifique dans les troubles fonctionnels digestifs. La Revue de Médecine Interne 18, suppl 2 (poster)

Crivat M, Simoneau G, Kodjo A, Blondon H, Dumitrescu L, Vittecoq D, Bergmann JF (1997)
Intestinal permeability and absorptive capacity in patients infected with human immunodeficiency virus. Gastroenterology 112 (4): A954

Crivat M, Simoneau G, Kodjo A, Blondon H, Dumitrescu L, Vittecoq D, Bergmann JF (1997b) Permeabilité intestinale et capacité d'absorption chez les patients infectés par le VIH. Méd Chirurg Digest 26 (6): 265

Kevorkian JP, Seroux C, Deharbe S, Salord JM, Bergmann JF (1997a) Prophylaxis of anaphylactoid reaction to antituberculous drugs. Ann Pharmacother 31: 373-374

Kevorkian JP, Halimi C, Le Dref O, Kedra W, Mundler O, Bergmann JF, Drouet L, Beaufils P, Segrestaa JM, Soria C (1997b) XVIth congress of the International Society on Thrombosis and Haemostasis. Florence, Italy, June. D-dimers plasma levels for monitoring treated acute thromboembolic venous disease. Thromb Haemostasis suppl (abst)

Kodjo A, Mouly s, Blondon H, Benelhadj S, Chassany O, Caulin C, Bergmann JF (1997) Temps de transit dans l'intestin grêle: des prélèvements salivaires peuvent-ils remplacer la scintigraphie. Gastroenterol Clin Biol 21: A 187

Kodjo A, Crivat M, Blondon H, Trout H, Dumitrescu L, Vittecoq D, Dohin E, Goerhs JM, Bergmann JF (1997) Digestive absorption of saquinavir in AIDS patients with severe diarrhea or wasting syndrome. Gastroenterology 112(4): A1016 (abst)

Centre de Pharmacologie Clinique de l'Hôpital Necker - Paris
The Clinical Pharmacology centre depends on Association Claude Bernard which provides two clinical research assistants and fundings. Studies are performed in the field of blood pressure and heart rate variability at the hospital. A close relation exists with the pharmacology laboratory of the faculty (located next to the hospital) in which computer work is performed with the help of institutional scientists. Foreign physicians or scientists may apply for a one-year grant offered by

Association Claude Bernard (usual deadline 15 April). A total of five permanent staff run the clinical and experimental research work. There are presently two PhD students and one postdoctoral fellow.

References

Constant I, Girard A, Le Bidois J, Villain E, Laude D, Elghozi JL (1995) Spectral analysis of systolic blood pressure and heart rate after heart transplantation in children Clin Sci 88: 95-102

Girard A, Meilhac B, Mounier-Vehier C, Elghozi, JL (1995) Effects of beta-adrenergic blockade on short-term variability of blood pressure and heart rate in essential hypertension. Clin Exp Hypertension 17: 15-27

Januel B, Laude D, Elghozi JL, Escourrou P (1995) Effect of autonomic blockade on heart rate and blood pressure in sleep apnea syndrome. Blood Pressure 4: 226-231

Laude D, Goldman M, Escourrou P, Elghozi JL (1993) Effect of breathing pattern on blood pressure and heart rate oscillations in man. Clin Exp Pharmacol Physiol 20: 619-626

Laude D, Weise F, Girard A, Elghozi JL (1995) Spectral analysis of systolic blood pressure and heart rate oscillations related to respiration. Clin Exp Pharmacol Physiol 22: 352-357

Laude D, Girard A, Consoli S, Mounier-Vehier C, Elghozi JL (1998) Anger expression and cardiovascular reactivity to mental stress: a spectral analysis approach. Clin Exp Hypertension, in press

Mounier-Vehier C, Girard A, Consoli S, Laude D, Vacheron A, Elghozi JL (1995) Cardiovascular reactivity to a new mental stress test: the maze test. Clin Auton Res 5: 145-150

Weise F, Laude D, Girard A, Zitoun P, Siché JP, Elghozi JL (1993) Effects of the cold pressor test on short-term fluctuations of finger arterial blood pressure and heart rate in normal subjects. Clin Auton Res 3: 303-310

Weise F, London G, Guerin AP, Pannier BM, Elghozi JL (1995a) Effect of head-down tilt on cardiovascular control in healthy subjects: a spectral approach. Clin Sci 88: 87-93

Weise F, London G, Pannier BM, Guerin AP, Elghozi JL (1995b) Effect of haemodialysis on cardiovascular rhythms in end-stage renal failure. Kidney Int 47: 1443-1452

Hôpital Pitié-Salpêtrière
Research programme
– Pharmacokinetic-pharmacodynamic modeling and dose-response relationships
– Drug development and clinical research in psychiatric and neurologic disorders: amyotrophic lateral sclerosis, depression, schizophrenia

- Drug development and clinical research in cardiovascular disease (heart failure), in endocrinology (diabetes)
- Pharmacovigilance
- Drug dependence: smoking cessation studies

Training/Teaching programme
- Pharmacology programme for medical students
- University specialized courses: pharmacokinetics and neuro-psychopharmacology
- Clinical and research facilities: phase I unit for studies in healthy volunteers
- Pharmaco-chemistry unit for drug dosages in plasma or other physiological fluids
- Connections with the unit for clinical investigation, which is a unit where clinical studies on patients from different departments from the Pitié-Salpêtrière Hospital can be informed.

Staff: two professors, five doctors

Application procedures: to become full time pharmacologist in the department, applicants must have followed specialized courses in pharmacology and clinical pharmacology, published papers in international journals, and finally have go through a PhD thesis.

References

Lacomblez L, Bensimon G, Leigh PN, Guillet P, Meininger V, for the Amyotrophic Lateral Sclerosis/Riluzole Study Group II (1996) Dose-ranging study of riluzole in amyotrophic lateral sclerosis. Lancet 347: 1425-1431

Lechat Ph, Escolano S, Golmard JL, Lardoux H, Witchitz S, Henneman JA, Maisch B, Hetzel M, Jaillon P, Boissel JP, Mallet A on behalf of the CIBIS investigators (1997) Prognostic value of bisoprolol-induced haemodynamic effects in heart failure during the Cardiac Insufficiency Bisoprolol study (CIBIS). Circulation, 96: 2197-2205

Mentré F, Pousset F, Comets E, Plaud B, Diquet B, Montalescot G, Ankri A, Mallet A, Lechat Ph (1998) Population pharmacokinetic-pharmacodynamic analysis of fluindione in patients. Clin Pharmacol Ther 63: 1 (in press)

Radat F, Berlin I, Spreux-Varoquaux O, Elatki S, Ferreri M, Puech AJ (1996) Initial monoamine oxidase-A inhibition by moclobemide does not predict the therapeutic response in patients with major depression. Psychopharmacology 127: 370-376

Warot D, Berlin I, Patat A, Durrieu G, Zieleniuk I, Puech AJ (1996) Effects of befloxatone, a reversible selective monoamine oxidase-A inhibitor, on psychomotor function and memory in healthy subjects. J Clin Pharmacol 36: 942-950

Hôpital Robert Debré
The division of Clinical Pharmacology opened in 1988. It is located at the Hôpital Robert Debré in a paediatric hospital of 450 beds, and obstetric department of 60 beds and out- patient clinics. All the paediatric specialities are present, including neonataology, nephrology, intensive care medicine, immunology, surgery, etc.

Three departments of basic research (INSERM: Institut National de la Santé Et de la Recherche Médicale) are in close relation with our department. Inserm U.120 is active in developmental pharmacology. In addition, a paediatric Centre of Clinical Investigations of six beds, exclusively to clinical investigations in children opened in January 1993. It is the only centre of this kind in France.

The Department of Clinical services
The concentrations of numerous drugs are monitored. Our analytical methods include radioimmunology and radioenzymology, liquid and gas chromatography, gas chromatography with mass spectrometry. Individual dose adjustments are performed for some of the drugs, based on individual pharmacokinetic data.

The maternity clinic provides antenatal counselling for physicians treating pregnant women exposed to drugs or chemicals. Long-term follow-up of neonates is carried out during the first year of life.

The division is active both in clinical research and basic research. The clinical studies are conducted in various divisions of the hospital and in the Centre of Clinical Investigations. The fellow will participate in the protocol design, study execution and interpretation of results. Several patient populations are currently under investigation: children with cystic fibrosis, children in Intensive Care and children with cancer, neonates. The basic research is focused on three main areas: pharmacogenetics of drug metabolizing enzymes; pharmacokinetics with emphasis on individual dose adjustments and population approaches.

A number of formal courses are offered by the Division
– Certificat de Pharmacologie Générale (Faculté de médecine Lariboisière – Saint Louis)
– Diplôme d'Etudes Approfondies (DEA) de Pharmacologie Expérimentale et Clinique

- Diplôme d'Etudes Approfondies (DEA) de Pharmacochimie Moléculaire, Pharmacologie Moléculaire et Métabolisme.

As of October 1997, the staff of the Division consisted of nine members.

In order to be enrolled in our post doctoral training programme, the candidate should have a competent MD, PhD or PharmD degree and should usually have completed pediatric (or other) specialty training.

The duration of the programme is one year for the Diplôme d'Etudes Approfondies (DEA) and three years for the Thèse de Sciences de la Vie et de la Santé (DEA required).

Applicants should submit a curriculum vitae, a transcript of undergraduate and postgraduate courses taken and two letters of reference to the head of the department of Perinatal and Pediatric Pharmacology. In a covering letter, applicants should indicate their areas of interest and career objectives. Training programmes start 1 October. Applications for the DEA should be made before 1 May.

Send your application to: Professor Evelyne Jacqz-Aigrain

References

Jacqz-Aigrain E, Bennasr S, Desplanques L, Peralma A (1994) Les risques d'intoxication grave liés à l'administration de quinine. Arch Pédiatr 1: 14-19

Jacqz-Aigrain E (1996) Fetal pharmacology and therapy. In: Intensive care in childhood. A challenge to the future (Update in intensive care and emergency medicine No. 25), Eds Springer Tibboel D, Van der Voort E, 365-374

Jacqz-Aigrain E, Burtin P (1996) Clinical pharmacokinetics of sedatives in neonates. Clin Pharmacokinet 31(6): 423-443

Jacqz-Aigrain E, Montes C, Brun Ph, Loirat C (1994a) Cycloporine pharmacokinetics in nephrotic and kidney transplanted children. Eur J Clin Pharmacol 47: 61-65

Jacqz-Aigrain E, Bellaich M, Faure C, Andre J, Rohrlich P, Baudouin V, Navarro J (1994b) Pharmacokinetics of intravenous omeprazole in children. Eur J Clin Pharmacol 47: 181-185

Jacqz-Aigrain E, Bessa E, Medard Y, Mircheva Y, Vilmer E (1994c) Thiopurine methyltransferase activity in a French population: HPLC assay conditions and effects of drugs and inhibitors. Br J Clin Pharmacol 38: 1-8

Jacqz-Aigrain E, Panserat S, Sica L, Krishnamoorthy R (1995) Molecular genetics of cytochrome pp450 IID. Clin Rev Allerg Immunol 13: 211-221

Jacqz-Aigrain E, Guillonneau M, Rey E, Macher MA, Montes C, Chiron C, Loirat C (1997a) Pharmacokinetics of the S(+) and R(-) enantiomers of vigabatrin during chronic dosing in a patient with renal failure. Br J Clin Pharmacol 44: 183-185

Jacqz-Aigrain E, Nafa S, Medard Y, Bessa E, Lescoeur B, Vilmer E (1997b) Pharmacokinetics and distribution of 6-mercaptopurine administered intravenously in children with lymphoblastic leukaemia. Eur J Clin Pharmacol 53(1): 71-74

Panserat S, Mura C, Gerard Y, Vincent-Viry M, Galteau MM, Jacqz-Aigrain E, Krishnamoorthy R (1994) DNA haplotype-dependent differences in the amino acid sequence of debrisoquine 4-hydroxylase (CYP2D6): evidence for two major allozymes in extensive metabolisers. Hum Genet 94: 401-406

Saint-Antoine University Hospital – University Pierre et Marie Curie - Paris VI

Research programme
– CYP450 dependent drug metabolism and drug - drug interactions: in vitro and in vivo studies (supported by grants from Hepatox Network PHRC, BIOMED II and INSERM)
– Effects of drugs on ventricular repolarization and risk of torsade de pointes: studies in normal subjects and in patients - correlations with electrophysiologic studies in anesthetized dogs.
– Pharmacokinetic - pharmacodynamic studies in cardiovascular pharmacology.
– Influence of PGP - dependent drug transport in pharmacokinetics and pharmacodynamics
– Drug-induced hepatotoxicity studies: clinical and pharmacoepidemiological studies (supported by grants from Hepatox Netword-PHRC, MIOMD II and Agence Française du Médicament).
– Monitoring of clinical trials with cardiovascular drugs: anti-anginal drugs and beta-blockers in congestive heart failure.

Training and teaching programme: experimental and clinical pharmacology for medical students; post-doc training programme on methodology of clinical trials; national diploma on formation of clinical research assistants; participation in inter-university PhD teaching programme on clinical pharmacology; participation in inter-university teaching programme on pharmacoepidemiology.

Clinical and research facilities: in Saint-Antoine University Hospital, the Pharmacology Department includes: (1) Unit of Clinical Pharmacology with four instrumented investigation beds; (2) Unit of Therapeutic Drug Monitoring with HPLC, immuno-enzymatic, and automatic analysers and pharmacokinetics modelling; (3) Regional centre of Pharmacovigilance and pharmaco-epidemiology in charge of adverse drug reactions diagnostic and documentation; (4) Clinical trial monitoring and audit centre; (5) CIBIS II trial medical centre; (6) Invitro drug metabolism laboratory; (7) Methodological Support Unit for clinical trials (8) Unit of Cardiac Electrophysiology.

The Pharmacology Department is also in charge of the Clinical Investigation Centre of Saint Antoine University Hospital, a five-bed facility open to clinicians and researchers of the hospital.

Staff: two professors of clinical pharmacology, three full-time assistant professors one full-time assistant, three full time MDs and two part-time MDs.

Application procedures: European GCP and guidelines.

References

Becquemont L, Ragueneau I, Le Bot MA, Riche C, Funck-Bretano C, Jaillon P (1997a) Influence of the CYP1A2 inhibitor fluvoxamine on tacrine pharmacokinetics in humans. Clin Pharmacol Ther 61: 619-627

Becquemont L, Lecoeur S, Simon T, Beaune Ph, Funck-Bretano C, Jaillon P (1997b) Glutathione S-transferase Q genetic polymorphism might influence tacrine hepatotoxicity in Alzheimer's patients. Pharmacogenetics 7: 251-253

Copie X, Pousset F, Lechat Ph, Jaillon P, Guize L, Le Heuzey JL and the Cardiac Insufficiency Bisoprolol Study (1996) Effects of b-blockade with bisoprolol on heart rate variablility in advanced heart failure: analysis of scatterplots of RR intervals at selected heart rates. Am Heart 132: 369-375

Demolis JL, Funck-Brentano C, Ropers J, Ghadanfar M, Nichols DJ, Jaillon P (1996a) Influence of dofetilide on QT interval duration and QT interval dispersion at various heart rates in humans. Circulation 94: 1592-1599

Demolis JL, Charransol A, Funck-Bretano C, Jaillon P (1996b) Effects of single oral dose of sparfloxacin on ventricular repolarization in healthy volunteers. Brit J Clin Pharmacol 41: 499-503

Demolis JL, Martel C, Funck-Bretano C, Sachse A, Weimann HJ, Jaillon P (1997) Effects of tedisamil, atenolol and their combination on heart rate and rate-dependent QT interval in healthy volunteers. Br J Clin Pharmacol 44: 403-409

Funck-Bretano C, Becquemont L, Leneveu A, Roux A, Jaillon P, Beaune P (1997) Inhibition by omeprazole of proguanil metabolism: mechanism of the interaction in vitro and prediction of in vivo result from the in vitro experiments. J Pharmacol Exp Ther 280: 730-738

Kevorkian JP, Michel C, Fofmann U, Jacqz-Aigrain E, Kroemer HK, Peraldi MN, Eichelbaum M, Jaillon P, Funck-Bretano C (1996) Assessment of individual CYP2D6 activity in extensive metabolizers with renal failure. Clin Pharmacol Ther 59: 583-592

Lechat P, Escolano S, Golmard JL, Lardoux H, Witchitz S, Henneman JA, Maisch B, Hetzel M, Jaillon P, Boissel JP, Mallet A and CIBIS investigators (1997) Prognostic value of bisoprolol induced haemodynamic effects in heart failure during the cardiac insufficiency bisoprolol study (CIBIS). Circulation 96: 2197-2205

Madjlessi-Simon T, Mary-Krause M, Fillette F, Lechat P, Jaillon P (1996) Persistent transient myocardial ischaemia despite b-blockade predicts a higher risk of adverse cardiac events in coronary patients. JACC 27: 1586-1591

Hôpital Saint-Louis - Centre for Clinical Investigations
St Louis Hospital is a multidisciplinary university affiliated hospital particularly devoted to haematology, Oncology, Transplantation, Dermatology, Gastroenterology, Intensive Infections diseases (AIDS) care.

Research programme
- Oncology: phase I, II, III of new cytotoxics, pharmacokinetics of new drugs supportive care of cancer, pharmacological interactions, new hormonal therapies in breast cancer, new approaches in the treatment of cancer gene therapies which do not necessitate a specific confinement.
- Haematology: monoclonal antibody treatment in non-Hodgkin's lymphoma, new drugs and antibodies in acute myeloid leukemia, new approaches in the treatment of leukaemias
- Immunology: immunity adjuvant for cancer (melanoma and breast cancer).
- Infectious medicine: especially in HIV patients (new medicines, new associations, supportive cares, new treatment of opportunistic infections).
- Epidemiology and genetics genes involved in familial naevi (study of 250 families), genes involved in colon cancer, Crohn disease.
- Dermatology: treatment of psoriasis, Kaposi sarcoma, melanoma.
- Gastroenterology: chronic inflammatory bowel diseases: pathogenesis and new treatments.
- Nephrology: genetic studies on graft rejection.

Training programme: internship and residency programmes in clinical pharmacology and therapeutic education (DESC). Training programme in clinical pharmacology (Diplôme interuniversitaire de formation des investigateurs aux essais cliniques: DIU FIEC) and oncology pharmacology.

Teaching programme: medical students teaching, DPRBM (diploma necessary to start PhD programmes in pharmacology), nurse's teaching programme: research in nurse care, educational programme on the basis of clinical trials (continuing education for nurses).

Clinical and research facilities
The centre for Clinical Investigations is located 1 minute walking distance from the intensive care unit ward. Since 1995, it has obtained the authorizations to perform biomedical research without individual benefit (physiology, physiopathology, epidemiology, genetics, pharmacodynamics and pharmacokinetics) delivered by the French sanitary authorities. It has access to the French National File for biomedical research volunteers. CNIL gave a favourable advice for computerized nominatives data (health volunteers). The department is affiliated with the CIC to help in protocol set up and evaluation.

Four patient rooms are available (fully equipped for clinical management and emergency: cardiac monotoring, arterial pressure monitoring tensiometer, oxygenotherapy, oximetry, aspiration and all materials for resuscitation).

A nurse room with a laminar air flow hood (to prepare cytotoxics and other medicines). A laboratory room with: vertical laminar air flow hood, pH meter, two refrigerated centrifuges, water bath, -20°C freezer. A -80°C freezer with an emergency procedure in case of failure, a room to keep medical charts and case report file during 15 years, a room for data monitoring and data capture.

Staff: one professor, one assistant professor, one senior staff member, one secretary, four nurses, one ward sister and one pharmacist.

References
Blum L, Pellet C, Morel p, Calvo F, Lebbe C (in press) Clinical and biological response to antiprotease therapy in Kaposi sarcoma patients. AIDS
Bourrat E, Lebbe C, Calvo F (1994) Etoposide for treating the hypereosinophilic syndrome. Ann Int Med 121: 899-900
Chevillard S, Validire P, Marie JP, Faussat AM, Barbu V, Bayle C, Benard J, Bonnal C, Boutonnat J, Calvo F, Charrier J, Clary A, Colosetti P, Danel-Moore L, Decremoux P, Delvincourt C, Finat-Duclos F, Genne Ph, Kataki A, Kouyoumdjian JC, Lacave R, Maugard C, Merlin JL, Mousseau M, Pinguet F, Quillien V, Raphael M, Richard B, Verrelle P, Robert J (1997) French multicentric evaluation of mdr1 gene expression by RT-PCR in leukemi and solid tumours. Standardization of RT-PCR

and preliminary comparisons between RT-PCR and immunohistochemistry in solid tumours. Leukaemia 11: 1095-1106

Costa Da Cunha C, Lebbe C, Rybojad M, Agbalika F, Ferchal F, Rabian C, Vignon-Pennamern MD, Calvo F, Morel P (1996) Long term follow-up of non HIV kaposi sarcoma treated with low dose recombinant interferon alpha 2b. Arch Dermatol 132: 327-331

De Cremoux P, Gluckman E, Podgorniak MP, Menier C, Thierry D, Calvo F, Socie G (1996) Decreased IL 1-beta and TNF alpha secretion in long-term bone marrow culture supernatant from Fanconi's anaemia patients. Eur J Haematol 57: 202-207

Giacchetti S, Cornez N, Eftekhari P, Awada A, Cuvier C, Bleiberg H, Hidvegi E, Berger F, Gerard B, Giroux B, Marty M, Calvo F, Piccart M (1998) Phase I clinical trial of the Olivacine S16020. AACR Annual Meeting. March 28-April 1. New Orleans, LA (Abstract)

Lan Tran P, Weinbach J, Opolon P, Linares-Cruz G, Reynes JP, Gregoire A, Kremer E, Durand H, Perricaudet M (1997) Prevention of bleomycin induced pulmonary fibrosis after adenovirus-mediated transfer of the bacterial bleomycin resistance gene. J Clin Invest 99: 608-617

Lebbe C, De Cremoux P, Rybojad M, Costa Da Cunha C, Morel P, Calvo F (1995) Herpes virus like sequences in patients with endemic and classic Kaposi sarcoma. Lancet 395: 761-762

Le Moyec L, Tatoud R, Degeorges A, Calabrese C, Bauza G, Eugene M, Calvo F (1996) Proton nuclear magnetic resonnance spectrostrospic reveals cellular lipids involved in resistance to adriamycin and taxol by the K562 leukaemia cell line. Cancer Res 56: 3461-3467

Paul C, Giacchetti S, Pinquier L, Flageul B, Dubertret L, Calvo F (in press) Cutaneous effects of G-CSF in healthy volunteers. Arch Dermatol

Sancrajrang S, Denoulet P, Tatoud G, Millot G, Calvo F, Fellous A (in press) Estramustin resistance in human prostate carcinoma cells is associated with modified tubulin expression pattern. Biochem Pharmacol

Hôpital Saint-Vincent de Paul - Université René Descartes (Paris V)
Research and training programme
- Clinical research : pharmacokinetic and pharmacodynamic studies, clinical trials in children, lactating mothers and pregnant women.
- Basic research : drug metabolism during maturation, hormonal regulation and influence of cytokines on drug metabolizing enzymes.
- Training programme: 1 year training with formal courses on basic and clinical pharmacology and a clinical study or experiment to perform (DEA de Pharmacologie Clinique et Expérimentale).

Clinical and research facilities
- One investigation bed
- One laboratory for analytical pharmacology (HPLC, GC-MS)

- One laboratory for experimental research
  Staff: one professor, four doctors

Application procedures
May 1st to July 1st, curriculum vitae, transcript of undergraduate and postgraduate courses taken, two letters of reference, covering letter indicating areas of interest and career objectives.
  Inquiries: Professor Gérard Pons

References
Bellissant E et al. (1997) The triangular test to assess the efficacy of metoclopramide in gastroesophageal reflux. Clin Pharmacol Ther 61: 377-384
Pariente-Khayat A et al. (1997) Isoniazid acetylation metabolic ratio during maturation in children. Clin Pharmacol Ther (in press)
Tran A et al. (1997) Influence of Stiripentol on P450-mediated metabolic pathways in humans in vitro/in vivo comparison and calculation of in vivo inhibition constants. Clin Pharmacol Ther (in press)
Vauzelle-Kervroëdan F et al. (1996a) Pharmacokinetics of the individual enantiomers of vigabatrin in neonates with uncontrolled seizures. Br J Clin Pharmacol 42: 779-781
Vauzelle-Kervröedan F et al. (1996b) Non-invasive in vivo study of the maturation of CYP IIIA in neonates and infants. Eur J Clin Pharmacol 51: 69-72
Vauzelle-Kervroëdan F et al. (1997) Equivalent antipyretic activity of ibuprofen and paracetamol in febrile children. J Pediatr (in press).

Poitiers
Research and training programme
- study of effects of psychotropic drugs on human psychomotor performance and memory
- training in general pharmacology for medical students and in clinical pharmacology for postgraduate MD

Research facilities: clinical pharmacology research are performed in a specialized unit using classic methods in human psychopharmacology (Leed's psychomotor testers, reaction time recorders, multipsy apparatus).

Our staff
One professor of pharmacology, head of the clinical pharmacology unit and of the regional drug survey centre (Professor B. Vandel).

One full time practitioner (Practicing Hospitalier) (Dr MC Perault).
One full time assistant working both at the University and the hospital.
Two residents.
Two students on stay to our hospital unit.

Application procedures
Contact either B Vandel or MC Perault.

References
Danjou P, Court L, Feuerstein C, Vandel B, Rosenzweig P (1993) Anxiolytics and electrogenesis: alpidem effects on waking EEG and sleep architecture. In Imidazopyridines in Anxiety Disorders: A novel Experimental and Therapeutic Approach, edited by G Bartholini, M Garreau, PL Morselli, and B Zivkovic, Raven Press, Ltd., New York pp. 133-142

Ledinghen V, Mannant PR, Foucher J, Perault MC, Barrioz T, Ingrand P, Vandel B, Silvain C, Beauchant M (1996) Non Stéroidal antiinflammatory drugs and variceal bleeding: A case-control study. J Hepatol 24: 570-573

Patat A, Perault MC, Vandel B, Ulliac N, Zieleniuk I, Rosenzweig P (1995a) Lack of interaction between a new antihistamine, mizolastine and lorazepam on psychomotor performance and memory in healthy volunteers. Br J Clin Pharmacol 39: 31-38

Patat A, Perault MC, Vandel B, Danjou PH, Brohier S, Zieleniuk I, Rosenzweig P (1995b) Assessment of the interaction between a partial agonist and a full agonist of benzodiazepine receptors, based on psychomotor performance and memory, in healthy volunteers. J Psychopharmacol 9 (2): 91-101

Perault MC, Bouquet S, Chapelle C, Chevallier P, Montay G, Chakroun H, Guillet PH, Sicard B, Perault MC, Enslen M, Chauffard F, Vandel B, Tachon P (1996) The effects of 600 mg of a slow release caffeine on mood an alertness. Aviation, Space and Environmental Med 67 (No. 9): 859-862

Vandel B (1994) Pharmacokinetic and pharmacodynamic study of suriclone imipramine interaction in man. Fundam Clin Pharmacol 8: 251-255

Vandel S, Bertschy G, Perault MC, Sandoz M, Bouquet S, Chakroun R, Guibert S, Vandel B (1993) Minor and clinically unsignificant interaction between toloxatone and amitriptyline. Eur J Clin Pharmacol 44: 97-99

Reims
Research programme (1997-1998):
- Nyctochemeral variations of blood metanephrines and normetanephrines for the screening of phaeochromocytoma.
- Pharmacokinetics of morphine after administration into the peridural space.

- Clinical pharmacokinetics of alcohol.
- Kinetics of carbamylated haemoglobin in acute renal failure.
- Functional and morphological study of vascular allografts after cryoconservation.
- Therapeutic evaluation of the association of pyrimethamine with sulphadoxine for the treatment of congenital toxoplasmosis

Training and teaching programme
The Department of Pharmacology is approved for the following training:
- For medical and pharmacy students: certificate of biology-biochemistry (to be a graduate in biology)
- For students in pharmacy: certificates of pharmaceutical sciences (biomedical and industrial pharmacy; hospital pharmacy and for communities; specialized pharmacy).
- Certificate of pharmacokinetics and drug metabolism
- Certificate of pharmacokinetics and drug metabolism
- Certificate of biological toxicology
- Certificate of clinical pharmacology and therapeutic assessment
- Pharmacovigilance for general practitioners

Clinical and research facilities
- Pharmacokinetic Centre: laboratory equipement such as gas chromatography with mass spetrometry (GC/MS: 2), gas chromatography (GC: 6), high performance liquid chromatography (HPLC: 8). analysers: Hitachi 704 (1), TDX Abbot (1), TDX FLX Abbot (1), IMX Abbot (2), Berilux (1), ES 600 Boehringer (1), Elecsys Boehringer (1), Immulite (1), Cobas Mira Plus (1). Atomic absorption spectrometry (flame and graphite furnace): Perkin Elmer 5000 (1), Varian Spectra A 300 plus (1). Spectrophotometry: Schimadzu UV 2100 (1); spectrofluorimetry: Perkin Elmer 204 (1). Analytical service develops new, fully validated analytical methods. We perform all types of studies: single and repeated dose, oral and parenteral dosing routes. Agreement from the Agence du Medicament.
- Pharmacodynamic Centre: contains a cardiovascular laboratory equipped with the latest advances in medical techniques (J. Elaerts, Professor of Cardiology; P. Nazeyrollas, MD).

Contains an endocrinology and metabolism evaluation centre (J. Caron, professor of endocrinology)

Clinical research facilities: performs early phase I-II-III studies.

Staff: three full professors, one assistant professor, one physician, three pharmacists, 22 laboratory assistants, 22 supervisors and five secretaries.

References

Bouvier N, Millart H (1997) Relation between selenium deficiency and 3,5,3'-triodothyronine (T3). Ann Endocrinol 58: 310-315

Brezillon S, Zahm JM, Pierrot D, Caillard D, Hinnrasky J, Millart H, Klossek JM (1997) ATP depletion induces a loss of respiratory epithelium functional integrity and downregulates CFTR (cystis fibrosis transmembrane conductance regulator) expression. J Biol Chem (in press)

Devillier Ph, Millart H, Advenier Ch (1997) Leucotriene antagonists: their interest in asthma. Rev Méd Brux 18: 279-285

Hoizey G, Vistelle R, Lamiable D, Millart H, Gourdier B, D'Arbigny P (1997) Determination of gacyclidine enantiomers in human plasma by gas chromatography-mass spectrometry using selected ion monitoring. J Chromatogr B 704: 167-174

Jolly DH, Poitrinal P, Millart H, Kariger E, Blanchard F, Collery Ph, Choisy H (1993) Blood zinc, copper, magnesium, calcium, aluminium and manganese concentrations in patients, with or without Alzheimer type dementia. Trace Elements in Medicine 10: 192-195

Millart H, Durlach V, Durlach J (1995) Red blood cell magnesium concentrations: analytical problems and significance. Magnesium Res 8: 65-76

Nazeyrollas P, Metz D, Jolly D, Elaerts J (1997) Use of transthoracic doppler echocardiography to predict acute pulmonary embolism. Cardiol Rev 14: 21-24

Nicolle E, Devillier P, Delanoy B, Durand C, Bessard G (1996) Drug monitoring of nalbuphine: placental transfer and estimated pharmacokinetics in the newborn. Eur J Clin Pharmacol 49: 485-489

Trenque T, Barre J, Lamiable D, Tillement J-P (1994) Linear pharmacokinetics of a new inotropic agent. Arzneimittelforschung 44: 471-474

Trenque T, Marx C, Quereux C, Leroux B, Dupouy D, Dorangeon PH, Choisy H, Pinon JM (1997) Human maternofoetal distribution of pyrimethamine-sulphadoxine. Br J Clin Pharmacol (in press)

Rennes

Research and training programme

In the experimental field, two ongoing programmes are officially supported: (1) CNS drug development on cell death is based on techniques such as in vivo microdialysis, central neurotransmitters measurements, trophic factors, behavioural pharmacology (Dr D Bentué Ferrer; Dr JM Reymann); (2) vascular pharmacology devoted to the determination of the biochemical compounds involved in the vascular tone, and the role of endothelium in different vessels strips (Dr D Pape).

In the clinical field, phase I, II and III studies are the core of the clincial research with special involvement in PK/PD studies, methodology, computerized testing of CNS drugs (Psychometry, Q.EEG...), drug safety. The main recent topics are the following: drugs for memory; antidepressants; antidementia compounds, GI tract drugs; antihypertensive.

Training programme: graduated students and post-docs are involved in both these fields. They come from France and abroad under the condition of a sound background in pharmacology. Possibilities for thesis (PhD) are offered within the department.

Clinical and research facilities: the department in Rennes is fully operational thanks to facilities at our disposal in the Pharmacology hospital ward (three units: methodology; pharmacovigilance; drug monitoring; and four beds for investigations); moreover, in 1989, for our Pharmacology department, BIOTRIAL SA (Director JM Gandon), was established, offering the highest standard in clinical pharmacology (30 beds; four biostratisticians; independent building on the site, 200 m^2). Permanent and closed links have been established with the various departments of the medical school as well as private physicians or those from other surrounding cities. In 1996, a new unit of Pharmacoepidemiology will open (O Zekri).

The University: the department is included in the University of Rennes I, where the whole spectrum of scientific research is present and is punctually of great help. Medicine, Dentistry and Pharmacy are located on the same site facilitating direct collaborations. The teaching of pharmacology is at a high standard not only for undergraduate students but mainly in the Master of Experimental and Clinical Pharmacology which is attended roughly by 30 students per year. Some exchange programmes have been established with Ireland (Galway, Professor Leonard), Canada (Montreál, Professor O'Hayon), Germany (Witten), USA (Cleveland, Professor Whitehouse).

The staff: At the hospital: seven permanent pharmacologists: head (H Allain), Methodology (E Belissant), Biology (D Bentué-Ferrer; D

Pape), Behavioural Pharmacology (JM Reymann), Drug Safety (C Bénéton), Gastroenterology (L Siproudhis).

At BIOTRIAL SA: 40 permanent persons. Head (J.M. Gandon), phase I (A Patat), PK/PD models (F Le Coz), Experimental (P Lacroix).

Application procedures: any application must be mailed to Professor Allain by medical doctors, pharmacists, biologist in the minimal possession of a diploma of Pharmacology. Positions for internship are available. June is the annual deadline for application. Students may have housing and daily facilities on the site.
Inquiries to Professor Hervé Allain

References
Allain H, Delahaye C, LE Coz F, Guillemault C, Blin P, Decombe R, Martinet JP (1991) Postmarketing surveillance of zopiclone insomnia. Sleep 14: 408-413
Allain H, Lieury A, Brunet-Bourgin F, Mirabaud C, TreboN P, Le Coz F, Gandon JM (1992) Antidepressants and cognition: comparative effects of moclobemide, viloxasine and maprolitine. Psychopharmacology 106: S56-S61
Allain H, Lieury A, Gandon JM (1993a) Psychopharmacology of memory components. Hum Psychopharmacol vol 4, Edited by I. Hindmarch and PD Stonier Johns Wiley & Sons Ltd. pp 143-164
Allain H, Belliard S, De Certaines J. Bentué-Ferrer D, Bureau M, Lacroix P (1993b) Potential Biological Targets for Anti-Alzheimer Drugs. Dementia 1993; 4: 347-352
Allain H, Patat A, Lieury A, Le Coz F, Janus C, Ménard G, Gandon JM (1995) Comparative study of the effects of zopiclone (7,5 mg), zolpidem, flunitrazepam and a lacebo on nocturnal cognitive performance in healthy subjects in relation to pharmacokinetics. Eur Psychiatry 10 (suppl 3): 129s-135s
Bellissant E, Thuillez C, Pussard E, Giudicelli JF (1992) Systemic and regional haemodynamic effects of zabicipril in healthy volunteers. Clin Pharmacol Ther 51: 308-319
Allain H, Lieury A, Belliard S, Caldwell M, Patat A, Gandon JM (1996) Effect of drugs on mnestic performance: a methodological approach. Hum Psychopharmacol 11: 11-19
Bellissant E, Benichou J, Chastang C (1994a) A comparison of methods for Phase II cancer clinical trials: advantages of the triangular test, a group sequential method. Lung Cancer 9: 10 (suppl l) S105-S115
Bellissant E, Thuillez C, Richer C, Pussard E, Giudicelli JF (1994b) Non-invasive assessment of regional arteriolar and arterial dilating properties of lisinopril in healthy volunteers. J Cardiovasc Pharmacol 24: 500-508
Patat A, Gandon JM, Durrieu G, Raoul P, Le Coz F, Beck A, Allain H (1995) Effects of single and multiple doses of a new reversible MAO-A inhibitor, befloxatone, on psychomotor performance and memory in healthty subjects. Hum Psychopharmacol 10: 111-125

Rouen

Research Programme: Phase I studies.
Evaluation of new cardiovascular treatments in healthy volunteers and patients with cardiovascular disease on: systemic and regional haemodynamics; sympathetic activity heart rate variability; mechanical properties of large arteries, endothelial function. New drug assays. Pharmacokinetic/pharmacodynamic analysis.

Training teaching programme
Internship programmes (Faculty of Medicine and Pharmacy), introductory courses in biomedical research (DPRBM). PhD programmes in cardiovascular pharmacology.

Clinical and research facilities
Three beds for clinical investigations. Techniques: heart rate and arterial pressure (cuff, oscillometry, photoplethysmography), variability of heart rate and arterial pressure (Anapres), cardiac output (bioimpedance), capillary flow (laser Doppler), large artery diameter (echotracking angiometers), regional blood blow (Doppler), pulse wave velocity, arterial tonometry, vascular echography, ambulatory blood pressure monitoring, biochemical measurements: catecholamines, serotonin (HPLC), cGMP (Elisa). Plasma concentration of drugs for pharmacokinetic/pharmacodynamic analysis and for toxicology, routine drugs analysis.

Staff: one professor, one associate professor, one doctor in pharmacology, one MD, one resident and two interns in pharmacology, two technicians and one secretary.

References

Joannidès R, Richard V, Moore N, Godin M, Thuillez C (1995a) Influence of sympathetic tone on mechanical properties of muscular arteries in humans. Am J Physiol 268: H794-H801

Joannidès R, Haefeli WE, Linder L, Richard V, Bakkali El H, Thuillez C, Lüscher TF (1995b) Nitric oxide is responsible for flow-dependent dilatation of human peripheral conduit arteries in vivo. Circulation 91: 1314-1319

Joannidès R, Richard V, Haefeli WE, Linder L, Lüscher TF, Thuillez C (1995c) Role of basal and stimulated release of nitric oxide in the regulation of radial artery caliber in humans. Hypertension 26: 327-331

Joannidès R, Bakkali El H, Richard V, Benoist A, Moore N, Thuillez C (1997a) Evaluation of the determinants of flow-mediated radial artery vasodilatation in humans. Hypertension 19 (5 & 6): 813-826

Joannidès R, Moore N, Iacob M, Compagnon P, Plan D, Thuillez C (1997b) A comparison of the effects of short-acting nifedipine, amlodipine and diltiazem at rest and during tilt and exercise in healthy volunteers. Br J Pharmacol (in press)

Joannidès R, Bakkali El H, Le Roy F, Rivault O, Godin M, Moore N, Fillastre JP, Thuillez C (1997c) Altered flow-dependent vasodilatation of conduit arteries in maintenance haemodiolysis. Nephrol Dial Transplant 12: 2623-2628

Joannidès R, Moore N, Iacob M, Compagnon P, Bacri AM, Thuillez C (1997d) Divergent effects of verapamil and amlodipine at rest and during exercise. J Hypertens 15 (suppl. 5): S1-S5

Joannidès, Richard V, Haefeli WE, Benoist A, Linder L, Lüscher TF and Thuillez C (1997e) Role of nitric oxide in the regulation of the mechanical properties of peripheral conduit arteries in humans. Hypertension 30: 1465-1470

Moore N, Fresel J, Joannidès R, Compagnon P, Thuillez C (1994) A comparison of the haemodynamic effects of Urapidil, Prazosin, and Clonidic in healthy volunteers. Blood Pressure 3 (Suppl.4): 7-12

Thiberville L, Compagnon P, Moore N, Bastian G, Richard MO, Hellot MF, Vincent C, Kannass MM, Dominique S, Thuillez C, Nouvet G (1994) Plasma 5-fluorouracil and a-fluoro-b-alanin accumulation in lung cancer patients treated with continuous infusion of cisplatin and 5-fluorouracil. Cancer Chemother Pharmacol 35: 64-70

Saint-Etienne
Unité de Pharmacologie Clinique - Hôpital Bellevue
Research progamme
Population pharmacokinetic and pharmacodynamic analyses and pharmacokinetic - pharmacodynamic relationship studies, controlled clinical trials (Phases I, II, III and IV), performed on antithrombotic agents.

Training and teaching programme
Pharmacokinetic/pharmacodynamic modelling, methodology, good clinical practices, statistical analysis, and meta-analysis for controlled clinical trials. Prescription, use and management of antithrombotic agents.

Clinical and research facilities
Department of internal medicine: twenty beds. Specialized in venous thromboembolism (phase II, III and IV studies).
    Clinical pharmacology unit: six beds qualified to do phase I studies. A network of 15 computers.

Staff: one PU-PH de Pharmacologie Clinique, one MCU-PH de Pharmacologie Clinique, one PH de Médecine Interne, two Ingénieurs Statisticiens, six Attachés de Recherce Clinique, two ARC Managers, one Technicienne de Recherche, two Secrétaires.

References

Cambus JP, Beguin S, Hemker HC, Mismetti P, Decousus H, Boneu B (1998) Endogenous thrombin potential and heparin monitoring: in vitro and in vivo studies in healthy volunteers and patients presenting veinous thromboembolism. Thromb Haemostas (in press)

Conchonnet P, Mismetti P, Reynaud J, Laporte-Simitsidis S, Tardy-Poncet B, Boissier C, Rambaud C, Decousus H (1994) Fibrinolysis and elastic compression: no fibrinolytic effect of elastic compression in healthy volunteers. Blood Coag Fibr 5: 949-953

Decousus H, Leizorovicz A, Parent F, Page Y, Tardy B, Girard P, Laporte S, Faivre R, Charbonnier B, Barral FG, Huet Y, Simonneau G for the PREPIC Study Group (1998) A clinical trial of vena cava filters in the prevention of pulmonary embolism in patients with proximal deep vein thrombosis. N Engl J Med (in press)

Girard P, Laporte-Simitsidis S, Mismetti P, Decousus H, Boissel JP (1995) Influence of confounding factors on designs for dose-effect relationship estimates. Stat Med 14: 987-1005

Leizorovicz A, Simonneau G, Decousus H, Boissel JP (1994) Comparison of efficacy and safety of low molecular wieght heparins and unfractionated heparin in initial treatment of deep venous thrombosis: a meta-analysis. Br Med J 309: 299-304

Mismetti P, Laporte-Simitsidis S, Tardy B, Queneau P, Decousus H (1993) Prophylactic treatment of post-operative deep venous thrombosis in orthopaedic surgery of the hip with oral anticoagulant. Clin Trials Meta-Analysis 28: 227-240

Mismetti P, Reynaud J, Tardy B, Simitsidis S, Scully M, Goldwyn C, Queneau P, Decousus H (1995) Chrono-pharmacological study of once daily curative dose of a low molecular weight heparin (200 IU antiXa/kg of Dalteparin) in healthy volunteers. Thromb Haemostas 74: 660-666

Simonneau G, Charbonnier B, Decousus H, Planchon B, Ninet J, Sie P, Silsiguen M, Combe S (1993) Subcutaneous low-molecular-weight heparin compared with continous intravenous infractionated heparin in the treatment of proximal deep vein thrombosis. A multicenter randomised trial. Arch Int Med 153: 1541-1546

Tardy B, Tardy-Poncet B, Laporte-Simitsidis S, Mismetti P, Decousus H, Guyotat D (1997) Evolution of blood coagulation and fibrinolysis parameters after abrupt versus gradual withdrawal of acenocoumarol in patients with venous thromboembolism: A double-blind randomized study. Brit J Haematol 96: 174-178

Tardy B, Tardy-Poncet B, Viallon A, Lafond P, Reynaud J, Page Y, Guyotat D, Bertrand JC (1998) Rapid and classic D-Dimères ELISA test in clinical suspicion of venous thrombo-embolism: unusefulness in elderly patients. Thrombo Haemostas (in press)

Central Laboratory of Pharmacology and Toxicology – Pharmacovigilance Centre

Research programme
- Drug monitoring and analytical process
- Cytochrome P450 drug metabolism
- Pharmacokinetics
- Epidemiological studies on drug use and drug safety

Training and teaching programme
- Pharmacokinetic/Pharmacodynamic modelling (PK/PD)
- Principles of drug metabolism
- Stable isotopes in pharmacological studies
- Epidemiological concepts in pharmacovigilance
- Good clinical practice
- Phase I studies

Clinical and research facilities;
Analytical labaoratory (HPLC, CPG, MS), software package for pharmacokinetic data modeling, a network of 150 GP for epidemiological or pharmacovigilance studies, six beds qualified to do phase I studies. Staff: one PU-PH in Pharmacology, two PH in Pharmacology, one assistant, four or five laboratory technicians, two secretaries.

References

Bertholon P, Convers P, Lachheb N, Guy C, Martin C, Ollagnier M, Michel D (1997) Sémiologie vestibulaire centrale prépondérante par interaction carbamazépine et dextropropoxyphène. Presse Méd 26 no 35: 1675-1677

Gaillard Y, Gay-Montchamp JP, Ollagnier M (1993) Simultaneous screening and quantitation of alpidem, zolpidem, buspirone and benzodiazepines by dual-channel gas chromatography using electron-capture and nitrogen-phosphorus detection after solid-phase extraction. J Chromatogr 622: 197-208

Gaillard Y, Gay-Montchamp JP, Ollagnier M (1994) Détection et dosage du méthanol, de l'éthanol et de l'éthylène-glycol dans les milieux biologiques par chromatographie en phase gazeuse. Toxicorama V no. 4: 39-42

Guy C, Dzviga C, Genot A, Patural F, Ollagnier M (1995) Hypersensibilité sous SINTROM7. Responsabilité du Rouge Cochenille A. Thérapie 50: 483-484

Guy C, Rousset H, Cartry O, Lauers A, Ollagnier M (1996) Fièvre sous médifoxamine. La Presse Méd 25 (3): 127

Moore N, Noblet C, Joannides R, Ollagnier M, Imbs JL, Lagier G (1993) Cough and ACE inhibitors. Lancet 341: 61

Moore N, Noblet C, Kreft-Jais C, Lagnier G, Ollagnier M, IMBS JL (1994) The French pharmacovigilance database: 8 years of use for hypothesis testing. European Medicine Research, GN Fracchia (Ed). IOS Press

Moore N, Noblet C, Kreft-Jais C, Lagier G, Olagnier M, Imbs JL (1995) La banque de cas du système français de pharmacovigilance: quelques exemples d'exploitation. Thérapie 50: 557-562

Moore N, Kreft-Jais C, Begaud B, Noblet C, Andrejak M, Haramburu F, Ollagnier M (1997) Hypoglycaemia associated with the use of ACE inhibitors and other drugs: a case - non case study in the French pharmacovigilance system database. Br J Clin Pharmacol 44 (5): 513-518

Olagnier M, Guy C, Beyens MN, Montmartin Ph (1995) Safety of influenza vacine: a prospective study on 741 patients with the collaboration of a GP network. Poster présenté au 11th International Conference of Pharmacoepidemiology, Montréal, Canada 27-30 Août. Pharmacoepidemiology and Drug Safety 4: Suppl 1

Strasbourg

Department of Hypertension, Vascular Diseases and Clinical Pharmacology, University Hospital Strasbourg.

Research and training programme: renovascular physiology and pharmacology, hypertension, renin-angiotensin system.

Clinical and research facilities: Department of hypertension, vascular diseases and clinical pharmacology, University Hospital Strasbourg. In- and out-patients; cardiovascular and renal investigations in hypertension, atherosclerosis and target organs.

Pharmacovigilance centre, Institute of Pharmacology, CJF INSEAM, Faculty of Medicine Strasbourg.

The University: Pharmacology, cardiovascular pharmacology: medical students

Post-graduated diploma in clinical pharmacology, including research training (1 year)

National diplomas in pharmacology: pharmacoepidemiology (one seminary); clinical development of drugs (one seminary) European course in pharmaceutical medicine (ECPM): workshop on pharmacovigilance.

Staff: Research: Imbs JL MD (professor of clinical pharmacology), Bousquet P MD (Professor of Fundamental Pharmacology), De Jong W MD (Professor of Pharmacology), Helwig JJ PhD (Research Director), Barthelmebs M PhD (Research Director), Stephan D MD (Professor of Clinical Pharmacology), Grima M PhD (Assistant Professor

of Pharmacology), Clinic: Imbs JL, Stephan D, Welsch M MD (Senior Clinician).
Application procedures: Professor Imbs

References

Barthelmebs M, Grima M, Imbs JL (1995) Ramipril-induced decrease in renal lithium-excretion in the rat. Br J Pharmacol 116: 2161-2165

Barthelmebs M, Krieger JP, Grima M et al. (1996) Vascular effects of [Arg8] vasopressin in the isolated perfused kidney. Eur J Pharmacol 314: 325-332

Massfelder T, Stewart AF, Endlich K et al. (1996a) Parathyroid hormone-related protein detection and interaction with NO and cyclic AMP in the renovascular system. Kidney Int 50: 1591-1603

Massfelder T, Helwig JJ, Stewart AF (1996b) Parathyroid hormone-related protein as a cardiovascular regulatory peptide. Endocrinology 137: 3151-3153

Michel B, Stephan D, Grima M et al. (1993) Effects of one-hour and one-week treatment with ramipril on plasma and renal brush border angiotensin converting enyme in rat. Eur J Pharmacol 242: 237-243

Michel B, Grima M, Stephan D et al. (1994) Plasma renin activity changes in tissue angiotensin converting enzyme. J Hypertension 12: 577-584

Stephan D, Billing A, Krieger JP et al (1995) Cyclosporine A impairs endothelium-dependent relaxation in isolated rat kidney. J Cardiovasc Pharmacol 26: 859-868

Toulouse

Research and training programme

We are currently working on clinical neuropharmacology, autonomic pharmacology and pharmacoepidemiology and pharmacovigilance. Since 1990, we have also been developing a regional centre of Pharmacodependence under the auspice of the Agence du Médicament. We are also involved in Cochrane collaboration. We have a ward of clinical neuropharmacology in the Department of Neurology and another special ward for general clinical pharmacology in the hospital clinical investigation centre.

References

Andreu N, Damase-Michel C, Senard JM, Rascol O, Montastruc JL (1997) A dose-ranging study of selegiline in patients with Parkinsons's disease: effect on platelet monoamine oxidase activity. Mov Disord 3: 293-296

Bagheri H, Picault P, Schmitt L, Houin G, Berlan M, Montastruc JL (1994) Pharmacokinetic study of yohimbine and its pharmacodynamic effects on salivary secretion in patients treated with tricyclic antidepressants. Br J Clin Pharmacol 37: 93-96

Barbe P, Stich V, Galitzky J, Kunesova M, Hainer V, Lafontan M. Berlan M (1997) In vivo increase in beta-adrenergic lipolytic response in subcutaneous adipose tissue of obese subjects submitted to a hypocaloric diet. J Clin Endocrinol Metab 82, 1: 63-69

Galinier M, Senard JM, Valet P, Arias A, Daviaud D, Glock Y, Bounhoure JP, Montastruc JL (1994) Cardiac bêta-adrenoceptors and adenylyl cyclase activity in human left ventricular hypertrophy due to pressure overload. Fundam Clin Pharmacol 8: 90-99

Lapeyre-Mestre M, Damase-Michel C, Adams P, Michaud P, Montastruc JL and community pharmacists of the Midi-Pyrénées (1997) Falsified or forged medical prescriptions as an indicator of pharmacodependence: a pilot study. Eur J Clin Pharmacol 52: 37-39

Lemozit JP, Petit de la Rhodiere G, Lapeyre-Mestre M, Montastruc JL (1996) A comparative study of adverse drug reactions reported through hospital and private medicine 41: 166-168

Llau ME, Durrieu G, Tran MA, Senard M, Rascol O, Montastruc JL (1996) A study of dopaminergic sensitivity in Parkinson's disease: comparison in 'de novo' and levodopa-treated patients. Clin Neuropharmacol 5: 420-427

Montastruc JL, Rascol O, Senard JM, Rascol A (1994) A randomised controlled study comparing bromocriptine to which levodopa was later added, with levodopa alone in previously untreated patients with Parkinson's disease: a 5-year follow-up. Neurol Neurosurg Psychiatry 57: 1034-1038

Montastruc P, Damase-Michel C, Lapeyre-Mestre M, Puget C, Damase L, Hurstel JF, Graille V, Montastruc JL (1995) A prospective intensive study of adverse drug reactions in urban general practice. Clin Drug Invest 10: 117-122

Muratet C on behalf of the Service Medical Interentreprises de la Région de Toulouse, Lapeyre-Mestre M, Montastruc JL (1995) Study on the regular use of drugs in workers over 50 years of age. Clin Drug Invest 1: 1-7

Tours
Research and training programme

The centre is a clinical pharmacology with its three activities, i.e. teaching, research and help to patient care. There are three units: (1) A laboratory for drug measurements (2) pharmaco- vigilance centre (national system) (3) Clinical evaluation of drugs (trials) and pharmacoepidemiology.

As Professor E Autret is a paediatrician, the centre is especially focused on: paediatric pharmacology, drug trials in children, evaluation of drug safety in children and in the fetus

Since 1995 we have organized an Inter-University Diploma of paediatric and therapeutic pharmacology (five universities in France).

References

Autret E, Dutertre JP, Barbier P, Jonville AP, Pierre F, Berger C (1993a) Parental opinion about biomedical research in children. Dév Pharmacol Ther 20: 64-71

Autret E, Dutertre JP, Breteau M, Jonvill AP, Furet Y, Laugier J (1993b) Pharmacokinetics of paracetamol in infant and neonate after administration of propacetamol chlorhydrate. Dev Pharmacol Ther 20: 129-134

Autret E, Breart G, Jonville AP, Courcier S, Lassale L, Goerhs JM (1994a) Comparative efficacy and tolerance of ibuprofen syrup and acetaminophen syrup in children with pyrexia associated with infectious diseases and treated with antibiotics. Eur J Clin Pharmacol 46: 197-201

Autret E, Jonville AP, Dutertre JP, Bertiere MC, Robert M, Averous M, Couet W (1994b) Plasma levels of oxybutynine chloride in children. Eur J Clin Pharmacol 46: 29-33

Autret E, Reboul-Marty J, Henry-Launois B et al. (1997a) Evaluation of ibuprofen versus aspirin and paracetamol on efficacy and comfort in children with fever. Eur J Clin Pharmacol 51; 5: 367-371

Autret E, Radal M, Jonville-Bera AP, Goehrs JM (1997b) Isotrétinoïne (Roaccutane7) chez la femme en âge de procréer: insuffisance de suivi des recommandations de prescription. Ann Dermatol Venereol 124: 518-522

Autret E, Berjot M, Jonville-Bera AP, Aubry MC (1997c) Anophtalmia and agenesis of optic chiasma associated with adapalene gel in early pregnancy. Lancet 350: 339

Dutertre J, Billaud EM, Autret E, Chantepie A, Olivier J, Laugier J (1993) Inhibition of angiotensin converting enzyme with enalapril maleate in infants with congestive heart failure. Br J Clin Pharmacol 35: 528-530

Jonville-Bera AP, Autret E, Laugier J (1995) Sudden infant death syndrome and diphtheria-tetanus-pertussis-poliomyelitis vaccination status. Fundam Clin Pharmacol 9; No. 3: 263-270

Jonville-Bera AP, Autret E, Galy-Eyraud C, Hessel L (1996a) Aseptic meningitis following mumps vaccine. A retrospective survey by the French Regional Pharmacovigilance Centres and by Pasteur-Mérieux Sérums & Vaccins. Pharmacoepidemiology and drug safety 1996; 5: 33-37

Jonville-Bera AP, Autret E, Galy-Eyraud C, Hessel L (1996b) Thrombocytopenic purpura following measles, mumps and rubella vaccination. Ped Infec Dis J 15: 44-48

Sitbon P, Laffon M, Lesage V, Furet P, Autret E, Mercier C (1996) Lidocaine plasma concentrations in pediatrics patients after providing airway topical anesthesia from a calibrated device. Anesth Analg 82: 1003-1006

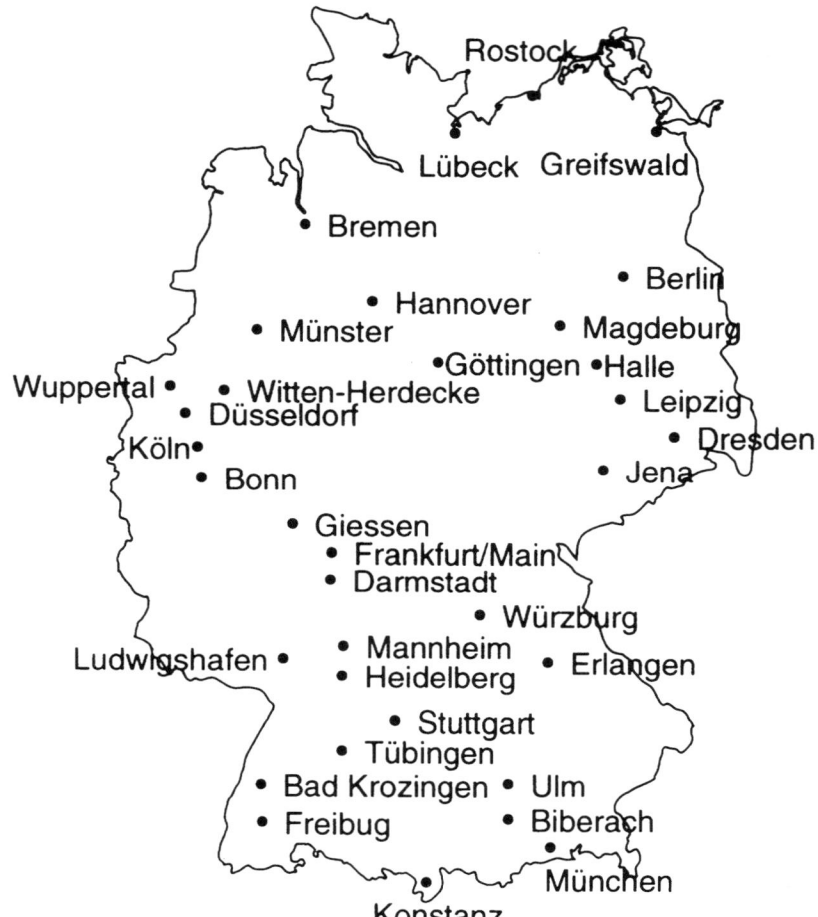

Germany

The German Medical Association has recognized Clinical Pharmacology as a specialty in medicine, but the discipline has developed rather slowly and evolved from experimental pharmacology rather than from internal medicine. There are presently 17 independent departments of clinical pharmacology, namely at the universities of Berlin (2), Bonn, Dresden, Erlangen, Frankfurt/Main, Göttingen, Greifswald, Hannover, Heidelberg, Jena, Leipzig, Magdeburg, Mannheim, München, Rostock and Tübingen. Ten units are affiliated with departments of pharmacology, internal medicine or other clinical disciplines at the universities of Düsseldorf, Freiburg, Giessen, Halle, Köln, Lübeck, Münster, Ulm, Witten/Herdecke and Würzburg. In addition, there are Institutes of Clinical Pharmacology in Stuttgart and Bremen and a division of Clinical Pharmacology at the Cardiology Clinic in Bad Krozingen and at the Institute of Aerospace Medicine of DLR in Köln. Many pharmaceutical companies such as Bayer, Boehringer Ingelheim, Boehringer Mannheim, BYK Gulden, Glaxo, Hoechst, Knoll, Merckle, Schering, Thomae as well as Tropon have clinical pharmacology units of their own in Germany. Furthermore, there are several contract research organizations running clinical pharmacology units.

Doctors who want to become specialists in clinical pharmacology must first obtain their MD degree and then enter a 5-year training programme. The programme includes 4 years in clinical pharmacology at an approved department or unit in clinical pharmacology. At least 1 year must be spent in clinical medicine. One year must be spent in experimental pharmacology or toxicology or basic science. There is a compulsory exam after 5 years and after successfully passing that, the candidate becomes a specialist in clinical pharmacology.

In medical school, clinical pharmacology is taught by clinical pharmacologists during the fourth and fifth year, and also during the sixth year of practical clinical training. Clinical pharmacology is part of the state examination.

The German Society for Experimental and Clinical Pharmacology and Toxicology (DGPT) was founded in 1920 and officially registered in 1921 as the German Society of Pharmacology (DPhG). The Section of Clinical Pharmacology of the DGPT was founded during the 12th Spring meeting in 1971. From the beginning of 1997 the DGPT was restructured into three sections 'Pharmacology', 'Clinical Pharmacology' and 'Toxicology' all under one mutual roof in order to guarantee the individual support of all three subjects. At the end of 1997, the Section of Clinical Pharmacology had 572 members. The goal of the DGPT is to represent scientifically the subject pharmacology and toxicology as well as the subject clinical pharmacology in their entirety, and to promote their total appearance and cooperation in research, science and literature as well as to look after and present their special interests in regard to the health system and their public appearance. The task of the section clinical pharmacology is to improve the situation for clinical pharmacology in Germany and to maintain an appropriate training in clinical pharmacology in collaboration with the societies for other clinical disciplines. There is a second organization for clinical pharmacology, namely the German Society for Clinical Pharmacology and Therapeutics (GKPharm) founded in 1990. The major aim of the Society is to arrange scientific meetings and to organize workshops on drug safety, pharmacokinetics, drug information systems and pharmacoepidemiology. Most clinical pharmacologists in Germany are members of the DGPT and/or of the GKPharm, which also has about 450 members. The first chair in clinical pharmacology was established in Berlin in 1967. In the EACPT, the DGPT is represented by Professor Dr Jochen Kuhlmann, and GKPharm is represented by Professor Dr Ivar Roots. Both the section and the society have very close relationships to the German Drug Regulation Agency and to the pharmaceutical industry.

Although clinical pharmacology is reasonably well established in Germany, the discipline needs to become even stronger. It is the hope that each German university with a medical faculty (36) should have its own unit in clinical pharmacology in order to improve both teaching and practical drug use at the undergraduate as well as the postgraduate level. Besides, a stronger position for clinical pharmacology in general health care would be desirable.

The governmental regulations are available on request at the Ministery of Health (Deutchherrenstrasse 87, D-53177 Bonn). A report on clinical pharmacology in Germany prepared by Dr. Giesela Gieselmann is available on request at the Secretariat of the Research Council (Brohler Strasse 11, D-50968 Köln).

Addresses

Bad Krozingen
Professor E Jähnchen
Herz-Zentrum Bad Krozingen
Abt. Klinische Pharmakologie
Südring 15
D-79189 Bad Krozingen
Phone: +49 7633 402 525
Fax: +49 7633 402 425

Berlin
Professor D Ganten
Institut für Klinische Pharmakologie
Universitätsklinikum Benjamin Franklin
Freie Universität Berlin
Hindenburgdamm 30
D-12200 Berlin

Professor W.M. Herrmann
PAREXEL GmbH
Spandauer Damm 130
D-14050 Berlin

Professor B Müller-Oerlinghausen
Forschergruppe Klinische Psychopharmakologie
Freie Universität Berlin
Univ.-Klinikum Benjamin Franklin
Psychiatrische Klinik und Poliklinik
Eschenallee 3
D-14050 Berlin
Phone: +49 30-8445-8648/9
Fax: +49 30 8445-8797
E-mail: bmoe@zedat.fv-berlin.de

Professor M Paul
Institut für Klinische Pharmakologie
Universitätsklinikum Benjamin Franklin
Freie Universität Berlin
Hindenburgdamm 30
D-10117 Berlin

Phone: +49 3028 025318
Fax: +49 3028 025318

Professor I Roots
Institut für Klinische Pharmakologie
Universitätsklinikum Charité
Humboldt-Universität zu Berlin
Schumannstr. 20/21
D-10098 Berlin
Phone: +49 30 28 02 53 18
Fax: +49 30 28 02 51 53

Dr W Seifert
Schering AG
Institut für klinische Pharmakologie
Sellerstrasse 31
D-13342 Berlin-Wedding
Phone: +49 304 6815156
Fax: +49 304 6811451

Biberach
Dr W Feuerer
Dr Karl Thomae GmbH
Abt. Klinische Forschung
D-88397 Biberach
Fax: +49 7351 542181

Dr CAPF Su
Dr Karl Thomae GmbH
Abt. Klinische Forschung
Fachbereich Klinische Forschung
Birkendorfer Strasse 65
D-88397 Biberach
Phone: +49 7351 544418
Fax: +49 7351 542181
Email: peter.su@hid.de

Bonn
Professor K von Bergmann
Universität Bonn

Abt. f. Klinische Pharmakologie
Sigmund-Freud-Str. 25
D-53127 Bonn
Phone: +49 228 2870
Fax: +49 228 2876094
E-mail: vonbergmann@uni-bonn.de

Bremen
Professor PS Schönhöfer
Institut für Klinische Pharmakologie
Zentralkrankenhaus
St. Jürgen-Str. 1
D-28205 Bremen
Phone: +49 421 4973562
Fax: +49 421 4973326

Darmstadt
Merck KGaA
Klinsiche Forschung
D-64293 Darmstadt
Phone: +49 6151 722756
Fax: +49 6151 722000
Homep: www.merck.de

Dresden
Professor W Kirch
Institut für Klinische Pharmakologie
Medizinische Fakultät
Technische Universität
Fiedlerstr. 27
D-01307 Dresden
Phone: +49 0351 458 2815
Fax: +49 0351 458 4341

Frankfurt
Professor N Rietbrock
University Hospital Frankfurt
Institute of Clinical Pharmacology
Theodor-Stern-Kai 7
D-6059o Frankfurt am Main
Phone: +49 69 6301 6423
Fax: +49 69 6301 7617
E-mail: harder@em.uni-frankfurt.de

Freiburg
Dr M Seiberling
Biodesign GmbH Quintiles Innovex
Leiter Phase 1 Services
Clinical Pharmacology Unit
Obere Hardtstr. 8-16
D-79114 Freiburg
Phone: +49 761 45410
Fax: +49 761 454155

Göttingen
Professor C Gleiter
Georg-August-Universität Göttingen
Zentrum für Phamakologie und Toxicologie
Abteilung Klinische Pharmakologie
Robert-Koch-Str. 40
D-37075 Göttingen
Phone: +49 551 395770
Fax: +49 551 349652
Homep: regulus.PharBP.Med.
Uni-Goettingen.DE/ Klinphar/
projekt.htm#Auftrag

Greifswald
Professor W Siegmund
Insitut für Klinische Pharmakologie
Ernst-Moritz-Arndt-Universität
Loefflerstrasse 23d
D-17487 Greifswald
Phone: +49 3834 865632
Fax: +49 3834 865631
E-mail: siegmuw@rz.uni-greifswald.de

Grünstadt
Professor PW Lücker GmbH
Institut für Klinische Pharmakologie
Bobenheim
Richard-Wagner-Str. 20
D-67269 Grünstadt
Phone: +49 6359 8990
Fax: +49 6359 899 226
E-mail: ikp@ikp.de
Homep: www.ikp.de

Halle
Professor W Sziegoleit
Inst. f. Pharmakologie & Toxikologie
Abt. Klinische Pharmakologie
Martin-Luther-Universität
Magdeburger Strasse
D-06112 Halle

Hannover
Professor JC Frölich
Medizinische Hochschule Hannover
Institut für Klinische Pharmakologie
D-30623 Hannover
Phone: +49 511 532 2820
Fax: +49 511 532 2750

Heidelberg
Professor I Walter-Sack
Universitätsklinikum
Medizinische Klinik und Poliklinik
Abt. Klinische Pharmakologie
Bergheimer Str. 58
D-69115 Heidelberg
Phone: +49 6221 56-8742
Fax: +49 6221 56-4642
E-mail: Ingeborg_Walter-Sack_at_med
@med.uni-heidelberg.de

Professor E Haefeli
Division of Clinical Pharmacology
and Pharmacoepidemiology
Department of Medicine
University of Heidelberg
Bergheimer Strasse 58
D-69115 Heidelberg
Phone: +49 6221 56-8740 or 8741
Fax: +49 6221 56-4642
E-mail: walteremilhaefeli@med.uni-heidelberg.de

Professor Klein/Dr W Tetzloff
IPHAR Institut
Arnikastrasse 4
D-85635 Höhenkirchen/Siegertsbrunn
Phone: +49 8102 8080
Fax: +49 8102 4007
E-mail: iphar@t-online.de

Ingelheim
Dr SW Adamus
Boehringer Ingelheim Pharma KG
Human Pharmacology Centre
P.o. Box 200
Binger Str 173
D-55216 Ingelheim
Phone: +49 6232 773212
Fax: +49 6132 774550

Jena
Professor A Hoffmann
Klinikum der Friedrich-Schiller-Universität Jena
Institut f. Klinische Pharmakologie
Bachstrasse 18
D-07740 Jena
Phone: +49 3641 937774
Fax: +49 3641 937788
E-mail: ahoffmann@landgraf.med.uni-jena.de

Konstanz
Dr W Wurst
Leiter Medizinische Forschung
Byk Gulden
Lomberg Chemische Fabrik GmbH
Postfach 10 03 10
D-78403 Konstanz
Phone: +49 7531 84-0
Fax: +49 7531 842474

Köln
Professor U Fuhr
Institut for Pharmacology of the University at Cologne
Clinical Pharmacology
Glueler Strasse 24
D-50931 Köln
Phone: +49 221 478 5230
Fax: +49 221 478 5022
E-mail: uwe.fuhr@medizin.uni-koeln.de

Professor R Gerzer
DLR-Institut für Luft- und Raumfahrtmedizin
Linder Höhe
D-51126 Köln
Phone: +49 2203 601 3115
Fax: +49 2203 695 211
E-mail: rupert.gerzer@dlr.de

Dr R Horstmann
Troponwerke GmbH und Co. KG
Neurather Ring 1
D-51063 Köln
Phone: +49 221 6472324
Fax: +49 221 6472353
E-mail: rolf.horstmann.rh@bayer-ag.de

Leipzig
Professor R Preiß
Universität Leipzig
Inst. f. Klinische Pharmakologie
Härtelstr. 16-18
D-04107 Leipzig
Phone: +49 341 9724650
Fax: +49 341 9724659

Magdeburg
Professor FP Meyer
Institut für Klinische Pharmakologie
Medizinische Fakultät
Otto-von-Guericke-Universität
Leipziger Strasse 44
D-39120 Magdeburg
Phone: +49 391 671 3060
Fax: +49 391 671 3062
E-mail: uwe.troeger@medizin.uni-magdeburg.de
Homep: www.med.uni-magdeburg.de/image\e24htm

Mannheim
Dr G Neugebauer
Department of Clinical Pharmacology
Boehringer Mannheim GmbH
Sandhofer Str. 116
D-68305 Mannheim
Phone: +49 621 759 2263
Fax: +49 621 759 4724
E-mail: guenter_neugebauer@bmg.boehringer-mannheim.com

Professor M Wehling
Institut für Klinische Pharmakologie
Fakultät für Klinische Medizin
Mannheim
Ruprecht-Karls-Universität Heidelberg
Theodor-Kutzer-Ufer 1-3
D-68135 Mannheim
Phone: +49 621 383 4057 or 4058
Fax: +49 621 383 2024

München
Dr R Eberhardt
PHARMALOG Institut für Klinische Forschung GmbH
Herrmann-Schmid-Str 10
D-80336 München
Phone: +49 89 544637-0
Fax: +49 89 544637-50
E-mail: Pharmalog@t-online.de
Homep: www.pharmalog.com

Professor Dr W Zieglgänsberger
Max-Planck-Institut für Psychiatrie
Klinisches Institut
Kraepelinstr. 10
80804 München
Phone: +49 89 306 22350
Fax: +49 89 306 22402
E-mail: wzg@mpipsykl.mg.de
Homep: www.mpipsykl.mpg.de

Regensburg
Professor H Grobecker
University of Regensburg
Department of Pharmacology and Clinical Pharmacology
Universitätsstrasse 31
D-93053 Regensburg

Phone: +49 941 943 -
Fax: +49 4764 4765

Rostock
Professor B Drewelow
Universität Rostock
Medizinische Fakultät
Institut für Pharmakologie und
Toxikologie
Schillingallee 70
D-18057 Rostock

Professor A Riethling
Universität Rostock
Medizinische Fakultät
Institut für Pharmakologie und
Toxikologie
Schillingallee 70
D-18057 Rostock

Sigmaringen
Professor Herbert Maier-Lenz
Dean Dpt. Pharmatechnology
FH Albstadt-Sigmaringen
Hochschule Für Technik und Wirtschaft
Anton-Günther-Strasse 51
D-72488 Sigmaringen
Phone: +49 7571 732 243/242
Fax: +49 7571 732 250

Stuttgart
Professor M Eichelbaum
Dr. Margarete Fischer-Bosch
Institute of Clinical Pharmacology
Auerbachstrasse 112
D-70376 Stuttgart
Phone: +49 711 8101 3700
Fax: +49 711 8592 95
E-mail: michel.eichelbaum@ikp-stuttgart.de

Tübingen
Professor TH Lippert
University Tübingen
Section of Clinical Pharmacology in
Gynecology and Obstetrics
Department OB/GYN
Schleichstrasse 4
D-72076 Tübingen
Phone: +49 7071 298 4801
Fax: +49 7071 29 4801
E-mail: klin-pharm-ufk@uni-tuebingen.de

Ulm
Professor J Rosenthal
Universität Ulm
Sektion Pharmakotherapie
Oberer Eselberg
D-89081 Ulm

Wiesbaden
Professor Dr.med. G Belz
Zentrum für Kardiovaskuläre Pharmakologie GmbH
Alwinenstr. 16
D-65189 Wiesbaden

Wuppertal
Dr PA Thürmann
Philipp Klee-Institut für Klinische Pharmakologie
Arrenberger Strasse 20
D-42117 Wuppertal
Phone: +49 202 394 5601
Fax: +49 202 394 5602
E-mail: Petra.Tuermann@klinikum-wuppertal.de

Professor J Kuhlmann
Institute of Clinical Pharmacology
Bayer AG
Business Group Pharma
Pharma Research Centre
Building 429
D-42096 Wuppertal
Phone: +49 202 368 509
Fax: +49 202 364 115
E-mail: JOCHEN.KUHLMANN.JK@bayer-ag.de

Training Centres in Germany

Bad Krozingen

Research and training programme: phase I, II and III studies on cardiovascular drugs, especially antianginal, vasodilatory, antiarrhythmic, anticoagulant and antiplatelet drugs.

Authorization for full training (5 years) in clinical pharmacology.

Research facilities: the Department of Clinical Pharmacology is part of the Heart Centre (255 beds). The Clinical Pharmacology unit has 12 beds for research and laboratories for haemodynamic and analytical measurements. The head of the department is Professor of Pharmacology and Clinical Pharmacology at the University of Mainz. The Department has four academic employees (three MDs, one PhD), one clinical monitor, three technical assistants, one secretary, two to three MD or PhD students.

References

Breslin E, Posvar E, Olson S, Trenk D, Jähnchen E (1996) A pharmacokinetic and pharmacodynamic comparison of intravenous quinaprilat and oral quinapril. Clin Pharmacol Ther 36: 414-421

Buschmann M, Wiegand A, Schnellbacher K, Bonn R, Rehe A, Trenk D, Jähnchen E, Roskamm H (1993) Comparison of the effects of two different galenical preparations of glyceryl trinitrate on pulmonary artery pressure and on the finger pulse curve. Eur J Clin Pharmacol 44: 451-456

Kovarik JM, Müller EA, Gaber M, Johnston A, Jähnchen E (1993) Pharmacokinetics of cyclosporine and steady-state aspirin during coadministration. J Clin Pharmacol 33: 513-521

Ruf G, Trenk D, Jähnchen E, Roskamm H (1994a) Determination of the antiischemic activity of nebivolol in comparison to atenolol. Int J Cardiol 43: 279-285

Ruf G, Gera S, Luu HG, Trenk D, De la Rey N, Löffler K, Schulz W, Jähnchen E (1994b) Pharmacokinetics and pharmacodynamics of ramipril and piretanide administered alone and in combination. Eur J Clin Pharmacol 46: 545-550

Russmann, S, Gohlke-Bärwolf Ch, Jähnchen E, Trenk D, Roskamm H (1997) Age-dependent differences in the anticoagulant effect of phenprocoumon in patients after heart valve surgery. Eur J Clin Pharmacol 52: 31-35

Stengele E, Winkler F, Jähnchen E, Trenk D, Petersen J, Roskamm H (1996a) Digital pulse plethysmography as non-invasive method to predict drug induced changes of left ventricular preload. Eur J Clin Pharmacol 50: 279-282

Stengele E, Ruf G, Jähnchen E, Trenk D, Löffler K, Schulz W, Roskamm H (1996b) Acute haemodynamic, antiischemic and antianginal effects of pirsidomine, a novel sydnonimine. A double-blind, placebo-controlled study in 48 patients with coronary artery disease. Am J Cardiol 77: 937-941

Trenk D, Seiler K-U, Buschmann M. Szathmary S, Benn, H-P, Jähnchen E (1993) Effect of concomitantly administered cimetidine or ranitidine on the pharmacokinetics of the 5-HT2-receptor antagonist ritanserin. J Clin Pharmacol 33: 330-334

Vogt D, Trenk D, Bonn R, Jähnchen E (1994) Pharmacokinetics and haemodynamic effects of ISDN following different dosage forms and routes of administration. Eur J Clin Pharmacol 46: 319-324

Berlin
Freie Universität Berlin

Structure: the Department of Clinical Pharmacology is located at the University Hospital Benjamin Franklin and is part of the Institute of Clinical Pharmacology and Toxicology of the Freie Universität Berlin. The current head of the department is Professor of Clinical Pharmacology at the Freie Universität and director of the Max-Delbrueck-Centre for Molecular Medicine at Berlin-Buch.

Research topics: research activities are focused on the development and analysis of cardiovascular disease models covering hypertension, cardiac hypertrophy, kidney damage, stroke, vascular damage, and neointima formation. One particular focus is the establishment and analysis of genetic models of hypertension in rodents. Methods applied include segregation analysis (e.g. establishment of congenic hypertensive rat strains), transgenic rat models, and knock-out mouse models (in close collaboration with the Max-Delbrueck Centre of Molecular Medicine at Berlin-Buch). Further research interests are focussed on the regulation and transcriptional control in vitro and in vivo of the endothelin system, renin angiotensin system, and NO system in cardiovascular cells and tissues under pathophysiological conditions.

Services: therapeutic drug monitoring (TDM) is performed for 11 drugs (aminoglycosides, vancomycin, theophylline, digitalis, anticonvulsants). In addition, plasma levels of vitamins B1, B12, and folic acid are determined. A drug therapy information service (phone +49-30-8445 2279/2289) for physicians and patients is provided. The departments is responsible for the scientific and administrative organization of the work of the local Ethics committee, which gives an opinion on approximately 200 clinical studies per year.

Training and teaching: the Department of Clinical Pharmacology can provide MD and PhD degrees and is fully licensed for the corresponding board certifications and offers the opportunity for 'habilitation'. Teaching of medical students include lectures ('Therapeutic Conferences' are held together with physicians of the Department of Internal Medicine) and topic-related seminars in clinical pharmacology in small teaching groups.

References

Hocher B, Liefeldt L, Thöne-Reineke C, Orzechowski HD, Distler A, Paul M (1996) Characterization of the renal phenotype in transgenic rats expressing the human endothelin-2 gene. Hypertension 28: 196-201

Kreutz R, Struk B, Rubattu S, Hubner N, Szpirer J, Szpirer C, Ganten D, Lindpaintner K (1997a) Role of the alpha-, beta-, and gamma-subunits of epithelial sodium channel in a model of polygenic hypertension. Hypertension 29: 131-136

Kreutz R, Struk B, Stock P, Hubner N, Ganten D, Lindpaintner K (1997b) Evidence for primary genetic determination of heart rate regulation: chromosomal mapping of a genetic locus in the rat. Circulation 96: 1078-1081

Liefeldt L, Schönfelder G, Stock P, Böcker W, Bohnemeier H, Langheinrich M, Orzechowski HD, van der Giet M, Ganten D, Paul M (1995) Transgene Tiermodelle in der Klinischen Pharmakologie am Beispiel der Hypertonieforschung. Klin Pharmacol Akt 6: 84-88

Orzechowski HD, Richter CM, Funke-Kaiser H, Kröger B, Schmidt M, Menzel S, Bohnemeier H, Paul M (1997) Evidence of alternative promoters directing isoform-specific expression of human endothelin-converting enzyme-1 mRNA in cultured endothelial cells. J Mol Med 75: 512-421

Paul M, Wagner J, Hoffmann S, Urata H, Ganten D (1994) Transgeneic rats: new experimental models for the study of candidate genes in hypertension research. Annu Rev Physiol 56: 811-829

Paul M, Zintz M, Böcker W, Dyer M (1995) Characterization and functional analysis of the rat endothelin-1 promotor. Hypertension 25: 683-687

Schönfelder G, John M, Hopp H, Fuhr N, van der Giet M, Paul M (1996) Expression of inducible nitric oxide synthase in placenta of women with gestational diabetes. FASEB J 10: 777-784

Forschergruppe Klinische Psychopharmakologie
The Research Group in Clinical Psychopharmacology at the Free University of Berlin is headed by Professor B Müller-Oerlinghausen and Professor WM Herrmann. Professor B Müller-Oerlinghausen and Professor WM Herrmann possess joint permission for running a 5-year training programme in clinical pharmacology. The clinical part of the training can be spent in the Department of Clinical Psychiatry, i.e. in the clinical wards or in the laboratories for clinical psychopharmacology, or clinical psychophysiology, or sleep medicine. Part of the

training can also be spent in the Department of Clinical Pharmacology of PAREXEL, mainly focusing on various kinds of assessments in healthy volunteers or patients within the context of phase I studies.

The Institute of Clinical Pharmacology - Schering AG
The Institute of Clinical Pharmacology is a function of Schering's Biological Development. Being a main department within a pharmaceutical company, our main task is to provide relevant information about new compounds in the drug development process.

Main areas of activities: planning of the clinical projects in an early preclinical stage

Planning, conducting and evaluating of phase I, clinical studies mainly in the areas of diagnostic/contract media/signal enhancers; hormone therapy; fertility control; cardiovascular diseases; degenerative neurological diseases and skin diseases according to the requirements of international drug development.

Structure: the staff counts 11 physicians, two information scientists, about 20 study nurses and servicing staff personnel of Schering's clinical pharmacology department.

The facility comprises among others up to 24 intensive care beds for general purposes; two Faraday cages for CNS research with EEG derivation; two psychometric units; one unit for studies with radio-labelled compounds; two units for gynaecological investigation including transvaginal ultrasound; one laboratory for skin methods, including ultrasound measurement of skin morphology, colourimetry, surface profile; 'hotel' beds for overnight stay.

Studies are conducted in so-called healthy subjects and patients (mainly in non-therapeutic indications).

Training and teaching: in connection with Berlin's academia, the institute can provide MD and PhD degrees and is fully licensed to train for the board certification (Art Fr Klinische Pharmakologie).

In co-operation with the clinical pharmacology of the medical school of Chariot Clinics, two seminars for clinical pharmacology are given per semester. Traditionally, Schering's ICP has been very dedicated in developing the area of Human Pharmacology, an activity that is now carried on by the society for Applied Human Pharmacology (http://ourworld.compuserve.com/homepages/agah/index.htm).

References

Lange L, Jaeger H, Seifert W et al (1992a) Good Clinical Practice. Bd. 1: Grundlagen und Strategie, Berlin, Heidelberg, New York: Springer, Konzepte in der Human-pharmakologie

Lange L, Jaeger H, Seifert W et al (1992b) Good Clinical Practice. Bd. 2: Praxis der Studien-durchführung. Berlin, Heidelberg, New York: Springer, Konzepte in der Human-pharmakologie

Lange L, Jaeger W, Seifert W et al. (1993) Pharmakodynamische Modelle güt die Arznei-mittelentwicklung. Berlin, Heidelberg, New York: Springer. Konzepte in der Human-pharmakologie.

Biberach

Dr Karl Thomae Gmbh, Abteilung Klinische Forschung

The centre offers research and training in phase I-IV research in the development of new drugs.

Points of emphasis are cardiovascular, antithrombotics, immunology and oncology. Not including phase I, 12 physicians and other personnel are on phase II-IV.

For phase I, the company maintains a centre with 36 beds and a staff of five physicians (three clinical pharmacologists, one cardiologist and one post-doc trainee for clinical pharmacology), nurses, household and administrative personnel. In co-operation with the pharmacokinetic and pharmacology units, the centre offers the whole range of phase I research. There is no vacancy at the moment. Inquiries should be directed to Dr W Feuere or Dr CAPF Su.

References

Degner FL, Narjes H, Tuerck D, Schepers C, Heinzel G, Su CAPF (1993) Lack of interaction between meloxicam 15 mg/day capsules and beta-acetyldigoxin 0.3 mg/day tablets in twelve healthy volunteers over a period of eight days. Klin Pharmakol Aktuell 4 (2): 23-24

Oosterhuis B, Storm G, Cornelisen PJG, Su CAPF, Sollie FAE, Jonkman JHG (1993) Dose-dependent uricosuric effect of ambroxol. Eur J Clin Pharmacol 44 (3): 237-241

Su CAPF, Heinigen PNM, van Lier JJ, van Bruin H, de Kirchgaessler KU, Cornelissen PJG, Jonkman JHG (1994) Pharmacodynamics of the AII antagonist BIBR0277SE, 95th Ann Mtg, American Society for Clinical Pharmacology and Therapeutics, New Orleans, March 30-April 1 1994, 205

Tuerck D, Su CAPF, Heinzel G, Busch U, Bluhmki E, Hoffmann J (1997) Lack of interaction between melozicam and warfarin in healthy volunteers. Eur J Clin Pharmacol 51 (5): 421-425

Vogt A, Essen R, von Tebbe U, Feuerer W, Appel KF, Neuhaus KL (1993) Impact of early perfusion status of the infarct-related artery on short-term mortality after thrombolysis for acute myocardial infarction: retrospective analysis of four German multicentre studies. J Am Coll Cardiol 21 (6): 1391-1395

Vogt A, Essen R, von Tebbe U, Feuerer W, Appel KF, Niederer W, Neuhaus KL (1994) Frequency of achieving optimal reperfusion with thrombolysis in acute myocardial infarction (analysis of four German multicentre studies). Am J Cardiol 74 (1): 1-4

Bonn

Research and training programme: phase I, II and III studies on lipid-lowering drugs, especially cholesterol synthesis, cholesterol absorption, cholesterol precursors, oxysterols, apolipoprotein turnover studies, biliary lipid secretion. Authorization for training in Clinical Pharmacology (4 years).

Research facilities: the head of the department is Director of the Department of Clinical Pharmacology, University of Bonn. The Department of Clinical Pharmacology has six beds for patients and is closely related to the Department of Internal Medicine (Gastroenterology, Hepatology, Oncology, Nephrology). The Department of Clinical Pharmacology has its own Outpatient Clinic (patients with hyper- and dyslipoproteinaemia and diabetes mellitus).

There is also a laboratory with gas chromatography, mass spectrometry, and high-liquid chromatography.

The department has five academics (four MD, one PhD), nurses, 52 technical assistants, one secretary, 10-14 MD or PhD students working for their thesis.

References

Becker M, Staab D, and von Bergmann K (1993) Treatment of severe familial hypercholesterolaemia in childhood with sitosterol and sitostanol. J Pediatr 122 (2): 292-296

Hahn C and von Bergmann K (1996) Relationship between the serum concentration of 7a-hydroxycholesterol and fecal bile acid excretions in humans. Scand J Gastroentrol 31

Hahn C, Reichel C, and von Bergmann K (1995) Serum concentration of 7a-hydroxycholesterol as an indicator of bile acid synthesis in humans. J Lipid Res 36: 2059-2066

Heinemann T, Axtmann G, and von Bergmann K (1993) Comparison of intestinal absorption of cholesterol with different plant sterols in man. Eur J Clin Invest 23 (12): 827-831

Lindenthal B and von Bergmann K (1994) Determination of urinary mevalonic acid using isotope dilution technique. Biol Mass Spectrom 23(7): 445-450

Lindenthal B, Simatupang A, Dotti MT, Federico A, Lütjohann D, and von Bergmann K (1996) Urinary excretion of mevalunic acid as an indicator of cholesterol synthesis. J Lipid Res 37: 2193-2201

Lütjohann D, Meese CO, Crouse JR 3rd, and von Bergmann K (1993) Evaluation of deuterated cholesterol and deuterated sitostanol for measurement of cholesterol absorption in humans. J Lipid Res 34(6): 1039-1046

Lütjohann D, Björkhem I, Beil UF and von Bergmann K (1995) Sterol absorption and sterol balance in phytosterolaemia evaluated by deuterium labelled sterols. Effect of sitostanol treatment. J Lipid Res 32:1861-1867

Schmidt J, Schmitt C, and von Bergmann K (1994) Serup concentration of 7a-hydroxycholesterol as an indicator of bile acid synthesis in humans. J Lipid Res 26(6): 352-360

Sudhop T, Lütjohann D, Ratmann C, Von Bergmann J, and von Bergmann K (1996) Differences in the response of serum lipoproteins to fenofibrate between women and men with primary hypercholesterolemia. Eur J Clin Pharmacol 50: 365-369

Bremen

The Institute of Clinical Pharmacology is structured as a service unit for the four central hospitals (community hospitals, about 3500 beds) and aims at

supplying qualified and independent drug information and therapeutic advice to the medical staff of the four central hospitals and other hospitals of the area.

– administering and advising the ethics committee of the state of Bremen.

– administering and advising the medicines committee of the central hospital pharmacy supplying seven hospitals (4500) beds in the area.

– visiting all intensive care units of the four central hospitals with pharmacotherapeutic rounds once a week.

– supplying therapeutic advice on drug-related problems, adverse drug events and individual therapeutic problems for GPs and the medical profession in the greater Bremen area by a special service phone, which is now increasingly used by out of area clients.

– offering training and teaching for interns and students of our teaching hospitals and also specifically for GPs of the region on therapeutic strategies and drug treatment.

– advising state and federal institutions (parliament, administration)

on problems of drug safety, drug-induced diseases and drug legislation.
- advising/supporting hospital units and medical staff on performing clinical studies according to the GCP rules and ascertaining high quality standards.

Research activities
Drug-induced diseases, monitoring, detecting, describing, reporting to authorities. The institute runs a hospital based system for detecting serious drug-induced events such as cause of hospitalization (about 2% of all admissions). Special emphasis is placed on drug-induced immunotoxic disease which amount to 40% of all serious drug-induced events. All events are reported to the responsible authorities, in addition to informing a network of mutual information run by a German drug bulletin.

Further research activities are aimed at improving the quality of independent drug information and drug therapy (internal and external quality assessment) in hospitals and for GPs.

Staff
The head of the institute is Professor of Pharmacology at the Medical Academy in Hannover. The institute has four medical employees.

References
Lelgemann M, Wille H, Trauernicht G, Skornicka H, Bethge H, Wärtzig HR (1998) Olanzapin: Erste Beobachtung einer Hyperglykämie wie unter Clozapin. Internist 5-168

Schönhöfer PS, Werner B, Tröger U (1997a) Drug points: ocular damage associated with proton pump inhibitors. Br Med J 314: 1805

Schönhöfer PS, Wille H, Lelgemann M, Poppenberd B, Weber D, Kröhn JR, Auerswald G (1997b) Das Bremer Erfassungssystem für arzneimittelbedingte Erkrankungen: Antikonvulsiva-Hypersensitivitätssyndrom nach Carbamazepin. Internist Praxis 37: 195-199

Werner B, Wille H, Spehn J (1997) Aus dem Bremer Erfassungssystem für arzneimittel-bedingte Erkrankungen: Naproxen-induzierte Pneumonitis. Internist Praxis 37: 657-660

Wille H, Werner B, Kardalinos V (1997) Aus dem Bremer Erfassungssystem für arzneimittelbedingte Erkrankungen: Endokardfibrose unter Ergot-Alkaloiden. Internist Praxis 37: 377-380

Darmstadt

Research and training programme
Phase I-IV predominantly in the cardiovascular and CNS areas at MERCK KGaA, Clinical Research and Development Pharma,

The phase I unit includes 10 beds and laboratories for pharmacodynamic and pharmaco-kinetic measurements. The staff consists of 20 coworkers (five MDs and one PhD). The Department also works in collaboration with external academic institutions and contract research organizations.

References

Achenbach H, Hohnerjäger P (1995) Monitoring of nilvadipine treatment in 23770 hypertensive patients. Int J Risk Saf Med 7: 17-31

Breithaupt-Grögler K, Butzer R, Ungethüm W, Belz G (1997) Pharmacodynamic and -kinetic interactions of imidapril with bisoprolol, nilvadipine and hydrochlorothiazide. Eur J Clin Pharmacol 52 Suppl. A 130

Erb K, De Mey C, Roll S, Köhnlein A, Ungethüm W, Leopold G, Belz G (1994) Cardiovascular effects of bimakalim, diltiazem and their combination in healthy volunteers. Eur J Clin Pharmacol 47: A 98

Harder S, Thürmann PA, Ungethüm W (1997) PK - PD modelling with the ACE - inhibitor imidapril in hypertensive patients. Clin Pharmacol Ther 62: 18

Hoogkamer JFW, Kleinbloesem CH, Nokhodian A, Ouwerkerk MJA, Lankhaar G, Ungethüm W, Kirch W (1997) Pharmacokinetics of imidapril and its active metabolite imidaprilat following single dose and during steady state in patients with impaired liver function. Eur J Clin Pharmacol 51: 489-491

Leopold G. Arzneimittelinteraktionen. p 121-138 (Chapter 7)

Leopold G. Kombinationstherapie und Kombinationspräparate. P 198-203 (Chapter 11)

Leopold G. Therapiekonzepte bei Schmerzen, p 507-513 (Chapter 17)

Leopold G (1996) Schmerzbehandlung mit stark wirksamen Analgetika, p 543-559 (Chapter 19) in Rietbrock N, Staib A, Loew D (editors). Klinische Pharmakologie, 3. edition, Steinkopff Verlag, Darmstadt

Leopold G, Kutz K(1997) Bisoprolol: pharmacokinetic profile. Rev Contemp Pharmacother 8: 35-43

Millerioux L, Gualamo V, Caplain H, Ungethüm W, Mignot A, Duvauchelle T (1996) Pharmacokinetic interaction study between cimetidine and imidapril at steady state in 12 normal healthy volunteers. Eur J Drug Metab Pharmacokin (special issue): 136-137

Staib A, Schwalbe J, Leopold G. Die Verschreibung von Arzneimitteln - Das ärztliche Rezept, p 30-45 (Chapter 2)

Dresden

The research and training programme at the Institute for Clinical

Pharmacology at the University of Technology in Dresden involves a 5-year training programme to become a specialist in clinical pharmacology (see also the chapter on clinical pharmacology in Germany).

Clinical and research facilities: two cardiovascular laboratories, two gastrointestinal pharmacology laboratories, one psychopharmacology laboratory, one pharmacoepidemiology department, four analytic laboratories, one clinical research unit: six beds including cardiovascular monitoring, one library.

Number of students (1996) = 1137 (including medical, dentist and public health students)

Staff: 23 persons in total: two Professors, eight MDs, two PhDs (Chemists), nine medical professionals, two secretaries.

References

Berndt A, Gramatté T, Oertel R, Teerhag B, Richter K, Kirch W (1995) Day-night variations in the renal excretion of the antiarrhythmic agent tiracizine its metabolites. Chronobiol Int 12: 135-140

Gramatté T, Oertel R, Teerhag B, Kirch W (1996) Direct demonstration of small intestinal secretion and site-dependent absorption of the b-blocker talinolol in humans. Clin Pharmacol Ther 59: 541-549

Hinrichsen H, Kirch W (1995) Cardiovascular effects of H2-receptor antagonists. J Clin Pharmacol 35: 107-116

Hinrichsen H, Halabi A, Fuhrmann G, Kirch W (1993) Dose-dependent heart rate reducing effect of nizatidine, a histamine H2-receptor antagonist. Br J Clin Pharmacol 35: 461-466

Kirch W, Schafii C (1996) Misdiagnosis at a University Hospital in four medical eras: Report on 400 cases. Medicine (Baltimore) 75: 29-40

Kleinbloesem C, Siepmann M, Kirch W (1995) Haemolysis on intravenous administration of a new calcium antagonist. J Cardiovasc Pharmacol 25: 855-858

Krönig B, Pittrow DB, Kirch W, Welzel D, Weidinger G (1997) Different concepts in first-line treatment of mild-to-moderate essential hypertension: comparison of a low-dose reserpine-thiazide combination with nitrendipine monotherapy. Hypertension 29: 651-658

Mescheder A, Ebert U, Halabi A, Kirch W (1993) Changes in the effects of nizatidine and famotidine on cardiac performance after pretreatment with ranitidine. Eur J Clin Pharmacol 45: 151-156

Oertel R, Richter K, Ebert U, Kirch W (1996) Determination of scopolamine in human serum by gas chromatography-ion trap tandem mass spectrometry. J Chromatography Biomed Appl B 682: 259-264

Siepmann M, Kleinbloesem C, Kirch W (1995) Dose-dependence of the digoxin-calcium antagonist interaction. Br J Clin Pharmacol 39: 491-496

Frankfurt am Main

The Institute of Clinical Pharmacology at the University Hospital Frankfurt has a broad research programme in the field of cardiovascular and neurological pharmacology, the application of pharmacokinetic-pharmacodynamic models and drug utilization as well as GCP-adherent conductance of clinical studies (phase I-III). The laboratory facilities comprise GC and HPLC. A phase I-unit with six beds is part of the institution.

The Frankfurt University Hospital has about 1200 beds and a medical school with about 1500 students. Medical focus are haematological and oncological diseases, special services include BMT and transplantation surgery.

Inquiries to: Sebastian Harder, MD, PhD, Institute of Clinical Pharmacology.

References

Bode H, Brendel E, Ahr G, Fuhr U, Harder S, Staib AH (1996) Investigation of the nifedipine absorption in different parts of the human gastrointestinal tract. Eur J Clin Pharmacol 50: 213-217

Hailer NP, Blaheta RA, Harder S, Scholz M, Encke A, Markus BH (1994) Modulation of adhesion molecule expression on endothelial cells by verapamil and other Ca-channel blockers. Immunobiology 191: 38-51

Harder S, Thürmann PA (1997): Pharmacokinetic and pharmacodynamic interaction trial after repeated oral doses of imidapril and digoxin in healthy volunteers. Br J Clin Pharmacol 43: 475-480

Harder S, Brei R, Caspary S, Merz PG (1993) Lack of a pharmacokinetic interaction between carvedilol and digitoxin or phenprocoumon. Eur J Clin Pharmacol 44: 583-586

Harder S, Baas H, Bergemann N, Demisch L, Rietbrock S (1995a) Concentration/effect relationship of levodopa in patients with Parkinsons's disease after oral administration of an immediate release and a controlled release formulation. Br J Clin Pharmacol 39: 39-45

Harder S, Baas H, Rietbrock S (1995b) Concentration-effect relationship of levodopa in patients with Parkinson's disease. Clin Pharmacokinet 29: 243-256

Harder S, Thürmann PA, Hellstern A, Benjaminov A (1996) Pharmacokinetics of trapidil, an antagonist of platelet derived growth factor, in healthy subjects and in patients with liver cirrhosis. Br J Clin Pharmacol 42: 443-449

Thürmann P, Harder S, Kirchmaier CM (1995) Influence of piroxicam coadministration on pharmacodynamic parameters and the plasma concentration/effect relationship of recombinant hirudin (CGP 39393). Eur J Clin Pharmacol 48: 241-247

Thürmann PA, Harder S, Steioff A (1997) Structure and activities of hospital drug committees in Germany. Eur J Clin Pharmacol (in press)

Woodcock BG, Abdel-Rahman MS, Wosch F, Harder S (1993) Effect of D,L-verapamil, verapamil enantiomers and verapamil metabolites on the binding of vincristine to a1-acid glycoprotein. Eur J Cancer 29: 559-561

Freiburg

The Phase I Clinical Pharmacology Unit belongs to the Quintiles Innovex (Biodesign) company and is located in Freiburg, Germany.

It performs phase I and early phase II studies in healthy subjects or special populations, such as postmenopausal women, diabetics, asthma, migraine, pollinosis patients, and hepatically/renally impaired patients.

It employs four physicians (two of whom clinical pharmacologists, one an internal specialist), 12 qualified nurses and male nurses, and further academic (four MSc, two MA) as well as specially trained staff for study planning, management, administration, co-ordination and biometrics.

This unit is mainly involved in studies with cardiovascular, CNS, gastrointestinal, analgesics, respiratory, and antibiotic agents; but it is also experienced in studies with hormones, antidiabetics, lipid lowering compounds, among others.

It has a wide range of pharmacodynamic facilities, including ECG monitoring via screen and ECG analysis; 12-lead ECG with automatic interval measuring; long-term Holter ECG over 24 hours; computer controlled ergometry; pulmonary function test with measurement of airway resistance; testing of fine motor response (pursuit rotor, tapping); EEG; gastroscopy; long-term gastric pH-metry; computer-aided psychometric test battery; pupillometry, rhinomanometry; impedance cardiography, and TILT test devices.

The head of the department is authorized for 3 years of training in clinical pharmacology.

References

Degen J, Wölke E, Seiberling M, Thomann P, Völter-Erhardt H (1997) Vergleichende Untersucheung zur relativen Bioverfügbarkeit und Pharmakokinetik von Estron nach oraler Gabe von veresterten Oestrogen als Drageeformulierung und als wässrige Suspension. Arzneimittelforschung 47 (I), Nr. 2

Hatorp V, Thomsen M, Seiberling M (1998) The pharmacokinetic profile of theophylline is not significantly altered by repaglinide co-adminstration. Excerpta Medica.

Hinderling PH, Tendolkar A, Dee CM, Barr WH, Seiberling M, Duerr H (1995) Single-dose interaction study of diprafenone HCl and propranolol HCl in healthy volunteers. J Clin Pharmacol 35: 721-729

Merz M, Seiberling M, Höxter G, Hölting M, Wortha HP (1997) Elevation of liver enzymes in multiple dose trials during placebo treatment: are they predictable? J Clin Pharmacol 37: 791-798

Skrumsager BK, Christensen JV, Snel S, Seiberling M (1995) Tolerability, safety and pharmacokinetics of single dose and multiple dosing of the selective D1 antagonist NNC 01-0687 in healthy subjects. Psychopharmacology 121: 294-299

Wölke E, Seiberling M, Schepers C, Roos U, Franke H, Bernhard I (1993) Investigation in healthy volunteers to evaluate serum concentrations and urinary excretions of aluminium, magnesium, calcium and phosphate after multiple administration of hydrotalcit (Talcid) suspension. Boll Chim Farmaceutico 132 (7): 234-240

Göttingen

The Department of Clinical Pharmacology at the University of Göttingen provides a number of services to the University Hospital and other surrounding hospitals. These services comprise a drug information hotline, therapeutic drug monitoring (antidepressants, anthelmintics, antiarrhythmic drugs). A further task is teaching of clinical pharmacology to medical students and training of MDs and PhDs for board certification. The head of the department is fully licensed for such training. The Department has a fully equipped eight-bed research facility where clinical research projects as well as contract research is being carried out in healthy volunteers and patients. The department has access to all clinical facilities at the university hospital. In addition, the department has a fully equipped laboratory for in vitro research and chemical analyses.

The head of the department serves on the local Ethics Committee and the hospital pharmacy board. The main topics of research are regulation of erythropoietin production in humans, pharmacology of morphine and its glucuronides and population pharmacokinetics. The entire list of recent publications is available at http://regulus.PharBP.Med.Uni-Goettingen.DE/Klinphar/projekt.htm// Auftrag

References

Gleiter CH, Farger G, Möbius HJ (1996) Pharmacokinetics of CGP 36 742, an orally active GABAB antagonist, in humans. J Clin Pharmacol 36: 428-438

Gleiter CH, Freudenthaler S, Delabar U, Eckhardt KU, Mühlbauer B, Gundert-Remy

U, Gleiter CH, Becker T, Schreeb KH, Freudenthaler S, Gundert-Remy U (1997a) Fenoterol but not dobutamine increases erythropoietin production in humans. Clin Pharmacol Ther 61: 669-676

Gleiter CH, Brause M, Delabar U, Eckardt KU (1997b) Evidence against a major role of adenosine in oxygen-dependent regulation of erythropoietin in rats. Kidney Int 52: 338-344

Gleiter CH, Becker T, Wenzel J (1997c) Erythropoietin production in healthy volunteers subjected to controlled hypobaric hypoxia: further evidence against a major role of adenosine. Br J Clin Pharmacol 44: 203-205

Gleiter CH, Schreeb KH, Goldbach S, Herzog S, Cunze T, Kuhn W (1998) Fenoterol increases erythropoietin concentrations during tocolysis. Br J Clin Pharmacol 45: 157-159

Löser SV, Meyer J, Freudentaler S, Sattler M, Desel C, Meineke I, Gundert-Remy U (1996) Morphine-6-O-D-glucuronide but not morphine-3-O-D-glucoronide binds to mu-, delta- and kappa-specific opioid binding sites in cerebral membranes. Naunyn-Schmiedebergs's Arch Pharmacol 354: 192-197

Meineke I, Schmidt W, Nottrott M, Schröder T, Hellige G, Gundert-Remy U (1997a) Modelling of nonlinear pharmacokinetics in sheep after short term infusion of cardiotoxic doses of imipramine. Pharmacol Toxicol 80: 266-271

Meineke I, Feltkamp H, Högemann A, Gundert-Remy U (1997b) Pharmacokinetics and pharmacodynamics of candesartan after administration of its pro-drug candesatan cilexetil in patients with mild to moderate hypertension, a population analysis. Eur J Clin Pharmacol 53: 221-228

Meineke I, Schreeb K, Kress I, Gundert-Remy U (1998) Routine measurement of fluoxetine and norfluoxetine by high-performance liquid chromatography with ultraviolet detection in patients under concomitant treatment with tricyclic antidepressants. Ther Drug Monit, in press

Osswald H (1996) Erythropoietin production in healthy volunteers subjected to controlled haemorrhage: evidence against a major of adenosine. Br J Clin Pharmacol 42: 729-735

Greifswald

Divisions
- Clinical pharmacology, clinical research unit (GCP-standard) drug analysis with GO, HPLC, MS, FPIA (GLP-standard) biometrics
- General pharmacology, molecular and biochemical pharmacology, isotope laboratory, cell laboratory, animal laboratory
- Working group: Therapeutic-toxicological service

Teaching staff: two clinical pharmacologists, four chemists, one biopharmacologist, one biochemist, one biologist, one pharmacist.

Lectures and courses for students of medicine and dentistry: 'General Pharmacology' and 'Clinical Pharmacology'. Lectures, seminars and courses for students of the Faculty of Mathematical and Natural Sciences (human biology, pharmacy, chemistry): lectures and courses 'General Pharmacology', 'Toxicology', Lectures 'Laboratory animals' and 'Basic Principles in Pharmacology'; Courses 'Clinical Pharmacology', 'Basic Methods of Drug Development', 'Biometrics in Pharmacology und Toxicology', 'Drug Analysis', 'Introduction in Animal Experiments'; video seminars 'Pharmacotherapy' and 'Alternative and Scientific Methods in Pharmacotherapy'.

Scientific Profile and Services
- Phenotyping:CYP2D6 (dextromethorphan or debrisoquine), CYP1A2 and NAT2 (caffeine), NAT2 (sulphamethazine).
- Genotyping: CYP1A1, CYP2C19, CYP2D6, CYP2E1, NAT2
- In vitro biotransformation: access to a liver bank with human and rat livers. The livers are characterized by 7-ethoxyresorufin O-deethylase, EROD YP1A1, CYP1A2 7-ethoxycoumarin O-deethylase, ECOD, CYP1A2, CYP2E1, 7-pentoxyresorufin, O-depentylase, PROD, CYP2B1/CYP2B6, dextromethorphan, O-demethylase, DXDM, CYP2D1/CYP2D6, 4-nitrophenol hydroxylase, NPH, CYP2E1, erythromycin N-demethylase, ERDM, CYP3A, procainamide N-acetyltransferase, NAT2, – Processes of signal transduction: proteinkinases A and C, Adenyl cyclase, iNOS (NO-synthase)
- Clinical studies: during the last few years, a large number of pharmacokinetic, bioequivalence and interaction and other human pharmacological studies have been done with several registered and new drugs. Usually, the analytical methods were developed and validated by our group.

References
Berndt A, Hoffmann C, Richter K, Oertel R, Vierkant A, Siegmund W (1995) Tiracizine disposition in healthy volunteers with reference to the debrisoquine oxidation phenotype. Br J Clin Pharmacol 40: 287-288
Hadašová E, Siegmund W, Walter R, Scheuch E, Franke G (1995) Effects of streptolysin O, picibanil (OK 432) and interferon a2A on cytochrome P-450-dependent monooxygenases and arylamine N-acetyltransferase in rat liver. Immunopharmacol Immunotoxicol 17: 283-300
Hadašová E, Cešková E, Zschiesche M, Franke G, Siegmund W, Zelenka M, Sláma J

(1996a) Genetic polymorphism of debrisoquin hydroxylation and sulphamethazine acetylation in patients with schizophrenia and endogenous depression. Br J Clin Pharmacol 41: 428-431

Hadašová E, Scheuch E, Franke G, Engels, Pác L, Engels C, Walter R, Siegmund W (1996b) Effects of LPS and its combination with L-NAME on the pharmacokinetics of procainamide in rats. Exp Toxic Pathol 48 (Suppl. II): 167-170

Hoffmann C, Focke N, Franke G, Zschiesche M, Siegmund W (1995) Comparative bioavailability of metronidazole formulations (Vagimid) after oral and vaginal administration. Int J Clin Pharmacol Ther 33: 232-239

Müller C, Siegmund W, Huupponen R, Kaila T, Franke G, Lisalo E, Zschiesche M (1993) Kinetics of propiverine as assessed by radioreceptor assay in poor and extensive metabolizers of debrisoquine. Eur J Drug Metab Pharmacokinet 18: 265-272

Siegmund W, Wölfle G, Franke G, Amon I (1993a) Effects of nocloprost on some mono-oxygenases of rat and human liver. Arzneimittelforschung 43: 1076-1078

Siegmund W, Scheuch E, Zschiesche M, Franke G, Stolz E, Amon I (1993b) Potential pharmacokinetic interactions of nocloprost clathrate with retarded theophylline and enteric coated diclofenac after single and repeated premedication in healthy volunteers. Int J Clin Pharmacol Ther Toxicol 31: 407-414

Siegmund W, Zschiesche M, Franke G, Amon I (1994) Pharmacokinetic interactions of nocloprost clathrate with acetylsalicylic acid. Int J Clin Pharmacol Ther Toxicol 32: 51-57

Walter R, Azazi M, Scheuch E, Hadašová E, Siegmund W (1996) Influence of selective serotonin reuptake inhibitors on the activities of various hepatic monooxygenases and of the arylamine N-acetyltransferase. Exp Toxicol Pathol 48 (Suppl. II): 433-436

Grünstadt

IKP Bobenheim GmbH

The Institute was founded in 1977 and it presently has a staff of 85 employees. We offer 21 years of experience with clinical phase I investigations, a ward with a capacity of 60 beds, generously equipped for a wide variety of clinical trials, non-invasive measurement techniques which, combined with our highly professional staff, enable us to handle almost all clinical pharmacological issues efficiently within the specified time scale. All studies are conducted according to German Medicines Act and EC-GCP or FDA-Standard. Two audits at IKP conducted by the US Food and Drug Administration (FDA) in 1991 and 1996 confirmed full compliance.

The managing director of the Institute is authorized to train postgraduates in the field of clinical pharmacology (3-year training period).

The department offers the following services: dose finding studies and first exposure of a new drug to humans; bioavailability and bioequivalence studies; pharmacodynamic studies; interaction studies; tolerability studies; studies with special volunteer group; stationary long-term studies.

Bioanalytic: since its foundation in 1977, the Bioanalytical Department of IKP has been specializing in chromatographic analysis of drugs and their metabolites in biological samples. After more than 20 years of analytical work with close contact with many clients of the national and international pharmaceutical industry, the number of validated analytical methods comes to more than 200 and the number of samples analysed, including validation, reaches over 60,000 annually. In 1991, an inspection by the US Food and Drug Administration was conducted at IKP GmbH. The Bioanalytical Department, which was also inspected, was found to be adequate. In 1992 and 1996, an independent inspectorate confirmed that our Bioanalytical Department complies with the regulations of Good Laboratory Practice and issued a GLP Certificate.

This department offers the following services: development of methods; validation of methods, determination of drug concentrations and metabolites in biological samples; drug release tests and tests for time to disintegration according to USP and German Pharmacopoeia; analysis under GLP standard; analytical reports.

Multi Centre Management Phase II-IV: in 1987, after IKP GmbH had been conducting clinical Phase I studies for 10 years, we extended our services to the complete range of phase II-IV studies. A main goal of our multicentric studies is exact planning and pursuit of projects to guarantee that they are completed within the required time scale. Besides time planning our cost planning and cost control enable a continuous and transparent flow of information to our sponsors. Our Clinical Research Associates are employed full-time and are trained in all practical and theoretical aspects of any future project. New employees go through a training period of 9 months in which they gain hands-on experience in all areas of the institute's work. The training concludes with a written and an oral examination.

This department offers the following services: scientific advice and trial planning; in-house 'Principal Investigator'; design of case report forms; preparation of applications for submission to ethics committees and legal authorities; acquisition of suitable trial centres; monitoring in accordance with EG-GCP guidelines and/or FDA-standard; central project management and study co-ordination; design of integrated final report; pharmacokinetic studies in the clinic with subpopulations (e.g. HIV patients) employing specially trained monitoring personnel; seminars for external Clinical Research Associates: seminars for clinical investigators; planning, organization and conduct of investigators' meetings; design of publications.

Data Management: we have conducted study related data management based on SAS, RS/1 and HoeRep for many years and could therefore gain a lot of experience in this field. Now, to keep pace in a continuously advancing field, we have obtained the SAS-Tool PH-Clinical. (The US Food and Drug Administration does not advise special software for the evaluation. However, all evaluations that are calculated with the SAS-system will be accepted without recalculation.)

This department offers the following services: statistical trial planning including sample size estimation; randomization; design of CRFs; data entry with electronic audit trail, coding; data cleaning/query management; evaluation including (pharmacokinetics, pharmacodynamics, safety); statistical report; data transfer/conversion.

Quality assurance: the Quality Assurance Unit of IKP GmbH supervises adherence to legal regulations as well as to national and international standards (German Medicines Act, ICH, GLP, FDA). By regular inspections, at any level of study planning, data reporting and processing, our academic staff members guarantee validity, integrity and reproducibility of the data from clinical phase I-IV investigations and bioanalytical studies. The structure and standards of the services are supported by an extensive SOP system.

This department offers the following services: support to establish your Quality Assurance system; support for the preparation of your specific SOPs; training of your employees; quality assurance in clinical phase I-IV studies from planning to study report; on-site audits in trial centres, system audits according to GCP (in pharmaceutical companies and in CROs (System audits according to GLP (in the bioanalytical laboratories).

Service centre: packaging and labelling: medication used for clinical trials requires special packaging and labelling (German Medicines

Act, pharmaceutical operation ordinance, PIC-GMP-guidelines, supplementary guidelines to GMP for clinical trial drugs). According to '13, section 1, German Medicines Act of August 24, 1976 (latest change on August 9, 1994) IKP GmbH is authorized to manufacture medication according to §2, section 1, German Medicines Act.

This department offers the following services: primary packaging of solid and oral administration, solid and non-oral administration; liquid and oral administration; secondary packaging and labelling of any primary packed medication.

Reporting and scientific consultation: this department specializes in pharmaceutical/clinical research and takes on the design and layout, and medical publications. From the basic concept to the graphical layout all texts are prepared in-house. The data material is based on the internally conducted phase I-IV studies as well as any other selected external studies. Careful and reliable treatment and continuous completion of the contracts are essential cornerstones for the co-operation with our sponsors. A main aim of our scientific and editorial work is to guarantee conclusive, consistent and clearly structured study results according to the sponsor's SOP or the ICH guidelines. Our clinical pharmacological knowledge is based upon many years of experience with clinical trials, dealing with drug formulations spanning the spectrum of indications. This is evident by the publication of more than 300 journal articles as well as lectures, poster displays, dissertations and the publication of a book.

This department offers the following services: integrated text and graphic processing on powerful work stations, word processing and layout, utilizing a choice of packages (MS Word 6.0, Lotus AmiPro 3.1); Internet search facilities to aid and enhance literature inquiries during the course of study protocol preparation; to oversee and process all formalities with authorities and ethics committees; study reports, editing, design and layout; expert reports on pharmacology/toxicology, pharmacokinetics, efficacy and tolerability for registration purposes, preparation of publications and lectures; translation of clinical pharmacological texts; data can be archived on optical data carriers on demand.

Hannover

The Department of Clinical Pharmacology at the Hannover Medical

School comprises the following staff: four physicians, one chemist, one chemist engineer, three laboratory assistance

Training: full 5-year course in clinical pharmacology

Our research programme focuses on:
- the role of nitric oxide in inflammatory joint diseases and the effects of non-steroidal anti-inflammatory drugs (NSAIDs) on the cyclooxygenase pathways.
- the distribution and the role of COX enzymes.
- the role of nitric oxide in the cardiovascular system.
- L-arginine nitric oxide pathway: role in atherosclerosis and therapeutic implications.

These topics are studied in vitro, animal and human experimentation. Studies are carried out according to GCP standards in phase I to III.

Service: drug information systems for physicians in private practice and in hospitals.

Drug monitoring and therapeutic recommendations.

Analytical facilities: dn-6-keto-PGF1a (by GC/MS-MS), dn-TxB2 (by GC/MS-MS)

PGE-MUM (by GC/MS-MS), 6-keto-PGF1 a (by GC/MS-MS), TxB2 (by GC/MS-MS)

PGE2 (by GC/MS-MS), LTE4 (by GC/MS-MS), LTB4 (by GC/MS-MS), NO2/NO3 (by GC/MS-MS), Cyclo-GMP (by RIA), Arginine (by HPLC), Asymmetric and symmetric, Dimethylarginine (by HPLC).

Analytical equipment: gas chromatograph-mass spectrometer (HP), gas chromatograph-mass spectrometer GC/MS-MS (Finnigan-MAT), 4 HPLC-instruments, GC/ECD

References

Bode-Böger SM, Böger RH, Alfke H, Heinzel D, Tsikas D, Creutzig A, Alexander K, Frölich JC (1996) L-arginine induces NO-dependent vasodilatation in patients with critical limb ischaemia - a randomized, controlled study. Circulation 93: 85-90

Bode-Böger SM, Böger RH, Kienke S, Junker W, Frölich JC (1996) Elevated L-arginine/ dimethylarginine ratio contributes to enhanced systemic NO production by dietary L-arginine in hypercholesterolemic rabbits. Biochem Biophys Res Commun 219: 598-603

Böger RH, Bode-Böger SM, Frölich JC (1996a) The L-arginine-nitric oxide pathway: role in atherosclerosis and therapeutic implications. Atherosclerosis 127:1 -11

Böger RH, Skamira C, Bode-Böger SM, Brabant G, von zur Mühlen A, Frölich JC (1996b) Nitric oxide may mediate the haemodynamic effects of recombinant growth hormone in patients with acquired growth deficiency. A double-blind, placebo-controlled study. J Clin Invest 98: 2706-2713

Böger RH, Bode-Böger SM, Thiele W, Junker W, Alexander K, Frölich JC (1997) Biochemical evidence for impaired nitric oxide synthesis in patients with peripheral arterial occlusive disease. Circulation 95: 2068-2074

Frölich JC (1996) Careers in pharmacology: the German perspective. TIPS 17: 47-49

Stichtenoth DO, Wagner B, Frölich JC (1997) Effects of meloxicam and indomethacin on cyclooxygenase pathways in healthy volunteers. J Invest Med 45: 44-49

Frölich JC (1997) A classification of NSAIDs according to the relative inhibition of cyclooxygenase isozymes. Trends Pharmacol Sci 18: 1-35

Stichtenoth DO, Selve N, Tsikas D, Gutzki FM, Frölich JC (1995) Increased total body synthesis of prostacyclin in rats with adjuvant arthritis. Prostaglandins 50: 331-340

Stichtenoth DO, Tsikas D, Gutzki FM, Frölich JC (1996) Effects of ketoprofen and ibuprofen on platelet aggregation and prostanoid formation in man. Eur J Clin Pharmacol 51: 231-234

Heidelberg

The Division of Clinical Pharmacology and Pharmacoepidemiology, Department of Medicine at the University of Heidelberg, is closely affiliated with the department of Internal Medicine. The staff comprises several senior physicians specialised in clinical pharmacology and internal medicine, postgraduate physicians and pharmacists. A senior chemist is in charge of the analytical laboratory.

Physicians are directly involved in patients' care, and in addition are on consultant service for special problems of drug therapy as well as for planning and performing drug trials in healthy individuals and in patients.

Scientific activities include proof-of-concept studies, phase I studies, participation in clinical drug projects (phase II and III studies), and focus on specific pharmacokinetic problems of drug metabolism and further aspects of drug disposition like drug interactions. Pharmacodynamic studies address questions of vascular drug effects and mechanisms of drug action and drug-drug interaction in vitro in human tissue and in vivo in healthy individuals as well as in patients. The main drugs of interest are metabolically active compounds, non-opioid analgesics, cardiovascular and anticoagulant drugs. Another major interest of the Division is the development and validation of electronic data bases providing information on the appropriate use of drugs and methods to increase drug safety.

Courses in clinical pharmacology are given by senior physicians, and are open for medical students and trainees as well. Application for a training in clinical pharmacology should follow the usual rules. A specific application form is not required.

References

Schweizer MWF, Brachmann J, Kirchner U, Walter-Sack I, Dickhaus H, Metze C, Kübler W (1993) Heart rate variability in time and frequency domains: effects of gallopamil, nifedipine, and metoprolol compared with placebo. Br Heart J 70: 252-258

De Vries JX, Walter-Sack I, Voss A, Forster W, Ilisistegui Pons P, Stoetzer F, Spraul M, Ackermann M, Moyna G (1993) Metabolism of benzbromarone in man: structures of new oxidative metabolites, 6-hydroxy- and 1'oxo-benzbromarone, and the enantioselective formation and elimination of 1'hydroxybenzbromarone. Xenobiotica 23: 1435-1450.

Walter-Sack I, de Vries JX, von Bubnoff A, Pfeilschifter V, Raedsch R (1995) Biotransformation and uric acid lowering effect of benzbromarone in patients with liver cirrhosis — evidence for active benzbromarone metabolites? Eur J Med Res 1: 16-20

Walter-Sack I, Klotz U (1996) Influence of diet and nutritional status on drug metabolism. Clin Pharmacokinet 31: 47-64

Wandel C, Böcker RH, Böhrer H, deVries JX, Hofmann W, Walter K, Kleingeist B, Neff S, Ding R, Walter-Sack I, Martin E (1998) Relationship between hepatic cytochrome P450 3A content and activity and the disposition of midazolam administered orally. Drug Metab Disp 26: 110-114

Bommer C, Werle E, Walter-Sack I, Keller C, Gehlen F, Wanner C, Nauck M, März W, Wieland H, Bommer J (1998) D-thyroxine reduces lipoprotein(a) serum concentration in dialysis patients. J Am Soc Nephrol 9: 90-96

Bauer TM, Ritz R, Haberthür Ch, Ha HR, Hunkeler W, Sleight AJ, Scollo-Lavizzari G, Haefeli WE (1995) Prolonged sedation due to accumulation of conjugated metabolites of midazolam. Lancet 346: 145-147

Schmassmannn-Suhijar D, Bullingham R, Gasser R, Schmutz J, Haefeli WE (1998) Rhabdomyolysis due to interaction of simvastatin with mibefradil. Lancet 351: 1929-1930

Schuerch LV, Linder LM, Grouzmann E, Haefeli WE (1998) Human neuropeptide Y potentiates (1-adrenergic blood pressure responses in vivo. Am J Physiol 275: H760-766

Rothen JP, Haefeli WE, Meyer UA, Wenk M (1998) Acetaminophen is an inhibitor of hepatic N-acetyltransferase 2 in vitro and in vivo. Pharmacogenetics 8: 553-559

Höhenkirchen-Siegertsbrunn
IPHAR Institut für klinische Pharmakologie GmbH

The IPHAR Institute was founded in 1976 and is one of the first clinical-pharmacological contract research organisations in Germany. IPHAR GmbH has been an independent subsidiary of the bioanalytic specialist MKL/McKnight Laboratories GmbH in Hamburg since 1993; a close working relationship exists between the two companies. Our facility in Höhenkirchen-Siegertsbrunn near Munich employs 33 staff members (including five physicians and 15 nurses) involved in clinical-pharmacological research. Our clinical-pharmacological services for drug development and evaluation distinguish themselves through a special medical-scientific orientation.

Strong Points of our service offering
- The IPHAR clinic has a total capacity of 40 beds (including an intensive-care area of four beds). Our infrastructure makes it possible to do both short-term, long-term and in-patient studies.
- Through close ties with Munich's university clinics, studies can be conducted on special groups and patients, both on an in- and outpatient basis.
- Our areas of expertise include: first administration on humans; pharmacokinetics: bioavailability and bioequivalence, dose proportionally, repeated dose studies and interaction studies; pharmacodynamics: cardiovascular system, algesiometry (different methods), ophthalmology, psychometry, abdominal sonography and blood circulation in the liver.
- Our bioanalytical services are performed in Hamburg at McKnight Laboratories GmbH and extend to a wide range of analytical methods.
- Our biometrics team performs data analyses (incl. new methods such as PK-PD modelling) in conformance with GCP guidelines and as required for certifications.
- Authorization for training in Clinical Pharmacology (3 years).

References
Appel S, Rüfenacht Th, Kalafsky G, Tetzloff W, Kallay Z, Hitzenberger G, Kutz K (1995) Lack of interaction between fluvastatin and oral hypoglycemic agents in healthy subjects and in patients with non-insulin-dependent diabetes mellitus. Am J Cardiology 76 (July 13)

Borum P, Eccles R, Tetzloff W, Van Cauwenberge P (1994) Can antihistamines relieve symptoms of the common cold? Am J Respiratory and Critical Care Medicine 149 (4): A602

Denzlinger C, Tetzloff W, Gerhartz HH, Pokorny R, Sagebiel S, Haberl C, Wilmanns W (1993) Differential activation of the endogenous leucotriene biosynthesis by two different preparations of granulocyte-macrophage colony-stimulating factor in healthy volunteers. Blood 81 (8): 2007-2013

Kovarik JM, Mueller EA, van Bree JB, Tetzloff W, Kutz K (1994) Reduced inter- and intraindividual variability in cyclosporine pharmacokinetics from a microemulsion formulation. J Pharm Sci 83 (3): 444-446

Kovarik JM, Mueller EA, Richard F, Tetzloff W (1997) Optimizing the absorption of valspodar, a P-glycoprotein modulator, part II: Quantifying its pharmacokinetic variability and refining the bioavailability estimate. J Clin Pharmacol 37 (11): 1009-1014

Mueller EA, Kovarik JM, van Bree JB, Tetzloff W, Grevel J, Kutz K (1994) Improved dose linearity of cyclosporine pharmacokinetics from a microemulsion formulation. Pharm Res 11 (2): 301-304

Rosak C, Ziegler D, Mehnert H, Schmidt K-H, Reichel G, Tetzloff W, Hermann R, Ruus P, Tritschler H-J, Ulrich H (1994) Lokale Verträglichkeit intravenöser a-Liponsäure. münchener Medizinische Wochenschrift 136 (10): 142-146

Rosenthal J, Bahrmann H, Benkert K, Baumgart P, Bönner G, Klein G, Neiss A, Schnelle K, Frohlich ED (1996) Analysis of Adverse Effects among patients with essential hypertension receiving an ACE inhibitor or a beta-blocker. Clin Pharmacol 87: 409-414

Scholze J, Klein G (1996) Equivalent blood pressure reduction and tolerability with controlled-release metroprolol 50 mg twice daily: a double-blind 8-week comparison in hypertensive patients. Clin Drug Invest 11 (6): 331-338

Tetzloff W, Dauchy F, Medimagh S, Carr D, Bär A (1996) Tolerance to subchronic, high-dose ingestion of erythritol in human volunteers. Regul Toxicol Pharmacol 24: S286-S295, Article No. 0110

Ingelheim

Research and training programme: phase I, II and III studies on antiasthmatics (anticholinergics, potassium-channel openers, leukotriene inhibitors) and CNS drugs (against stroke, against Alzheimer's disease, antidepressants). The institute is authorized for 3 years training in clinical pharmacology.

Research facilities: the institute has 30 investigational beds and 12 beds for an overnight stay. The main laboratories are: (a) lung function laboratory (whole-body plethysmography, spirometry, provocation methods); (b) cardiovascular laboratory (impedance cardiography, Laser-Doppler flowmetry, venous occlusion plethysmography);

(c) central nervous system (pharmaco-EEG, computerized psychometric laboratory, infrared TV pupillometry)

Staff: five physicians, one engineer, eight medical assistants, three secretaries, five auxiliary staff members.

Job applications can be sent to the head of the institute.

References

Adamus WS (1998) Pharmacodynamic methods for investigating anti-asthma drugs in healthy volunteers. Methods Find Exp Clin Pharmacol 20 (4) in press

Adamus WS, Leonard JP, Tröger W (1995) Phase I clinical trial with WAL 2014, a new muscarinic agonist for the treatment of Alzheimer's disease. Life Sci 56: 883-890

Brecht HM, Adamus WE, Heuer HO, Birke FW, Kempe ER (1991) Pharmacodynamics, pharmacokinetics and safety profile of the new platelet activation antagonist apafant in man. Arzneimittelforschung 41 (I): 51-59

Leonard JP, Ahlstich S, Lohmann HF (1992) Kognitive Vigilanzkontrolle im Pharmako-EEG: Eine effektive, aufgabenbezogene Methode. In Oldigs-Kerber J & Leonard JP (Hrsg), Pharmakopsychologie. Experimentelle und klinische Aspekte 265-284, Jena: Fischer

Leonard JP, Heinrich-Nols N, Roth TG (1996) Nocturnal psychometric assessment of the hypnotic activity of low and normal doses of brotizolam. Arzneimittelforschung 46 (I): 462-467

Oldigs-Kerber J, Adamus WS, Kitzinger M (1991) Zur Beeinflussung von verbalen Lern- und Gedächtnisprozessen durch Anticholinergica am Beispiel Scopolamin, ein pharmako-psychologischer Beitrag für die neuropsychologische Praxis. Zeitschrift für Neuropsychologie 1: 29-40

Schilling JC, Adamus WS (1991) Effects of a new analgesic on pupillary and neuroendocrine parameters in healthy subjects. Clin Pharmacol Ther 49: 132

Schilling JC, Adamus WS, Kuthan H (1990) Antihistaminic activity and side effect profile of epinastine and terfenadine in healthy volunteers. Int J Clin Pharmacol Ther Toxicol 28 (12): 493-497

Schilling JC, Adamus WS, Palluk R (1992a) Neuroendocrine and side effect profile of pramipexole, a new dopamine receptor agonist, in man. Clin Pharmacol Ther 51: 541-548

Schilling JC, Marini MP, Vidi A, Leonard JP, Rizzi CA, Daniotti S, Daniotti A (1992b) Tolerability and pharmacokinetics of single doses of DAU 6215 CL in healthy volunteers. Mechanisms and Control of Emesis 223: 173-174

Jena

Research and training programme: the Institute of Clinical Pharmacology is an independent department of the medical faculty of the university with applied clinical pharmacology research. Authorization for full training (5 years) in Clinical Pharmacology. The institute can provide MD degrees and is fully licensed to train MDs for their corresponding board certifications and habilitation. The Clinical Pharmacology unit has laboratories for analytical measurements and characterization of genetic polymorphism, study unit (four beds) for clinical research with healthy volunteers and patients; good collaborations with departments of the university hospitals; special therapeutic drug monitoring (TDM) with individualized dosage regimens.

Clinical and research facilities: phase I and IV studies; analytical chemistry (e.g. HPLC, GC, capillary electrophoresis, fluorimetry) for analysis of drugs and metabolites in different biological material; influence of drug therapy on different biotransformation reactions (phenotyping and interaction studies); molecular pharmacology and cell biology (characterization of genetic polymorphism of gene expression; characterization of signal transduction pathways concerning cytocine expression); investigation of influence of transdermal transport of drugs; research in field of pharmacoepidemiology and pharmacovigilance (adverse drug reactions, thromboembolic reactions after contraceptives, risk of urothelic and nephrotic cancers).

The university was founded in 1558, has 10 faculties and 11,116 students (15% medicine, 61.4% arts, economics and jurisprudence, 23.5% mathematics, technics and natural sciences.

Staff: The head of the department is professor of clinical pharmacology; four medical doctors (three of them are specialists of clinical pharmacology), three pharmacists and biologist, five technical assistants and one secretary, one MD student.

References

Endres HGE, Henschel L, Merkel U, Hippius M, Hoffmann, A (1996) Lack of pharmacokinetic interaction between dextromethorphan, coumarin and mephenytoin in man after simultaneous administration. Pharmazie 51: 46-51

Farker K, Schweer H, Vollandt R, Nassr N, Nagel U, Seyberth HW, Hoffmann A, Oettel M (1997) Measurements of urinary prostaglandins in young ovulatory women during the menstrual cycle and in postmenopausal women. Prostaglandins 54: 655-664

Hippius M, Henschel L, Sigusch H, Tepper J, Brendel E (1995) Pharmacokinetic interactions of nifedipine and quinidine. Pharmazie 50: 613-616

Hippius M, Uhlemann C, Smolenski U, Reissig S, Hoffmann A (1998) In vitro investigations of drug release and penetration-enhancing effect of ultrasound on transmembrane transport of flufenamic acid. Int J Clin Pharmacol Ther 36: 107-111

Hoffmann A, Kraul H, Burkhardt I (1997) Nilvadipine in hypertension – experience in ambulatory treatment. Int J Clin Pharmacol Ther 35: 195-203

Merkel U, Hoffmann A (1996) Inhibition of 7-ethoxyresorufindeethylase in mouse and human liver microsomes by flavonoids. Exp Toxicol Pathol 48: 274-279

Reimann IR, Karpinsky C, Hoffmann A (1993) Epidemiological data on drug use during pregnancy in Thuringia, East Germany. Int J Clin Pharmacol Ther 34: 80-83

Reimann IR, Meier-Hellmann A, Reinhart K, Hoffmann A (1997) Comments to consensus document. Once-daily dosing of aminoglycosides from N. Anaizi. A supplement to dosage and monitoring in critically ill patients. Int J Clin Pharmacol Ther 35: 397

Sigusch HH, Vogt S, Gruber U, Rienhardt D, Lang K, Surber R, Farker K, Müller S, Hoffmann A (1997) Angiotensin-I-converting enzyme DD genotype is a risk factor of coronary artery disease. Scand J Clin Lab Invest 57: 127-132

Weber A, Jäger R, Börner A, Klinger G, Vollanth R, Matthey K, Balogh A (1996) Can grapefruit juice influence ethinylestradiol bioavailability? Contraception 53: 41-47

Köln

University of Cologne/Universität Köln

The Department of Clinical Pharmacology of the Institute of Pharmacology of the University of Cologne has the following major current areas of research: drug metabolism, drug interactions, grapefruit juice effects, drug absorption and its variation along the human gastrointestinal tract, biosensors for cytochrome P450 enzymes, pharmacokinetics and pharmacodynamics of antineoplastic agents. Additionally, pharmacokinetic studies are conducted in collaboration with pharmaceutical companies. The training programme for clinical pharmacologists includes participation in twice weekly ward rounds at the intensive care unit of the internal medicine with a weekly seminar where cases of general pharmaco-therapeutic issues are discussed with clinical colleagues, and a weekly seminar within the clinical pharmacology unit. Facilities include a small ward for clinical studies (six beds available), HPLC, electrochemistry and genotyping equipment. The scientific collaborations with other departments of the University at Köln include: Clinic of Internal Medicine I (Head: V. Diehl); Clinic for Surgery (Head: A. H. Hoelscher).

Our current staff includes Professor Uwe Fuhr (physician), Dr Michael Zaigler (physician)

Dr Stephan Rietbrock (physician and mathematician), Dieter Barthold (technician) Iliana Tantcheva (physician, postgraduate student), Svane Beckmann (chemist, postgraduate student), Shiba Joseph (chemist, undergraduate student), Annelie Ben Othman (under-graduate student), Heiko Menzel (junior house officer).

The application procedure is not formalized; a CV and the area of interest are sufficient for the first contact.

Inquiries should be directed to Professor Uwe Fuhr.

References

Bode H, Brendel E, Ahr G, Fuhr U, Harder S, Staib AH (1996) Investigation of nifedipine absorption in different regions of the human gastrointestinal (GI) tract after simultaneous administration of 13Cand 12C-nifedipine. Eur J Clin Pharmacol 50: 195-201

Fuhr U, Kummert A (1995) The fate of naringin in man: a key to grapefruit juice – drug interactions? Clin Pharmacol Ther 58: 365-373

Fuhr U, Rost KL (1994) Simple and reliable CYP1A2 phenotyping by the paraxanthine/ caffeine ratio in plasma and in saliva. Pharmacogenetics 4: 109-116

Fuhr U, Klittich K, Staib AH (1993a) Inhibitory effect of grapefruit juice and the active agent naringenin on CYP1A2 dependent metabolism of caffeine in man. Br J Clin Pharmacol 35: 431-436

Fuhr U, Doehmer J, Battula N, Wolfel C, Flick I, Kudla C, Keita Y, Staib AH (1993b) Biotransformation of methylxanthines in mammalian cell lines genetically engineered for expression of single cytochrome P450 isoforms. Allocation of metabolic pathways to isoforms and inhibitory effects of quinolones. Toxicology 82: 169-189

Fuhr U, Staib AH, Harder S, Becker K, Liermann D, Schollnhammer G, Roed IS (1994) Absorption of ipsapirone along the human gastrointestinal tract. Br J Clin Pharmacol 38: 83-86

Fuhr U, Rost KL, Engelhardt R, Sachs M, Liermann D, Belloc C, Beaune P, Janezic S, Grant D, Meyer UA, Staib AH (1996a) Evaluation of caffeine as a test drug for CYP1A2, NAT2 and CYP2E1 phenotyping in man by in vivo versus in vitro correlations. Pharmacogenetics 6: 159-176

Fuhr U, Weiss M, Kroemer HK, Neugebauer G, Rameis H, Weber W, Woodcoc BG (1996b) Systematic screening for pharmacokinetic interactions during drug development. Int J Clin Pharmacol Ther 34: 139-151

Rietbrock S, Merz P-G, Fuhr U, Harder S, Marschner J-P, Loew D (1995) Absorption behaviour of sulpiride described using Weibull functions. Int J Clin Pharmacol Ther 33: 299-303

Staib AH, Fuhr U (1995) Drug absorption differences along the gastrointestinal tract in man: Detection and relevance for the development of new drug formulations. In: Kuhlmann J Weihrauch TR (eds.): Food-Drug interactions. Clinical Pharmacology, Vol 12. W. Zuckschwerdt Verlag, München, 34-56

DLR Institute of Aerospace Medicine

The Institute of Aerospace Medicine at DLR in Cologne, Germany, is especially equipped for conducting clinical studies. Due to tasks in Aviation Medicine, we have a specially equipped metabolic ward facility with a sleep laboratory that can house up to eight subjects. In this facility, which is a fully equipped Clinical Research Centre, we can, in addition to regular clinical studies, also focus on circadian rhythms and on sleep quality.

Studies on Astronauts require a large scenario for systems diagnostics possibilities including non-invasive cardiovascular diagnostics, lung function, metabolism and hormonal regulation mechanisms, bone formation, muscle and reflex functions, psychophysiological performance, etc. For all these tasks, we have specific experience and equipment including a cardiovascular research laboratory with seven beds and a research MRI with 4.7 Tesla.

Due to the necessity to do telemedical diagnosis in astronauts, we have also a major programme for telemedicine of the mobile patient and can perform home monitoring programmes for the ambulatory patient.

The Institute Head is approved for 3 years of training in Clinical Pharmacology.

References

Drummer C, Fiedler F, Bub A, Kleefeld D, Dimitriadis E, Gerzer R, Forssmann W-G (1993) Development and application of a urodilatin (CDD/ANP 95-126)-specific radioimmunoassay. Eur J Physiol 423: 372-377

Drummer C, Frank W, Heer M, Forssmann WG, Gerzer R, Goetz KL (1996) Postprandial natriuresis in humans: further evidence that urodilatin, not ANP, modulates sodium excretion. Am J Physiol 270: F301-F310

Heer M, Drummer C, Maass H, Röcker L, Baisch F, Gerzer R (1993) Long-term elevations of dietary sodium produce parallel increases in the renal excretion of urodilatin and sodium. Eur J Physiol 425: 390-394

Kentsch M, Drummer C, Gerzer R, Müller-Esch G (1995a) Severe hypotension and bradycardia after intravenous urodilatin infusion in patients with congestive heart failure. Eur J Clin Invest 25: 281-283

Kentsch M, Otter W, Drummer C, Peinke V, Theisen K, Müller-Esch G, Gerzer R (1995b) The dihydropyridine calcium channel blocker BAY t 7207 attenuates the exercise induced increase of plasma ANF and cyclic GMP in mild congestive heart failure. Eur J Clin Pharmacol 49: 177-182

Norsk P, Drummer C, Röcker L, Strollo F, Christensen NJ, Warberg J, Bie P, Stadeager C, Johansen LB, Heer M, Gunga H-C, Gerzer R (1995) Renal and endocrine responses in humans to an isotonic saline infusion during microgravity. J Appl Physiol 78: 2253-2259

Wolfram G, Meier U, Scheske U, Horn M, Drummer C, Spannagl M, Gerzer R (1996) Effect of organic nitrates on ex vivo platelet aggregation and fibrinolysis in man. Eur J Med Res 1: 1-8

Zange J, Müller K, Gerzer R, Wehling M (1996) Non-genomic effects of aldosterone on phosphocreatine levels in human calf muscle during recovery from exercise. J Clin Endocrinol Metab 81: 4296-4300

Kentsch M, Drummer C, Nötges A, Gerzer R, Müller-Esch G (1996) Neutral endopeptidase 24.11 may not exhibit beneficial haemodynamic effects in patients with congestive heart failure. Eur J Clin Pharmacol 51: 269-272

Knau B, Sturm C, Heim J-M, Fricke H, Emmerich B, Haas RJ, Gerzer R (1997) Particulate ANP-sensitive guanylyl cyclase in blood and bone marrow cells of patients with acute leukaemia. Eur J Med Res 2: 101-105

Troponwerke GmbH & Co. KG

The Department of Clinical Pharmacology at the Troponwerke in Köln is part of the Institute of Clinical Pharmacology of the Bayer AG in Wuppertal (see corresponding Bayer documentation) and also contains study areas, laboratories, measuring rooms, rooms for doctors and scientific teams and physical examination rooms.

The study areas have 12 beds for day as well as overnight studies, an intensive care room, three functional rooms for pharmacodynamic studies, day rooms for volunteers, and overnight accommodation for doctors and nursing staff.

The research conducted at the departments of pharmacodynamics in Wuppertal and Köln centres are around two main fields: development of new clinical pharmacological methods and establishment of existing methods for evaluating pharmacodynamic drug effects. These non-invasive techniques are applied in cardiovascular, respiratory tract, gastrointestinal tract and central nervous system drug research. The subdepartment of Biochemical Pharmacodynamics (Wuppertal only) has two main aims. The first is to develop standardized methods for charting the course of active substances as they undergo clinical testing. The second is to determine the biochemical effect of exogenous and endogenous factors on the organism. The Department of Clinical Pharmacokinetics (Wuppertal only) develops sensitive analytical methods for the determination of drug concentrations in the human body with much improved accuracy. Further progress in developing mathematical models for the use in pharmacokinetics and an integrated approach for pharmacokinetics and pharmacodynamics are interesting new research areas in this department. The Department of Biometry & Pharmacometry (Wuppertal only) is responsible for statistical evaluation for all preclinical studies and phase I studies.

The Department of Clinical Pharmacology at the facility in Köln has a staff of five MDs and 14 administrative and technical employees. The department is also responsible for organization and monitoring of externally (CRO, hospital) conducted clinical pharmacological studies. We can offer special training to achieve the degree of a 'Medical Doctor in Clinical Pharmacology' and 'Specialist in Human Pharmacology of DGPT (German Society of Experimental and Clinical Pharmacology and Toxicology, Wuppertal only)', respectively. The Institute of Clinical Pharmacology can provide MD and PhD degrees. Inquiries should be directed to Professor Dr Jochen Kuhlmann.

References

Beckermann B, Beneke M, Boettcher M, Dietrich H, Horstmann R, Seitz I (1993) Influence of formulation, food or antacids on the pharmacokinetics of BAY x 1005 in human volunteers. Naunyn-Schmiedeberg's Arch Pharmacol, Suppl to Vol 347, R 27

Boettcher M, Beneke M, Dietrich H, Horstmann R, Luedtke W, Seitz, I (1992a) Application to multifunctional image analysis system to static posturography in clinical pharmacology. Naunyn-Schmiedeberg's Arch Pharmacol, Suppl. to Vol 345, R 4

Boettcher M, Luedtke W, Beneke M (1992b) Optimisation of a dynamic pupillometric measuring method. Publications Health Care Research, Bayer, Ed.: Rosen-Edwards PA, Sci Inform Doc 61

Boettcher M, Hoeflich G, Luedtke W (1995) Concentration effect correlations between pupil reaction and serum levels of psychotropics. Pharmacopsychiatry 28: 167

De Vry J, Dietrich H, Glase TH, Heine H-G, Horvath E, Jork R, Maertins TH, Mauler F, Opitz W, Schohe-Loop R, Schwarz TH (1997) BAY x 3702: a highly potent and selective 5-HTIA receptor agonist with neuroprotective properties. Drug of the Future 22 (4) 341-349

Dietrich H, Horstmann R, Sietz I (1992) Arrhythmias in young healthy volunteers detected by cardiac monitoring in clinical pharmacological studies. Naunyn-Schmiedeberg's Arch Pharmacol, Suppl. to Vol 346, P 95

Dietrich H, Ritter W, Wingender W, Unger S, Ochmann K (1997) Cerivastatin – a new HMG-CoA reductase inhibitor – in combination with the antacid Mallox7: an investigation of safety and pharmacokinetics. 68th Meeting of the European Atherosclerosis Society (EAS), B Brugge, Mai 7-10, 1997. Int J of Research and Investigation on Atherosclerosis and Related Diseases, Vol 130

Horstmann R, Beckermann B, Seitz I, Dietrich H, Boettcher M, Lemm G, Beneke M (1993) Tolerability and pharmacokinetics of the new leucotriene synthesis inhibitor BAY x 1005. Naunyn-Schmiedeberg's Arch Pharmacol, suppl to vol 347, R 35

Schmidt N, Horstmann R, Kuhlmann J (1995) Influence of H2-Blocking Agents on

Safety, Tolerability and pharmacokinetics of BAY x 1005, a novel FLAP-inhibitor. Therapie (Suppl): 497, 1st Eur Associate Clin Pharmacol Ther, Paris, 27-30.9.1995

Schoellnhammer G, Beneke M, Boettcher M, Dietrich H, Horstmann R, Seitz I (1993) Absolute oral bioavailability of two preparations of ipsapirone hydrochloride. Pharmacopsychiatry 26: 199

Konstanz

Research and training

Responsibilities of the Medical Research Department include the planning, performing and reporting of clinical studies Phase I, II and III as required by the regulatory and registration authorities. The research fields include pneumology, gastroenterology, neurology, cardiology and oncology. The Medical Research Department, in conjunction with the Department of Pharmacology, is authorised to provide a full 5 year training in Clinical Pharmacology.

Research facilities

The Department of Medical Research is subdivided into four groups. One of these is Clinical Pharmacology which is concerned with phase I clinical studies. The other three groups deal with studies in different clinical indications and co-ordinate phase II and III clinical studies. These four clinically oriented groups co-operate closely with the departments of Biometry and Drug Metabolism and Pharmacokinetics. Such an organizational structure allows for fully integrated and independent evaluation of the performed clinical studies.

While most of the Phase I studies organised by the Clinical Pharmacology group are performed by Contract Research Organisations (CROs), about 20% are done in-house. The unit is equipped with four beds and consists of four medical doctors, two technical assistants, one clinical monitor and one secretary.

The three clinical research groups co-ordinate phase II and III clinical studies according to the Ich guidelines, with the aim to prepare an internationally acceptable dossier for regulatory authorities. Most of the drug developments deal with new chemical entities (NCE). The clinical research groups has a total of 18 academic employees (six MDs and 12 PhDs), seven clinical monitors and 11 assistants and secretaries.

References

Cazzola M, Spinazzi A, Santangelo G, Steinijans VW, Wurst W, Solleder P, Girbino G (1990) Acute effects of urapidil on airway response in hypertensive patients with chronic obstructive pulmonary disease. Multiple action antihypertensive therapy with special reference to alpha and 5-HT-receptors. Drugs 40 (suppl 4): 71-72

Gugler R, Hartmann M, Rudi J, Brod I, Huber R, Steinijans VW, Bliesath H, Wurst W, Klotz U (1996) Lack of pharmacokinetic interaction of pantoprazole with diazepam in man. Br J Clin Pharmacol 42: 249-252

Karck U, Dürr D, Du Bois A, Rathgeb F, Wurst W, Meerpohl H (1995) Phase I study of the multidrug resistance modifying compound dexniguldipine-HCL in combination with cyclophosphamide (FEC) in breast cancer. Breast Dis 8: 63-68

Liebau H, Solleder P, Müller H, Wurst W (1989) Long-term antihypertensive treatment with urapidil. Curr Opinion Cardiol 4 (suppl 4): 57-62

Schultz HU, Hartmann M, Steinijans VW, Huber R, Lühmann R, Bliesath H, Wurst W (1991/1996) Lack of influence of pantoprazole in the disposition kinetics of theophylline in man. Int J Clin Pharmacol and Ther. Vol 29, No. 9: 369-375/Vol 34 (suppl No.1): 51-57

Simon B, Müller P, Hartmann M, Bliesath H, Lühmann R, Huber R, Bohnenkamp W, Wurst W (1990) Pentagastrin-stimulated gastric acid secretion and pharmacokinetics following single and repeated intravenous administration of the gastric H^+, K^+-ATPase inhibitor pantoprazole (BY1023/SK&F96022) in healthy subjects. Gastroenterologie 9: 443-447

Solleder P, Haerlin R, Wurst W, Klingmann I, Mosberg H (1989) Effect of urapidil on steady-state serum digoxin concentration in healthy subjects. Eur J Clin Pharmacol 37: 193-194

Tebbe U, Wurst W, Neuhaus KL (1988) Acute haemodynamic effects of urapidil in patients with chronic left ventricular failure. Eur J Clin Pharmacol 35: 305-308

Ukena D, Boewer C, Oldenkott B, Rathgeb F, Wurst W, Sybrecht GW (1995) Tolerance, safety and kinetics of the new antineoplastic compound dexniguldipine-HCL after oral administration: A phase I dose escalation trial. Cancer Chemoth Pharmacol 36: 160-164

Leipzig

Research and training programme
- Pharmacokinetic investigation within phase I-IV studies.
- Basic research work in antineoplastic drug metabolism by the P450-isoenzyme family and MDR phenotype.
- Drug monitoring and toxicological screening as a service offer to clinical departments of the university, local hospitals and doctors' practices.
- Toxicological and pharmacotherapeutic consultation service.
- Teaching Clinical Pharmacology to students during the 7th, 8th and 9th term.

Research facilities: the Institute of Clinical Pharmacology is an independent department of the university. The department has four laboratories for analytical measurements (HPLC, GC, LC-MS, FPIA, RT-PCR) and one for cell culture. The head of the department is Professor of Clinical Pharmacology at the University of Leipzig. The department has six academic employees (three MDs, one colleague in specialization, two PhDs), four technical assistants, one secretary, two or three MD students.

References
Antonin KH, Bieck PR, Preiss R, Schenker U, Hastewell J, Fox R, MacKay M (1996) The absorption of human calcitonin from the transverse colon of man. Int J Pharmaceutics 130: 33-39

Dassow H, Ladusch M, Leiblein S, Köhler T, Helbig W, Preiss R (1996) Multidrug resistance: mdr1-mRNA- and P170-expression in adult leukemic patients and implications for therapy. J Kuhlmann, U Klotz (eds): Klin Pharmakol 14: Zuckschwerdt Verlag, 64-67

Dassow H, Lassner D, Remke H, Preiss R (1998) Modulation of p-glycoprotein-mediated multidrug resistance in a doxorubicin-resistant subline of the human lymphoblastoid cell line CCRF-CEM by phosphorothioate antisense oligonucleotides. Int J Clin Pharmacol Ther 36: 93-96

Preiss R (1998) P-glycoprotein and related transporters. Int J Clin Pharmacol Ther 36: 3-8

Preiss R, Teichert J, Preiss C, Kern J, Tritschler HJ, Ulrich H (1996) Untersuchungen zur Pharmakokinetik von alpha-Liponsäure (Thioctsäure) and Patienten mit diabetischer Polyneuropathie. Diabetes und Stoffwechsel 5: 17-22

Regenthal R, Künstler U, Junhold U, Preiss R (1997) Haloperidol serum concentrations and D2 dopamine receptor occupancy during low-dose treatment with haloperidol decanoate. Int Clin Psychopharmacol 12: 255-261

Schmidt R, Sorger D, Walter F, Schönfelder M, Preiss R (1996a) Cathepsin D in association with established prognostic factors in early recurrence of breast cancer. Onkologie 19: 176-180

Schmidt R, Sorger D, Walter F, Schönfelder M, Preiss R (1996b) PS2 protein, EGFR and cathepsin D in association with established prognostic factors in early recurrence of breast cancer. J Kuhlmann, U Klotz (eds.): Klin Pharmakol 14: Zuckschwerdt Verlag, 77-81

Teichert J, Preiss R (1997) High-performance liquid chromatography methods for determination of lipoic and dihydrolipoic acid in human plasma. Methods in Enzymology 279: Academic Press, 159-166

Magdeburg
Research areas: characterization of 'symptomatic' subjects by their dominating personality traits and under motivational, emotional and

immunological aspects (differential clinical psychoimmunopharmacology); influence of drugs. Early differentiation responders/non-responders in the treatment with neuroleptics and antidepressants. Cerebral information processing and immunology in healthy subjects and patients under the influence of anti-epileptics and their metabolites. Bioavailability studies.

Training programme: complete series of lectures and courses in clinical pharmacology (special pharmacology) in the fourth and fifth years of studies. Lectures in general studies. Industry-independent further training of physicians within the scope of the regional doctors' corporation. Intensive seminars to advance clinical research (jointly with Institute of Biometrics and Medical Informatics).

Medical care: consulting services for physicians of the clinical centre and the region.

Therapeutic Drug Monitoring (TDM) for drugs and metabolites. Evaluation of adverse drug reactions. Pharmacokinetic advisory service on the basis of individual "blood levels" determined from the TDM through population-kinetic data. Clinical toxicology (diagnostic analyses, detoxication control, drug abuse).

Clinical and research facilities: day-care unit (five places) for clinical studies in volunteers

Most advanced chemical analytical methods (HPLC, GC, GC-MS and the like).

The university: find more information on the homepage: http//www.uni-magdeburg.de/ index_eng.html (english)

Staff: six scientists (two physicians), nine technical staff members (two research nurses).

Application procedures: informal. The medical registration for physicians according to German or EC member law is required.

Inquiries: Professor FP Meyer

References

Darius J (1996) On-column gas chromatographic-mass spectrometric assay for metabolic profiling of valproate in brain tissue and serum. J Chromatogr B 682: 67-72

Darius J, Meyer FP (1996) Concentrations of valproate metabolites under therapeutic conditions. Exp Toxicol Pathol 48: 87-92

Martens J, Banditt P (1997) Simultaneous determination of midazolam and its metabolites 1-hydroxymidazolam and 4-hydroxy-midazolam in human serum using gas chromatography-mass spectrometry. J Chromatogr B 692: 95-100

Meyer FP (1996) Pharmacokinetic responses to caffeine in volunteers with higher scores for neuroticism. Psychopharmacology 126: 275 – 276
Meyer FP, Tröger U, Röhl F-W (1996a) Adverse nondrug reactions – an update. Clin Pharmacol Ther 60: 347 – 352
Meyer FP, Tröger U, Röhl F-W (1996b) Adverse nondrug reactions in healthy volunteers – personality, motivation, emotion. Naunyn-Schmiedeberg's Arch Pharmacol 353: R 144
Tröger U, Fritzsch C, Darius J, Gedschold J, Meyer FP (1996) Sulthiame-associated mild compensated metabolic acidosis. Int J Clin Pharmacol Ther 34: 542-545
Ulrich S, Isensee T, Pester U (1996a) Simultaneous determination of amitriptyline, nortriptyline and four hydroxylated metabolites in serum by capillary gas-liquid chromatography with nitrogen-phosphorus selective detection. J Chromatogr B 685: 81-89
Ulrich S, Neuhof S, Braun V, Martens J, Meyer FP (1996b) Oxazepam and carbamazepine as co-medication to haloperidol in acute schizophrenic patients: investigation of drug-drug inter-actions, metabolism and extrapyramidal adverse effects. Exp Toxicol Pathol 48: 404-409
Ulrich S, Meyer FP, Bogerts B (1996c) A capillary gas-liquid chromatographic method for the assay of the neuroleptic drug zotepine in human serum or plasma. J Pharm Biomed Anal 14: 441-444

Mainz

ZeKaPha GmbH – Centre of Cardiovascular Pharmacology

The Centre of Cardiovascular Pharmacology in Mainz and Wiesbaden was founded in 1977. Since then, this institution achieved and maintained a leading position in the field of cardiovascular clinical pharmacology. Close cooperations between ZeKaPha and the University academic institutions in Mainz and Frankfurt/Main have continuously contributed to the successful word of ZeKaPha. The objectives of ZeKaPha are to explore modes of actions/interactions not only of cardiovascular drugs in man in order to make their use even more easy and successful under our motto: explorando, sciendo, curatum (explore, research, cure)

Main topics of research are
Clinical pharmacology and especially pharmacodynamics and cardiovascular drugs. A broad spectrum of methods has been established to test the haemodynamic effects of drugs on the heart, and arterial/venous site of the circulation as well. One main focus of our research is the extension of principles from basic pharmacology to clinical pharmacology. Examples are dose-effect analyses and Schild's regression analysis,

i.e. the evaluation of dose-effect curves of agonists in the presence of different doses of antagonists. This principle was successfully applied in human studies on b-blockers, ACE inhibitors, angiotensin-II antagonists and others. In addition, during the last few years, there has been an engagement also in the field of rational phytotherapy.

Structure: ZeKaPha has all facilities and equipment to do clinical research including a ward with eight beds. The staff of about 15-20 members includes four board certified clinical pharmacologists (MDs) and physicians in training of board certification. Some of the methods established, in part developed by ZeKaPha are:

- Non-invasive determination of drug actions on the cardiovascular system by: systolic time intervals; echocardiography (2D, M-mode, CW- and PW-Doppler); dual-beam echoaortography; electrical impedance cardiography; applanation tonometry (sphygmocardiography according to O'Rourke); aortic pulse wave velocity; dorsal hand vein method (according to Aellig); venous occlusion plethysmography; aortic blood flow by rheography; Doppler ultrasound of supraaortic and intracranial arteries; Doppler ultrasound of distal arteries.
- Various methods to analyse dose-effect relations of agonists (i.e. adrenaline, isoprenaline, angiotensin-I and -II) and antagonists.
- Study ward for clinical research in healthy volunteers and patients (phases I-III).
- Study clinics for chronic ambulatory studies of interventions (experience up to 3 years of treatment).

Training and teaching: the ZeKaPha offers facilities for obtaining MD degrees via its co-operation with Universities. For board certification, a 3-year period is accepted by the chamber of Physicians of Rheinland-Pfalz, Mainz. The Centre organizes international conferences and presents abstracts and presentations in national/international conferences. The Centre has published more than 200 original papers and abstracts in peer reviewed journals and the scientists of ZeKaPha attend actively leading international conferences in the field.

References

Belz GG et al. (1997) Inhibition of angiotensin-II pressor response and ex vivo ang II radioligand binding by candesartan cilexetil and losartan in healthy human volunteers. J Hum Hypertens 11 (suppl 2): 45-47

Breithaupt-Grögler K et al. (1997) Protective effect of chronic garlic intake on elastic properties of aorta in the elderly. Circulation 96: 2649-2655

Goldberg MR et al. (1996) Differential effects of losartan and enalapril on local venous and systemic pressor responses to angiotensin I and II in healthy men. Clin Pharmacol Ther 59: 72-82

Nixdorff U et al. (1997) b-Adrenergic stimulation enhances left ventricular diastolic performance in normal subjects. J Cardiovasc Pharmacol 29: 476-484

Mannheim

Fakultät für Klinische Medizin Mannheim – Ruprecht-Karls-Universität Heidelberg

The Institute for Clinical Pharmacology at Mannheim was founded in 1995 and has developed to a competent clinical and basic research unit located in house within a university clinic.

The opportunities regarding training and research include a phase 1 unit with 12 beds equipped with an non-invasive ICU Monitoring system, clinical studies of phase 2-4 that are conducted in co-operation with the clinical departments of the university clinic and partners of the pharmaceutical industry. The institute also includes laboratories in which basic research is performed using methods of molecular biology (cloning, sequencing, expression, ATwo-HybridA), biochemistry (FPLC, radiobinding assays, SDS-PAGE/Western-Blot) and cell-physiology (cell culture, intracellular Ca^{2+}/pH-measurement, cAMP, cGMP assays). The main topics of research are rapid steroid effects and cardiovascular pharmacology.

The academic staff consists of five physicians, two biologists, one biometrician and one biotechnologist.

At the moment, four physicians are in training to become specialists in clinical pharmacology. The combination of front-line basic research and clinical research conducted in co-operation with and using all the facilities of a large university hospital offers broad and intensive training opportunities. Possible applicants can provide further information from the Head of the Institute, Professor Wehling.

References

Christ M, Eisen C, Aktas J, Theisen K, Wehling M (1993) The inositol-1,4,5-trisphosphate system is involved in rapid effects of aldosterone in human mononuclear leucocytes. J Clin Endocrinol Metab 77: 1452-1457

Christ M, Sippel K, Eisen C, Wehling M (1994) Non-classical receptors for aldosterone in plasma membranes from pig kidneys. Mol Cell Endocrinol 99: 31-34

Christ M, Meyer C, Sippel K, Wehling M (1995a) Rapid aldosterone signaling in vascular smooth muscle cells: involvement of the phospholipase C, diacylglycerol and protein kinase Ca. Biochem Biophys Res Commun 213: 123-129

Christ M, Douwes K, Eisen C, Bechtner G, Theisen K, Wehling M (1995b) Rapid effects of aldosterone on sodium transport in vascular smooth muscle cells. Hypertension 25: 117-123

Christ M, Rauen P, Klauss V, Krüger T, Frey A, Theisen K, Wehling M (1996) Spontaneous changes of heart rate, blood pressure, and ischemia-type ST-segment depressions in patients with hypertension without significant coronary artery disease: beneficial effects of b-blockade. J Cardiovasc Pharmacol 28: 755-763

Falkenstein E, Meyer C, Eisen C, Scriba P, Wehling M (1996) Full-length cDNA sequence of a progesterone membrane binding protein from porcine vascular smooth muscle cells. Biochem Biophys Res Commun 229: 86-89

Meyer C, Christ M, Wehling M (1995) Characterization and solubilization of novel aldosterone-binding proteins in porcine liver microsomes. Eur J Biochem 229: 736-740

Meyer C, Schmid R, Scriba PC, Wehling M (1996) Purification and partial sequencing of high-affinity progesterone-binding site(s) from porcine liver membranes. Eur J Biochem 239: 726-731

Wehling M (1997) Specific, nongenomic actions of steroid hormones. Annu Rev Physiol 59: 365-393

Zange J, Müller K, Gerzer R, Sippel K, Wehling M (1996) Nongenomic effects of aldosterone on phosphocreatine levels in human calf muscle during recovery from exercise. J Clin Endocrinol Metab 81: 4296-4300

Boehringer Mannheim GmbH

The Department of Clinical Pharmacology at Boehringer Mannheim is headed by Dr Günter Neugebauer. The Research and Training Programme includes drug development in the cardiovascular area, haematology, bone metabolism, diabetes, biotechnological compounds and 4 years approved training programme in clinical pharmacology. The facilities are 10 single bed room units, two study labs, phlebotomy room, clinical chemistry laboratory informatics/ biometrics group. The university staff consists of 15 people, including two part-time and six academic.

Applications should be addressed to Human Resources Department of Boehringer Mannheim GmbH.

References

DeMey C, Breithaupt K, Schloos J, Neugebauer G, Palm D, Belz GG (1994) Dose-effect and pharmacokinetic-pharmacodynamic relationships of the ß1-adrenoceptor blocking properties of various doses of carvedilol in healthy man. Clin Pharmacol Ther 55: 329-337

Fuhr U, Weiss M, Kroemer HK, Neugebauer G, Rameis H, Weber W, Woodcock BG (1996) Systematic screening for pharmacokinetic interactions during drug development. Int J Clin Pharmacol Ther 34: 139-51

Groop L, Neugebauer G (1996) Clinical pharmacology of sulphonylureas. Handbook of Exp Pharmacology – Vol. 119 Oral antidiabetics. Eds: Kuhlmann J, Puls W, Springer Verlag, 199-259

Martin U, von Möllendorff E, Akpan W, Kientsch-Engel R, Kaufmann B. Neugebauer G (1991a) Pharmacokinetics and haemostatic properties of the recombinant plasminogen activator BM 06.022 in healthy volunteers. Thromb Haemostasis 66: 569-574

Martin U, von Möllendorff E, Akpan W, Kientsch-Engel R, Kaufmann B. Neugebauer G (1991b) Dose-ranging study of the novel recombinant plasminogen activator BM 06.022 in healthy volunteers. Clin Pharmacol Ther 50: 429-436

Neugebauer G (1993) Pharmakokinetik und klinische Pharmakologie der Bisphosphonate, in Friedberg, Rüfer: Therapie von Knochenerkrankungen mit Bisphosphonaten. Fischer Verlag, 33-50

Neugebauer G, Neubert P (1991) Metabolism of carvedilol in man. Eur J Drug Metab Pharmacokin 16: 257-260

Neugebauer G, Gabor M, Reiff K (1992) Disposition of carvedilol enantiomers in patients with liver cirrhosis: evidence for disappearance of stereo-selective first-pass extraction. J Cardiovasc Pharmacol 19: S142-S146

O'Rourke NP, McClosky EV, Neugebauer G, Kanis JA (1994) Renal and non-renal clearance of clodronate in patients with malignancy and renal impairment. Drug Invest 7: 26 -33

München

Max-Planck-Institut für Psychiatrie – Klinische Neuropharmakologie

The group continuously focuses on interneuronal communication in the central nervous system. In this endeavour, studies are designed that combine molecular and cellular analyses with behavioural and pharmacological approaches and clinical studies. These interdisciplinary skills within the group will help to develop treatment and prevention strategies for patients with psychiatric and neurological disorders. Amino acid transmitter receptors are integral components of almost all circuitries studied so far in the central nervous system. At present, the attempt to integrate electrophysiological, anatomical and pathophysiological findings still awaits a higher level of molecular precision with regard to the localization of the various subunits of neurotransmitter receptors. We try to correlate the results of investigations by novel microscopic techniques developed in our group, advanced double-label in situ hybridization histochemistry, immunocytochemistry methods, metabolic mapping with the 2-DG (deoxyglucose)-method, single cell polymerase chain reaction combined with electrophysiology on individual neurones, differential display techniques and grain region-specific gene knockouts of L-glutamate (NMDA) receptor subtypes. The introduction of concepts of neuronal plasticity mediated via the activation of glutamatergic transmission in pain and addiction research has already led to important therapeutic consequences. Novel compounds and new regimens for drug treatment to prevent activity-dependent long-term changes are emerging. Our recent data suggest that the first anti-craving drug, acapprosate, which was recently approved in Europe for the treatment of alcoholism, preferentially interacts with NMDA receptor assemblies containing distinct splice variants, and quite specifically influences the transcription of receptor subunits substantially advance our understanding of the significance of glutamate and GABA neurotransmitter receptor diversity and their modulation by neurosteroids, cytokines and psychotropic drugs, and give us a greater insight into neuropathologies arising from disturbed function of these receptors.

Pharmalog Institut für klinsiche Forschung GmbH
The aim of the Pharmalog Institute for Clinical Research is the planning, performance, statistical evaluation and scientific report of phase I-IV studies in Germany, EU, East-Europe. The Pharmalog Institute for Clinical Research is an independent Clinical Research Organisation.

Research and training programme: phase I, II, III and IV trials on the following main indications/drugs: cardiovascular; rheumatology, analgesia; gastroenterology; angiology; dermatology, phlebology, topical agents; pulmonology, asthma; CNS, neurology/psychiatry; metabolism, diabetes mellitus; vaccine, endocrinology, antibiotics; urology/gynaecology/hormones; pharmaco-economics. Authorisation for training in clinical pharmacology: 2 years.

Structure and facilities: the head of the institute is a medical doctor, specialist in clinical pharmacology and specialist in laboratory medicine, the deputy is a medical doctor and specialist in paediatrics and children cardiology.

The following disciplines are covered by a staff of about 40 members (including external monitors): medical doctors, biologists, nutritionist, biochemists, statisticians, economists MD and PhD students, technical assistants.

Services (also for multinational multicentre trials): development of study protocols including statistical planning; Scientific consultant and 'Leiter der klinischen Prüfung' according to German Drug law; organization/logistic of studies; monitoring; study management; assessment of adverse events/safety management; risk/benefit assessment; data management and statistical evaluation; final scientific reports; publications.

Training/lectures on clinical research/clinical pharmacology.

References

Eberhardt R (1994) Cost-benefit-analysis in the healthcare system of the FRG – Cost-Effectiveness of prevention of NSAID-induced ulcers. Eur J Clin Pharmacol 47 (1)

Eberhardt R (1995a) Arzneimittelprüfung in Deutschland: noch sinnvoll und möglich. Marketing Report Gesundheit 1/1995 – Themen letter

Eberhardt R (1995b) Monitoring von klinischen Studien nach GCP – Übersicht unter Einbezug der 5. AMG-Novelle. Die pharmazuetische Industrie 57 (4): 295-298

Eberhardt R, Söhngen M (1996) Ein Handbuch für die Praxis. ECV-Verlag, Reihe Pharmind, Serie Dokumentation

Eberhardt R, Zwingers Th, Hofmann R (1995a) DMSO bei Patienten mit aktivierter Gonarthrose – eine doppelblinde, plaebokontrollierte Phase-III-Studie. Fortschritte der Medizin 113. Jg. 31: 38-42

Eberhardt R, Frank-Szentgyörgyi M, Brand A (1995b) Phytotherapie: wirksamkeit und Verträglichkeit einer Dulcamara-Zeitschrift für Dermatologie 181 (4) 202-207

Eberhardt R, Zwingers T, Gerbershagen H-U, Nagyivanyi P (1995c) Analgesic efficacy and tolerability of lysine-cloniximate versus ibuprofen in patients with gonarthrosis. Current Ther Res 56 (6)

Kori-Lindner C, Eberhardt R (1994) Kosten-Nutzen-Bewertungen von Arzneimitteln und pharmako-ökonomische Studien. Pharm Ind 56 (5)

Kori-Lindner C, Eberhardt R (1995) Pharmako-Ökonomie in Deutschland. Gesetzliche Vorgaben; Umsetzung in die Praxis: Eine grundsätzliche Übersicht. Pharma-Marketing J 2 Apr./Mai: 48-59

Kori-Lindner C, Berlin M, Eberhardt R, Hönig R, Hutt HJ, Rieder HP, Sieger C (1996) Pharmakoökonomie – Information der Fachgesellschaft der Ärzte in der Pharmazeutische Industrie e.V. die pharmazeutische Industrie 58 (12): 1069-1079

Regensburg

The Department of Pharmacology and Clinical Pharmacology of the University of Regensburg is headed by HF Grobecker, MD, Professor of Pharmacology and Clinical Pharmacology.

Staff: one associate professor of toxicology; two assistant professor of anaesthesiology; three technicians, postgraduate students and post-doctoral fellows: fluctuation between four and six persons.

Rooms: Ca. 800 m², including teaching rooms for students: ca. 240 qm2, pharmaceutical medical, dentistry students.

Research facilities: full equipment for research in experimental cardiovascular research, pharmacokinetic and pharmacodynamic studies in volunteers and patients, including five research beds, HPLC, assay laboratory for molecular pharmacology, etc. Close co-operation with intensive care unit of the Department of Anaesthesiology (Head: K. Taeger, MD, Professor of Anaesthesiology, University Hospital Regensburg).

Training programme: full time training for medical doctors to reach after examination the appointment as pharmacologists or clinical pharmacologists of Medical Association of Bavaria, Mühlbaurstrasse 16, D-81677 Munich, Germany.

University: all faculties are present, including a new university hospital with ca. 1500 beds.

Application procedure: please write to the head of the department and include a curriculum vitae with two or three selected references.

Stuttgart

Aim of the Dr Margarete Fischer-Bosch Institute of Clinical Pharmacology: in close collaboration with the departments of the Robert Bosch Hospital (RBK), the IKP works towards a better understanding of drug action in humans. The objective is to improve the safety and efficacy of drug therapy.

Main topics of research: basic and applied clinical research ('from the gene to the patient') is directed to drug metabolism and drug action and delineating the endogenous and exogenous factors underlying the large interindividual variability of drug response. Thereby, the scientific activities have recently been focused on three major areas: a) pain treatment with opioids, b) elderly patients – a risk population for drugs, c) metabolism and action of anticancer drugs.

Structure: the IKP has all laboratory facilities and equipment as well as a clinical research ward to perform a wide spectrum of in vitro and in vivo studies. The following disciplines are covered by a staff of about 60 members (including physicians, pharmacists, biochemists, chemists, biologist; postdocs as well as MD and PhD candidates)

- Analytical chemistry (e.g. HPLC,GLC, GC-MS, MS-MS, LC-MS,

capillary electrophoresis, NMR) for analysis of drugs and metabolites in different biological material.
- Synthetic chemistry to provide internal standards, reference compounds and stable isotopes.
- Biochemical pharmacology for in vitro systems (human tissue bank of liver, kidney and intestinal samples) to study drug metabolism in subcellular fractions.
- Molecular pharmacology and cell biology is used to investigate the regulation of drug-metabolizing enzymes, genetic defects and age-dependent actions of drugs; all modern methods (e.g. RFLP, PCR, Southern/Northern/Western blotting, differential display, gene cloning and sequencing) are available.
- Study unit for clinical research with patients and healthy volunteers.

Services: therapeutic drug monitoring (TDM) with individualized dosage regimens is provided for 16 different drugs (e.g. digitalis, anticonvulsants, aminoglycosides, theophylline, lithium, methotrexate); phenotyping for CYP2D6 and CYP2C19 is also routinely performed. A drug therapy information service (phone 'hot line': +49 0172 732 6500) is available to help physicians in case of drug problems.

Training and teaching: the IKP can provide MD and PhD degrees and is fully licensed to train MDs and PhDs for their corresponding board certifications and 'habilitation'. The IKP is part of the new co-operative centre of Clinical Pharmacology Tübingen/Stuttgart at the Medical School of the University of Tübingen and several members of the IKP teach basic, applied and clinical pharmacology.

References
Ammon E, Schäfer C, Hofmann U, Klotz U (1996) Disposition and first-pass metabolism of ethanol in humans: is it gastric or hepatic and does it depend on gender? Clin Pharmacol Ther 59: 503-513

Engel G, Hofmann U, Heidemann H, Cosme J, Eichelbaum M (1996) Antipyrine as a probe for human oxidative drug metabolism: Identification of the cytochrome P450 enzymes catalyzing 4-hydroxyantipyrine, 3-hydroxymethylantipyrine, and norantipyrine formation. Clin Pharmacol Ther 59: 613-623

Evert B, Eichelbaum M, Haubruck H, Zanger U (1997) Functional properties of CYP2D6 1 (Wild-type) and CYP2D6 7 (His324Pro) expressed by recombination baculovirus in insect cells. Naunyn-Schmiedeberg's Arch Pharmacol 355: 309-318

Fromm MF, Busse D, Kroemer HK, Eichelbaum M (1996) Differential induction of prehepatic and hepatic metabolism of verapamil by rifampin. Hepatology 24: 796-801

Mikus G, Trausch B, Rodewald C, Hofmann U, Richter K, Gramatté T, Eichelbaum M (1997) Effect of codeine on gastrointestinal motility in relation to CYP2D6 phenotype. Clin Pharmacol Ther 61: 459-466

Mürdter T, Sperker B, Kivistö K, McClellan M, Fritz P, Freidel G, Linder A, Bosslet K, Toomes H, Dierkesmann R, Kroemer H (1997) Enhanced uptake of doxorubicin from a glucuronide prodrug (HMR 1826) at the tumour site. Cancer Res 57: 2440-2445

Stüven T, Griese E-U, Kroemer HK, Eichelbaum M, Zanger UM (1996) Rapid detection of CYP2D6 null alleles by long distance and multiplex-polymerase chain reaction. Pharmacogenetics 6: 417-421

Treiber G, Ammon S, Klotz U (1997) Age-dependent eradication of Helicobacter pylori with dual therapy. Aliment Pharmacol Ther 11: in press

Tübingen

Research and training programme: gynaecological endocrinology, gynaecological oncology, hormone replacement therapy (osteoporosis, cardiovascular system, menopausal symptoms), clinical trials phase I-IV (e.g. testing new progestins, new application forms), oral contraception, development of new pharmaceutical concepts in the gynaecological area (e.g. SERMS, Selective Oestrogen Receptor Modulating Substances), drugs in pregnancy and lactation: official advisory function. Assessment of fetal and neonatal risks. Therapeutic drug monitoring in pregnancy and gynaecological oncology.

Clinical facilities: the section is part of the University Hospital, Department OB/GYN (unique in Germany!), menopause ambulance, interdisciplinary clinical facilities, e.g. specialised cardiologists for hormone replacement to treat cardiovascular diseases.

Research facilities: analytical laboratories for measuring biochemical parameters (RIA, EIA, HPLC), research laboratory for investigating cell cultures.

The University of Tübingen is a 500-year-old ancient university with a whole range of faculties.

Staff: head of the section: Professor, MD, medical specialist in obstetrics/gynaecology and in Clinical Pharmacology. Co-workers: one MD/PhD, chemist and medical specialist (endocrinologist) in Clinical Pharmacology, one PhD, chemist, three PhD, biochemists.

Application procedure: No special requirements.

Inquiries: to the head of the section.

References

Lippert TH, Armbruster FP, Seeger H, Mueck AO, Zwirner M, Voelter W (1996a) Urinary excretion of relaxin after estradiol treatment of postmenopausal women. Clin Exp Obstet Gynecol 23: 65-69

Lippert TH, Filshie GM, Mueck AO, Seeger H, Zwirner M (1996b) Serotonin metabolite excretion after postmenopausal estradiol therapy. Maturitas 24: 37-41

Lippert TH, Seeger H, Mueck AO, Hanke H, Haasis R (1996c) Effects of estradiol, progesterone and progestogens on calcium-influx in cell cultures of human vessels. Menopause 3(1): 33-37

Mueck AO, Seeger H, Wiesner J, Korte K, Lippert TH (1994) Urinary prostanoids in postmenopausal women after transdermal and oral oestrogen J Obstet Gynaecol 14: 341-345

Mueck AO, Seeger H, Lippert TH (1996a) Calcium antagonistic effects of natural and synthetic oestrogens – Investigations on a non-genomic mechanism of direct vascular action. Int J Clin Pharm Therap 34: 424-426

Mueck AO, Seeger H, Kaßpohl-Butz S, Teichmann AT, Lippert TH (1996b) Urinary cGMP excretion after hormone replacement therapy in postmenopausal women. Exp Clin Endocrinol Diabetes 104: 392-395

Mueck AO, Seeger H, Armbruster FP, Lippert TH (1997) Urinary excretion of insulin after estradiol treatment of postmenopausal women. Clin Exp Obstet Gynecol 1: 11-13

Seeger H, Mueck AO, Lippert TH (1997) Effect of estradiol metabolites on the susceptibility of low density lipoprotein to oxidation. Life Sciences 61: 865-868

Wuppertal

The Bayer Institute of Clinical Pharmacology

The Bayer Institute of Clinical Pharmacology of the Pharmaceutical Research Centre in Wuppertal contains study areas, laboratories, measuring rooms, rooms for doctors and scientific teams and physical examination rooms.

The study areas have 12 beds for 1-day studies, eight three-bed rooms for long-term studies, an intensive care room, four functional rooms for pharmacodynamic studies, day rooms for volunteers and overnight accommodation for doctors and nursing staff. Facilities were also installed for carrying out investigations with radiolabelled substances in humans. A second clinical pharmacology facility was established in Cologne at Tropon, one of Bayer's affiliated companies, increasing the capacity for long-term studies by another 12 beds. The research conducted at the departments of pharmacodynamics in Wuppertal and Cologne centres around two main fields: development of new clinical-pharmacological methods and establishment of existing methods for evaluating pharmacodynamic drug effects.

These non-invasive techniques are applied in cardiovascular, respiratory tract, gastrointestinal tract and central nervous system drug research.

The subdepartment of Biochemical Pharmacodynamics has two main aims. The first is to develop standardized methods for charting the course of active substances as they undergo clinical testing. The second is to determine the biochemical effect of exogenous and endogenous factors on the organism.

The Department of Clinical Pharmacokinetics develops sensitive analytical methods for the determination of drug concentrations in the human body with much improved accuracy. Further, progress in developing mathematical models for the use in pharmacokinetics and an integrated approach for pharmacokinetics and pharmacodynamics are interesting new research areas in this department.

The Institute of Clinical Pharmacology with the facility in Cologne has a staff of 38 MDs and PhDs and 94 administrative and technical employees. We can offer special training to achieve the degree of a 'Medical Doctor in Clinical Pharmacology' and 'Specialist in Human Pharmacology of DGPT (German Society of Experimental and Clinical Pharmacology and Toxicology)A, respectively.

The Institute can provide MD and PhD degrees. Inquiries should be directed to Professor Dr Jochen Kuhlmann.

References

Kuhlmann J (1995) Aufgaben und Ziele der Klinischen Pharmakologie. Arzneimitteltherapie, 13. Jahrgang, Heft 10: 289-240

Kuhlmann J (1997) Drug research: from the idea to the product. Int J Clin Pharmacol Ther Vol 35: 541-552

Mück W, Ahr G, Kuhlmann J (1995) Nimodipine: potential for drug-drug interactions in the elderly. Drugs Aging, 6: 229-242

Mück W, Tanaka T, Ahr G, Kuhlmann J (1996a) No interethnic differences in stereoselective disposition of oral nimodipine between Caucasian and Japanese subjects Int J Clin Pharmacol Ther 34: 163-171

Mück W, Breuel H-P, Kuhlmann J (1996b) The influence of age on the pharmacokinetics of nimodipine. Int J Clin Pharmacol Ther, 34: 293-298

Mück W, Ritter W, Ochmann K, Ahr G, Wingender W, Kuhlmann J (1997) Absolute and relative bioavailability of the HMG-CoA reductase inhibitor cerivastatin. Int J Clin Pharmacol Ther 35: 255-260

Schäfer HG, Ahr G, Kuhlmann J (1995) Pharmacokinetic development of quinolone antibiotics. Int J Clin Pharmacol Ther 33: 266-276

Schaefer HG, Staß H, Wedgwood J, Hampel B, Fischer C, Kuhlmann J, Schaad UB (1996) Pharmacokinetics of ciprofloxacin in pediatric cystic fibrosis patients. Antimicrob Agents Chemother 4: 29-34

Schaefer HG, Heinig R, Ahr G, Adelmann H, Tetzloff W, Kuhlmann J (1997) Pharmacokinetic-pharmacodynamic modelling as a tool to evaluate the clinical relevance of a drug-food interaction for a nisoldipine controlled-release dosage form. Eur J Clin Pharmacol 51: 473-480

Wensing G, Heinig R, Priesnitz M, Kuhlmann J (1994) Effect of BAY x 7195, an oral leucotriene-D4 receptor antagonist, on leucotriene-D4 induced bronchoconstriction in normal volunteers. Eur J Clin Pharmacol 47: 227-230

Wensing G, Heinig R, Kuhlmann J (1996) Pharmacodynamics and pharmacokinetics of BAY x 7195 aerosol, a new and selective receptor antagonist of cysteinyl-leucotrienes, in normal volunteers. Br J Clin Pharmacol 42: 171-178

Philipp Klee-Institute of Clinical Pharmacology, Klinikum Wuppertal GmbH

The Institute is integrated in the Klinikum Wuppertal GmbH, a teaching hospital with around 1200 beds, the major tasks are a Drug Information Service (DIS) and the collection of adverse drug reactions. Currently an intensified monitoring programme is conducted, collecting all ADRs, which are responsible for hospitalisation of our patients. Furthermore, ADRs occurring during the hospital stay are collected. A regional Drug Information Service for general practitioners is established, as well as a pharmacovigilance project.

Authorization for training in Clinical Pharmacology: currently for 1 year (preliminary).

Research facilities: the Institute has a clinical pharmacology unit with four beds for research, mainly studies on pharmacokinetics. At present, there is no laboratory facility.

The head of the department is the chair of Clinical Pharmacology of the University Witten/Herdecke. The Institute has two further academic employees (two MDs) and one secretary.

References

Gossmann J, Thürmann P, Bachmann R, Weller S, Kachel H-G, Schoeppe W, Scheuermann E-H (1996) Mechanism of angiotensin converting enzyme inhibitor-related anaemia in renal transplant recipients. Kidney Int 50: 973-978

Marschner JP, Thürmann P, Harder S, Rietbrock N (1994) Drug utilization review on a surgical intensive care unit. Int J Clin Pharmacol Ther 9: 447-451

Thürmann P, Harder S (1996) Criteria for the appropriate drug utilisation of immunoglobulin. Pharmaco Economics 9: 417-429

Thürmann P, Harder S, Kirchmaier CM (1995a) Influence of piroxicam coadministration on pharmacodynamic parameters and the plasma concentration/effect relationship of recombinant hirudin (CGP 39393). Eur J Clin Pharmacol 48: 241-246

Thürmann PA, Sonnenburg-Chatzopoulos C, Lissner R (1995b) Pharmacokinetics characteristics and tolerability of a novel intravenous immunoglobulin preparation. Eur J Clin Pharmacol 49: 237-242

Thürmann PA, Stepehns N, Heagerty AM, Kenedi P, Wiedinger G (1996) Influence of isradipine and spirapril on left ventricular hypertrophy and resistance arteries. Hypertension 28: 450-456

Thürmann PA, Harder S, Wolter K, Münck A-C, Fritschka E (1997a) Pharmacokinetics of the PDGF-antagonist trapidil in patients with and without renal impairment. Clin Nephrol 47: 99-105

Thürmann PA, Harder S, Steioff A (1997b) Structure and activities of hospital drug committees in Germany. Eur J Clin Pharmacol 52: 429-435

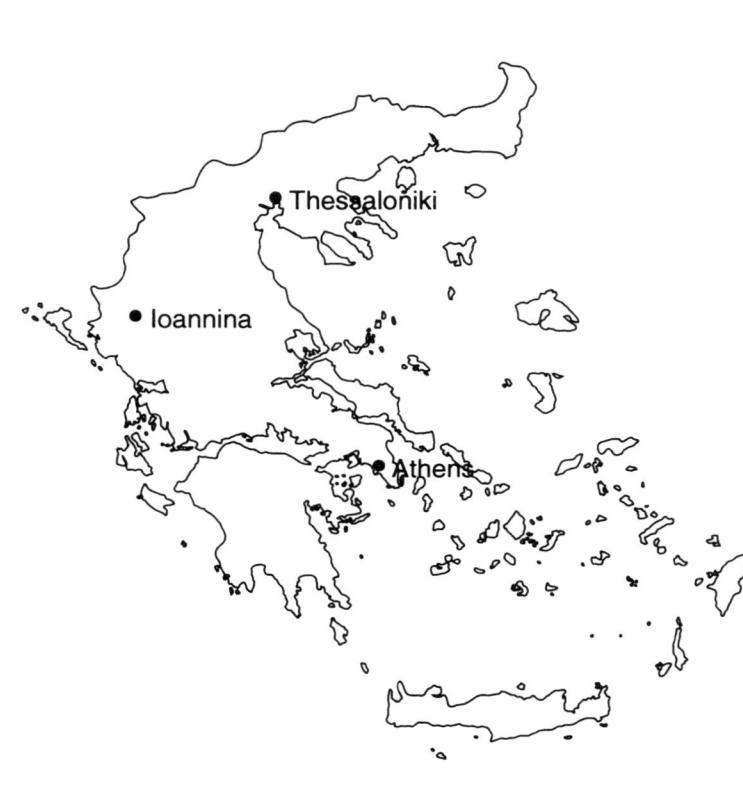

Greece

Teaching, research and service of clinical pharmacology at both undergraduate and postgraduate levels is well established at the National and Capodistrian University of Athens, despite the absence of its official recognition as an independent academic discipline or speciality yet. Basic pharmacology is taught to all medical students in the Greek universities, usually in the third year, by departments of experimental pharmacology where relative research on special subjects is also carried out. The medical school of the National and Capodistrian University of Athens includes a department of clinical therapeutics at Alexandra Hospital, where a section of clinical pharmacology was established in 1982. The section has a laboratory and direct responsibility for the clinical care of a 20 bed ward of the department of internal medicine and consultation responsibility for the university department of clinical therapeutics which are located at the same hospital. The section teaches medical students at both undergraduate and postgraduate levels, provides service and conducts research devoted to the subject.

The *undergraduate teaching – training course* (either in full or in part) organized by the section, is embedded (so far) in the obligatory courses mainly of therapeutics and internal medicine in the fifth and sixth year of medical studies and to a lesser degree in some elective courses of basic pharmacology in the third year of medical studies. This includes theoretical, laboratory and clinical teaching – training in the principles of the subject by using all the established methods – materials and focusing on clinical pharmacokinetics, drugs analysis, direct clinical, patient- and problem-oriented training in small groups and application of the section's 'Hospital Formulary' and 'Monitoring Programme' on partly self-directed basis.

The postgraduate training course, organized by the section, is a 3-year continuous full time course of full specialization in the subject which combines advanced theoretical, laboratory and clinical teaching – training in the principles of the subject in the same institution with involvement in laboratory, clinical care services, teaching and research (usually leading to an MD thesis). In addition to all established methods and materials used for training, emphasis is given on clinical pharmacokinetics, drug analysis, direct clinical, patient evaluation and problem-solving-oriented training in small groups and application of the section's 'Hospital Formulary' and 'Hospital Monitoring Program' on partly self- directed basis. Trainees are medical graduates and either specialized or specializing in internal medicine trainees after the second year of their specialization who combine both trainings in the same hospital. The course is also suitable for continuing education.

The section's *research activities* focus on: its 'Hospital Intensive Monitoring of Adverse Reactions and Drug Utilization Programme' (established in 1991) which is an integrated hospital programme of continuous research in drug usage and drug-induced diseases. The programme is using all the methods of the discipline (patient evaluation, clinical pharmacokinetics, level monitoring – evaluation, individualization, literature evaluation, drug epidemiology, statistics) for the diagnosis, treatment, documentation and prevention of drug related problems, diseases or interactions in hospital practice as a service, teaching and research tool and clinical pharmacokinetic studies of new and established drugs.

The *service function* of the section is provided at three levels: at hospital level, which includes taking direct care and providing pharmacotherapy and drug problem consultation service as well as drug information service to hospital patients, editing (1994) the first *hospital formulary* of the country, conducting utilization – cost surveys, monitoring and investigating adverse reactions and interactions, evaluating pharmacotherapy of individual patients and information – education programmes, carrying out laboratory analysis of drugs, monitoring and evaluating drug levels, providing consultation for clinical trial protocols, and participating in regular local pharmacotherapy symposia for practising doctors at a regional revel, by making all the section's services accessible on demand to out patients and to all the other health sector physicians (Social Insurance Foundation, etc.) and, *at national level*, by playing a leading role in the development of the national pharmacovigilance system as member of the national scientific advisory committee (so far), by serving as national investigator of serious adverse reactions (so far) and by playing an important advisory role on national drug withdrawal measures based on the results of the section's 'Hospital Monitoring Programme'.

Similar activities are in progress in the medical school of Thessaloniki, where clinical pharmacologists are involved in research activities on special subjects or drugs and to a lesser degree in undergraduate teaching of clinical pharmacology which is also included in the obligatory courses or elective courses of some departments of internal medicine or of basic pharmacology. Their service functions are usually a combination of private practice and hospital practice of subjects related to their main clinical or laboratory specialities, e.g. hypertension and bacteriology. Drug level measurement services which are provided by some hospitals are performed usually by laboratory specialists of related subjects. Adverse drug reaction monitoring services which will be provided in collaboration with the national pharmacovigilance system are developing slowly, and it is hoped that their recent participation in the national advisory pharmacovigilance committee will enforce these activities.

In the other five medical schools of the country, there have not been developed similar activities yet. Apart from the universities, there are some more clinical pharmacologists who are working either in the national health system and national drug regulatory organization or private clinical or laboratory practice with responsibilities related to their main speciality or service who maintain their interest in clinical pharmacology by carrying out research in special subjects. There are also a number of interested medical graduates and some young promising scientists of related subjects who after their specialist training would enforce the development of the speciality in our country. These scientists as well as any other practising physician in the country have access on demand to the special clinical pharmacological services provided by a few hospitals.

Despite the unofficial profile of the speciality in the country, the number of clinical pharmacologists is increasing steadily. The requirements for becoming a specialist is a degree in medicine and 3 years specialist training. Specialist training includes combined advanced training in clinical pharmacology laboratory (1 year) and clinical pharmacology and therapeutics clinical training (2 years). The laboratory training includes training in laboratory principles and methods of drug analysis, clinical pharmacokinetics and special techniques for service and research. The clinical training includes training in basic clinical service and specialist clinical service in clinical pharmacology and therapeutics principles with service, teaching and research involvement. Trainees could be either graduates of medicine or specializing in internal medicine trainees who can start the specialist training after the second year of their specialization in internal medicine. Specialists in internal medicine or related subjects could also be trained. The recommended but not compulsory parts of the specialist course are: internal medicine or related specialization (full or in part), experimental or basic pharmacology training, drug regulation training and MD thesis in clinical pharmacology or basic pharmacology. For the time being, the full specialist course is undertaken by the section of clinical pharmacology of the university department of clinical therapeutics and the department of internal medicine at Alexandra Hospital. Four specialists have already been trained and some more are in the training process. The course is partly funded by the National Drug Regulatory Organization which is affiliated to the Ministry of Health. Foreign scientists can be accepted for 1-year short-training but no funds are available for them.

As far as the participation of clinical pharmacologists in the rest of the central national services i.e. drug registration, control of clinical trials, and national formulary, these areas have been limited due to a small number of well trained specialists. The National Drug Regulatory Organization, which is affiliated to the Ministry of Health, is for the time being in charge of these functions. Poor is also the participation of clinical pharmacologists in clinical trials of new drugs or international multicentre trials.

The Greek Society of Pharmacology, founded in 1985, has a Clinical Pharmacology Section where most of the clinical pharmacologists of the country are members. It serves as the national forum for collaboration with all interested bodies in the development of the discipline at national level, for designing the national strategy, for organizing national or international scientific meetings and for the presentation of the results of research within this field.

In summary, despite the absence of its recognition as an independent discipline or speciality yet and the small number of specialists, clinical pharmacology in Greece has played a leading role (1) in developing its functions in the form of a section affiliated to an established academic department, (2) in establishing the undergraduate training in the subject mainly in the clinical phase (last 2 years) and to a lesser degree in the preclinical phase of the course of medical studies, (3) in establishing postgraduate training for specialization in the subject of medical graduates and internal medicine trainees (suitable also for continuing education), (4) in establishing its research programme (Hospital Intensive Monitoring) as the 'keystone' of service, teaching and research (interrelated) functions not only at local or national level (developmental model for universities, district hospitals) and (5) in providing its expertise in the subject for the integrated development of the discipline services at a national level in collaboration with the central national drug regulatory sector (e.g. national pharmacovigilance system).

In conclusion, for the development of the discipline or specialty: at *a national level* are needed

- Many more specialists and more interest in the national development of the discipline and speciality;
- Better use, co-ordination and support of the existing training courses and section (model);
- Reinforcement of the role and more active participation of specialists in every aspect of the services provided by the speciality at local, regional and central level; and
- at *international level*, more active participation in international education and research, programmes or studies.

Further information can be obtained from Associate Professor A. Iliopoulou

Addresses

Athens
Associate Professor Karageorgiou Haris
Athens University
Bacteriology, Clinical Pharmacology
Univ. Department of Experimental
Pharmacology
75 M. Asias qtr.
Athens 11527
Phone: +30 1779 6532
Fax: +30 1779 0841

Associate Professor Iliopoulou Angeliki
Therapeutics of Athens University
Internal Medicine
Section of Clinical Pharmacology
Alexandra Hospital
80 Vas. Sofias Souron Str.
Athens 11528
Phone: +30 1777 1731
Fax: +30 1777 1731
E-mail: ailiop@atlas.uoa.gr

Dr Paviou Haris
Cardiology, Clinical Pharmacology
St Savvas Oncology Hospital
32 Acheloou qtr.
Vrilissia 15235
Phone: +30 1640 9311
Fax: +30 1642 0146

Dr Dracoulis Nicolaos
Biochemistry, Clinical Pharmacology
25 Efroniou qtr.
Athens 16577
Phone: +30 1725 1805
Fax: +30 1684 3310

Dr Siouti Miranda
Physician, Clinical Pharmacology
National Drug Regulatory Organisation
284 Mesogion Av 155 62 Holargos
Athens 15562

Phone: +30 1654 9500
Fax: +30 1654 9585

Dr Vorropoulou Ourania
Specialties: Internal Medicine, Clin.
Pharmacology
Health Section of National Institute of
Technology
17 Aphroditis qtr. Kalamaki
17342 Athens
Phone: +30 1993 9743
Fax: +30 1995 5439

Dr Giannakopoulos George
Specialties: Internal Medicine
Clin. Pharmacology
Section of Clin. Pharmacology
Univ. Department of Clin. Therapeutics
and Department
Internal Medicine, Alexandra Hospital
80 Vas. Sofias qtr.
Athens 11528
Phone: +30 1777 1731
Fax: +30 1777 1731

Zervoudi Emella
Physician, Clin. Pharmacology
4 Lemesou qtr., Glyfada
Athens 17723
Phone: +30 1962 5124

Goutou Panayiota
Internal Medicine, Clin. Pharmacology
Section of Clin. Pharmacology
Univ. Department of Clin. Therapeutics
and Departmentof Internal Medicine
Alexandra Hospital
80 Vas. Sofias qtr.
Athens 11528
Phone: +30 1777 1731
Fax: +30 1777 1731

Ioannina

Dr Karabali Sofia
Internal Medicine, Clin. Pharmacology
19 Kaloudi qtr.
Ioannina
Phone: +30 6512 5346
Fax: +30 6513 1993

Thessaloniki

Associate Professor Nicolaidis Paul
Internal Medicine of Thessaloniki University
Nephrology, Clinical Pharmacology
Univ. Department of Internal Medicine
Ahepa Hospital
46-48 Mitropoleos qtr.
Thessaloniki
Phone: +30 3199 4615
Fax: +30 3199 4651

Associate Professor Boutis Lasaros
Exper. Pharmacology of Thessaloniki Univ.
Oncology, Clinical Pharmacology
Department of Internal Medicine
Theagenion Hospital
33 Tsimiski qtr.
Thessaloniki 54622
Phone: +30 3182 9212
Fax: +30 3184 5514

Associate Professor Makedou Areti
Dept of Paediatrics of Thessaloniki Univ.
Bacteriology- Biochemistry, Clin. Pharmacology
Lab of bacteriology
Univ. Dept of Paediatrics
Ahepa Hospital
7 Patriarchou Ioakim qtr.
Thessaloniki 54622
Phone: +30 3122 0553
Fax: +30 3123 8490

Associate Prof Zamboulis Chrysanthos
Internal Medicine of Thessaloniki Univ.
Specialties: Hypertension
Clin. Pharmacology
Univ. Department of Internal Medicine
Hippokration Hospital
5 Metropolitou Josef qtr.
Thessaloniki 54622
Phone: +30 3123 7643
Fax: +30 3189 2158

Assistant Professor Karagiannis Asterios
Internal Medicine of Thessaloniki University
Specialties: Hypertension
Clinical Pharmacology
Hippokration Hospital
Thessaloniki 54622
Phone: +30 3182 3595
Fax: +30 3189 2158

Dr Mamzoridou Ekaterini
Specialties: Paediatrics, Clinical Pharmacology
69 Tsimiski qtr.
Thessaloniki 54622
Phone: +30 3126 5732
Fax: +30 3127 1974

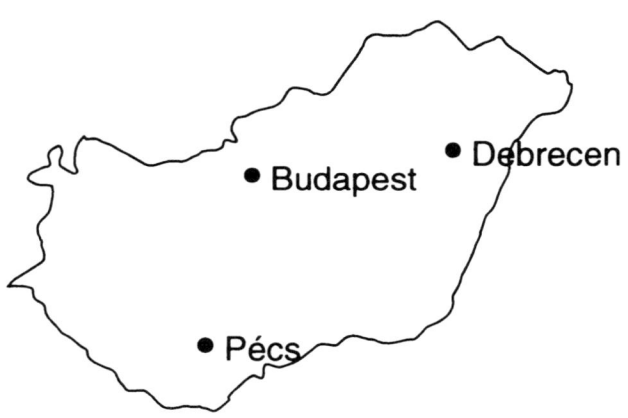

Hungary

Clinical pharmacology is recognized as a medical speciality in Hungary. Most of the candidates with clinical pharmacology as the only speciality work in the pharmaceutical industry. Candidates may also be specialists in clinical pharmacology as a supplement to one or even two other clinical specialities. The former ones become specialists in clinical pharmacology after 3 years of employment in the pharmaceutical industry followed by 1 year of training in a unit of clinical pharmacology. For candidates with a clinical speciality, two years in a unit of clinical pharmacology are required. Both lines of training end with a board exam. Haynal Imre University of Health is responsible for all postgraduate training and examination in Hungary. There are regular postgraduate courses in clinical pharmacology including the clinical and methodological aspects of the discipline. Most energy is put on the postgraduate training, but the Department of Clinical Pharmacology at Debrecen University also participates in the undergraduate training.

The Hungarian Society of Experimental and Clinical Pharmacology has about 500 members, some of whom are also members of the Society's Section of Clinical Pharmacology. Clinical pharmacologists in Hungary have very good relations with colleagues in related areas. The relationships, however, are based on institutions rather than the scientific societies. At the moment, there is only one department of clinical pharmacology in Hungary (at Debrecen University). However, much effort is being made to establish similar chairs in clinical pharmacology at Semmelweis University of Medicine and at Haynal Imre University of Health Sciences; both are located in Budapest.

The Minister of Welfare and the Minister of Education are both responsible for clinical pharmacology. Clinical pharmacologists have very good relations both with the Drug Regulation Agency (the National Institute of Pharmacy) and with the pharmaceutical industry.

Addresses

Budapest
Professor Csaba Farsang
St Imre Teaching Hospital
2nd Department of Medicine & Unit of
Clinical Pharmacology
H-1502 Budapest
PO Box 4
Phone: +36 1 203 3613
Fax: +36 1 203 3588

Professor B Gachályi
Haynal Imre University of Health
Sciences
Division of Clinical Pharmacology
H-1389 Budapest
P.O. Box 112
Phone: +36 1 270 4770
Fax: +36 1 270 4770
E-mail: osp@hiete.lib.hu

Debrecen
Professor F Hernádi
University Medical School of Debrecen
Clinical Pharmacology Research Centre
H-4012 Debrecen
P.O. Box 12
Phone: +36 52 411 600/5495
Fax: +36 52 314 912
E-mail:herfer@king.pharmacol.dote.hu

Pécs
Dr L Nagy
Pécs University of Medicine
1st Department of Medicine
H-7624 Pécs
Ifjúság út 13.
Phone: +36 72 311 122
Fax: +36 72 326 244

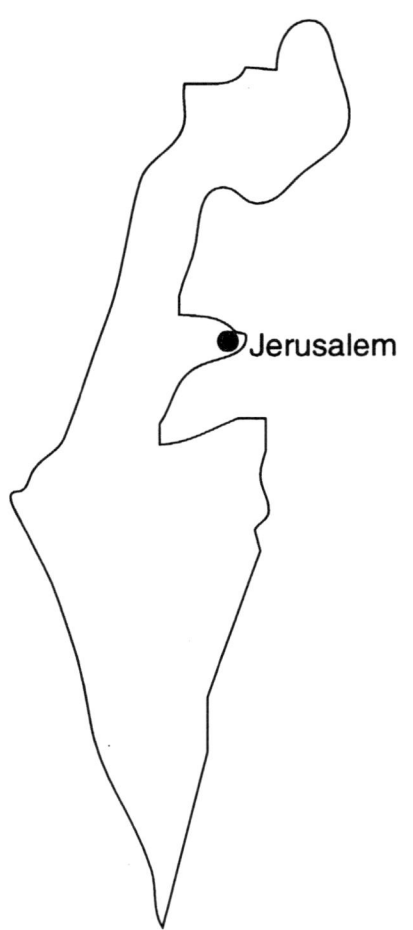

Israel

Clinical pharmacology became an independent medical speciality in May 1996. The authorization was given by the Scientific Council of Medicine, who according to the law is the body that provides board recognition in Israel (pending training and examination based on prior specialization in internal medicine, paediatrics or psychiatry). The national requirement to become a specialist in clinical pharmacology is 30 months of training at an authorized unit or department of clinical pharmacology according to the set syllabus. Right now, the Scientific Council is in the process of identifying those clinical pharmacologists who received their training abroad and who have already been active in the field for a number of years. This process will be followed by recognizing units or departments who shall be authorized to train clinical pharmacologists. Each unit or department must have at least two specialists in clinical pharmacology but also the facilities that are required to provide the training.

Clinical pharmacology has developed in close connection with the university teaching hospitals in Israel. The first unit was established in 1974. There are four medical schools in Israel: in Beersheba, Haifa, Jerusalem and Tel Aviv. At the four medical schools, there are at the moment 11 units of clinical pharmacology. Nine of the units are situated within departments of internal medicine and two are independent units. One of the independent units are responsible for undergraduate teaching in pharmacology. The units are run by physicians trained in either internal medicine, or basic pharmacology, or both and who have received training in clinical pharmacology abroad.

At the undergraduate level, clinical pharmacology is taught during the fourth year of the medical study. During the sixth and last year of the medical study, clinical pharmacology teaching is given in the form of seminars. Seminars or short courses in clinical pharmacology are also given as postgraduate courses. Trainees in clinical pharmacology are to spend up to 6 months in basic research.

All of the clinical pharmacology units have active research programs, and they also provide clinical service to hospitals. The clinical service includes therapeutic drug monitoring, drug information and adverse drug reaction monitoring.

Both health and academic authorities fully accept that clinical pharmacology is distinct from basic pharmacology. The Israel Society of Clinical Pharmacology has about 30 members. The Society arranges two scientific meetings each year.

Addresses

Jerusalem
Professor M Levy
Israel Society of Clinical Pharmacology
Clinical Pharmacology Unit
Hadassah University Hospital
P.O. Box 12000
91 120 Jerusalem
Fax: +972 2 6422384

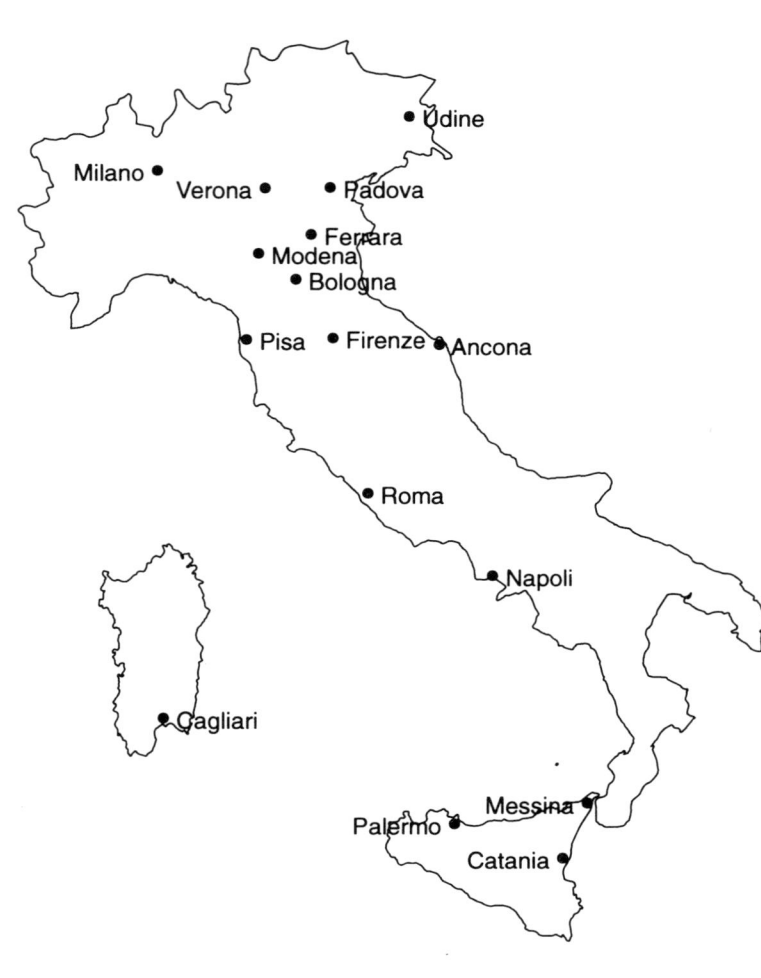

Italy

Clinical pharmacology is a subspeciality of pharmacology. The subspeciality of clinical pharmacology is available only to trainees with an MD degree, and the training takes place at postgraduate schools of pharmacology. The training lasts 4 years. The schools follow an EU indication and will issue a title recognized by the EU. There are presently 15 university hospitals that have a clinical pharmacology unit within the Italian Health Service.

The Italian Society of Pharmacology (SIF) has a Section of Clinical Pharmacology with about 70 members. The history of clinical pharmacology in Italy goes back to the late 1960s, where the first chair was established in Florence. The subsequent development was heterogenous, and the profile of each centre very much depended on local factors. Hospital positions in clinical pharmacology were often combined with toxicology. In 1983, 12 universities had developed a programme for clinical pharmacology. However, during the national revision of the medical curriculum (the so-called Tabella XVIII) in 1986, clinical pharmacology did not achieve a status as an independent discipline. Therefore, clinical pharmacology disappeared from all of the universities except in Florence, Modena and Padua. During the second revision of the medical curriculum in 1989, it again became possible for medical schools to plan a programme for teaching clinical pharmacology. As a result, 14 universities now have clinical pharmacology in their statutes. In addition, 19 universities started postgraduate schools in pharmacology with special programme for the subspeciality clinical pharmacology. Pharmacology including clinical pharmacology (corso integrato di farmacologia, area 13) is taught during the 5th year at medical schools.

The Minister of Health is politically responsible for clinical pharmacology. The Section for Clinical Pharmacology has developed guidelines for the function of clinical pharmacology units in hospitals. The section has also developed guidelines for teaching clinical pharmacology to both undergraduates and postgraduates in medical schools.

Addresses

Ancona
Professor L Rossini
Universitsà di Ancona
Via Tronto 10A
I-60020 Ancona
Phone: +39 71 22063066 (secretary)
       +39 71 2181028 (personal)
Fax: +39 71 22063067
E-mail: animo@popcsi.unian.it

Bologna
Professor E Ambrosioni
Università di Bologna
Policlinico Sant'Orsola
I-40100 Bologna
Phone: +39 51 6363242
Fax: +39 51 6363518

Cagliari
Professor GL Gessa
Department of Neurosciences 'B.B. Brodie'
University of Cagliari
Via Porcell, 4
I-09124 Cagliari
Phone: +39 70 6758417
Fax: +39 70 657237

Catania
Professor M Amico-Roxas
Università di Catania
V.le A. Doria, 6
I-95125 Catania
Phone: +39 95 330533
Fax: +39 95 333219
E-mail: roxas@dematel

Ferrara
Professor L Beani
Università di Ferrara
Departimento di Medicina Clinica e Sperimentale
Via Fossato di Mortara, 17-19
I-44100 Ferrara
Phone: +39 532 291203
Fax: +39 532 291205
E-mail: MCS@IFEUNIV.UNIFE.IT

Firenze
Professor L Zilletti
Università di Firenze
Viale G.B. Morgagni, 65
I-50134 Firenze
Phone: +39 55 411133
Fax: +39 55 4361613

Messina
Professor AP Caputi
Università di Messina
Piazza XX Settembre, 1
I-98122 Messina
Phone: +39 90 712533
Fax: +39 90 661029

Milano
Professor A Pontiroli
Ospedale S. Raffaele
Via Olgettina, 60
I-20132 Milano
Phone: +39 2 26432951
Fax: +39 2 26432951

Professor CR Sirtori
Institute of Pharmacological Sciences
Via Balzaretti 9
I-20133 Milano
Phone: +39 220 488303
Fax: +39 229 404961
E-mail: Cesare Sirtori@unimi.it

Dr G Tognoni
Istituto M. Negri
Via Eritrea 62
I-20157 Milano
Phone: +39 239 014468
Fax: +39 233 200049
E-mail: tognoni@irfmn.mnegri.it

Modena
Professor E Sternieri
Università di Modena
Via del Pozzo, 71
I-41100 Modena
Phone: +39 59 424064
Fax: +39 59 424069
E-mail: sternierei@unimo.it

Napoli
Professor L Annunziato
Area Funzionale di Farmacologia Clinica
Facoltà di Medicina e Chirurgia
University Frederico II
Via S. Pansini 5
I-80131 Napoli
Phone: +39 81 7463318
Fax: +39 81 7463323

Professor F Rossi
1st Farmacologia e Tossicologia
II Università di Napoli
Via Costantinopoli 16
I-80138 Napoli
Phone: +39 81 459802
Fax: +39 81 5665878

Padova
Professor M Ferrari
Università di Padova
Via Giustiniani, 2
I-35128 Padova
Phone: +39 49 8212340
Fax: +39 49 8754179
E-mail: farmclin@uxl.unipd.it

Palermo
Professor G Cannizzaro
Policlinico Giaccone
Via del Vespro, 129
I-90127 Palermo
Phone: +39 91 6553259
Fax: +39 91 6553212

Pisa
Professor M Del Tacca
Division of Pharmacology and Chemotherapy
Department of Oncology
University of Pisa
Via Roma, 55
I-56126 Pisa
Phone: +39 50 830148
Fax: +39 50 562020
E-mail: m.deltacca@do.med.unipi.it

Roma
Professor P Preziosi
Università Cattolica S. Cuore
L.go F. Vito
I-00168 Roma
Phone: +39 630 154253
Fax: +39 630 50159
E-mail: ibifa@rm.unicatt.it

Udine
Professor M Furlanut
University of Udine
P.le S. Maria della Misericordia, 3
I-33100 Udine
Phone: +39 432 559833
Fax: +39 432 559833
E-mail: furnalut@hydrus.cc.uniud.it
Homep: www.uniud.it/ifct/wel

Verona
Dr S Milleri
Glaxo-Wellcome
Via Fleming, 2
I-37135 Verona
Phone: +39 45 9218254
Fax: +39 45 9218193

Professor GP Velo
Università di Verona
Policlinico Borgo Roma
I-37134 Verona
Phone: +39 45 500408, 807 4899
Fax: +39 45 581111
E-mail: GPVelo@Farma.Univr.it
Homep: www.sfm.univr.it

Training Centres in Italy

Messina

Research and training programme
The Institute of Pharmacology is a specialized postgraduate medical institute of the Medical School of the University of Messina. The Institute is a centre for teaching, training and research in clinical and basic pharmacology. The Institute is involved in a wide range of research fields. Basic research is carried out in the cardiovascular and neuropharmacology fields. The Institute of Pharmacology's clinical scope of activity covers three areas
- pharmacoeconomy, pharmacoepidemiology and pharmacovigilance;
- pharmacokinetics of antidepressant and antipsychotic drugs;
- therapeutic drugs monitoring.

Several training opportunities and courses are run by the Institute of Pharmacology. They are: (1) specialist Trainee in Clinical Pharmacology and Medical Toxicology (4 years); (2) PhD Course in Experimental Medicine (4 years); (3) Postgraduate Course in Substance Misuse and Dependence (1 year); (4) Short Annual Courses on several aspects of new drugs and substances of abuse (1 year).

Clinical and research facilities
Several clinical and research facilities support the different research units that work in clinical pharmacology. The group of pharmacoeconomy, pharmacoepidemiology and pharmacovigilance through a computer network is involved in the analysis of adverse drugs reactions and in the evaluation of efficacious and costeffective methods for the prevention of pharmacological treatments. The Clinical Psychopharmacology group is active in the field of pharmacokinetics and pharmacogenetics of psychotropic drugs, mainly anti- depressants and antipsychotics, with particular interest to their clinical implications. The Therapeutic Drugs Monitoring unit evaluates through radioimmunoassay techniques serum ciclosporine levels for hospital departments and external patients. Moreover, the same unit determine the most common drugs of abuse for Addiction Treatment Services and Community Drug Teams.

The Institute has a specialist pharmacological library and an access to international bibliographic database.

Staff
The staff of the Institute of Pharmacology comprise a full professor, several associate professors lectures and fellows.

Milano
Center E. Grossi Paoletti – Niguarda Hospital
Research activities at the Center E. Grossi Paoletti, located in the Niguarda Hospital, one of the largest European City Hospitals, are focussed on the diagnosis and management of clinical conditions at high risk for cardiovascular disease. Among these, predominant are hyperlipoproteinaemias, but also thrombotic and other vascular diseases in the young. Clinical facilities in the Centre allow the clinical follow-up of some 5,000 patients with hyperlipidaemias or other metabolic disorders with a high cardiovascular risk. The major diagnostic procedures are based on:
- evaluation of the lipid/lipoprotein abnormalities with highly sophisticated technologies (ultracentrifugation, lipoprotein separation and apoprotein identification according to immunological, electrophoretic and other advanced physicochemical technologies);
- evaluation by non-invasive techniques of the conditions of the vascular tree, with special interest in the carotid intimamedia thickness evaluation (a technique originally developed at the Centre) and peripheral arterial compliance;
- determination of the thrombotic risk by all major platelet/coagulation procedures (aggregation, adhesion, fibrinolysis, etc.) in parallel with in vivo studies in volunteers and treated patients; studies on the enhanced thrombotic tendency in hypercholesterolemic patients;
- studies of apolipoprotein pathologies: the major contribution has been the discovery of the apolipoprotein A-IMilano mutant, the first mutation of human apolipoproteins;
- clinical effectiveness of different lipid lowering diets, particularly of the soy protein diet and of n-3 fatty acid enriched diets.
  The medical and laboratory staff of the Center is mainly composed of people with training in basic and clinical pharmacology. There

are four full-time clinicians, four full-time basic scientists and a large staff of pre- and postgraduate students. It also carries out research programs on
- modelling of drug pharmacokinetics in the elderly;
- P450 polymorphisms in patients with high cardiovascular risk and hyperlipidaemias.

The University of Milano recognizes this research activity as part of the student training in clinical pharmacology, for the School of Pharmacy.

Graduates willing to apply for research activities at the Center E. Grossi Paoletti may do so freely by writing to Professor Cesare Siriori.

References

Baldassarre D, Gianfranceschi G, Pazzucconi F, Sirtori CR (1995) Non-invasive assessment of unstimulated forearm arterial compliance in human subjects. Impaired vasoreactivity in hypercholesterolaemia. Eur J Clin Invest 25: 859-66

Calabresi L, Vecchio G, Longhi R, Gianazza E, Palm G, Wadensten H, Hammarström A, Olsson A, Karlström A, Sejlitz T, Ageland H, Sirtori CR, Franceschini G (1994) Molecular characterization of native and recombinant apo A-IMilano dimer. J Biol Chem 269: 32168-32174

Franceschini G, Cassinotti M, Vecchio G, Gianfranceschi G, Pazzucconi F, Murakami T, Sirtori M, D'Acquarica AL, Sirtori CR (1994) Pravastatin effectively lowers LDL cholesterol in familial combined hyperlipidemia without changing LDL subclass pattern. Arterioscler Thromb 14: 1569-1575

Franceschini G, Werba JP, D'Acquarica AL, Gianfranceschi G, Michelagnoli S, Sirtori CR (1995) Microsomal enzyme inducers raise plasma HDL-cholesterol levels in healthy controls but not in patients with primary hypoalphalipoproteinemia. Clin Pharmacol Ther 57: 434-440

Lovati MR, Manzoni C, Corsini A, Granata A, Fumagalli R, Sirtori CR (1996) 7S Globulin from soybean is metabolized in human cell cultures by a specific uptake and degradation system. J Nutr 126: 2831-2843

Pazzucconi F, Barbi S, Baldassarre D, Colombo N, Dorigotti F, Sirtori CR (1996) Iron-ovotransferrin preparation does not interfere with ciprofloxacin absorption. Clin Pharmacol Ther 59:418-22

Roma P, Gregg RE, Meng MS, Ronan R, Zech LA, Franceschini G, Sirtori CR, Brewer HB Jr.(1993) In vivo metabolism of a mutant form of apolipoprotein A-I, apo A-IMilano, associated with familial hypoalphalipoproteinemia. J Clin Invest 91: 1445-1452

Sirtori CR, Paoletti R, Mancini M, Crepaldi G, Manzato E, Rivellese A, Pamparana F Stragliotto E (1997) n-3 fatty acids do not lead to an increased diabetic risk in patients with hyperlipidemia and abnormal glucose tolerance. Am J Clin Nutr 65: 1874-1881

Soma MR, Donetti E, Parolini C, Sirtori CR, Fumagalli R, Franceschini G (1995) Recombinant apolipoprotein A-IMilano dimer inhibits carotid intimal thickening induced by perivascular manipulation in rabbits. Circ Res 76: 405-411

Tremoli E, Maderna P, Marangoni F, Colli S, Eligini S, Catalano I, Angeli MT, Pazzucconi F, Gianfranceschi G, Davi G, Stragliotto E, Sirtori CR, Galli C (1995) Prolonged inhibition of platelet aggregation following n-3 fatty acid ethyl ester administration to healthy volunteers. Am J Clin Nutr 61: 607-613

Vaccarino V, Borgatta A, Gallus G, Sirtori CR (1995) Prevalence of coronary heart disease risk factors in Northern-Italian male and female employees. Eur Heart J 16: 761-769

M Negri Institute

The institutional context of Clinical Pharmacology at the M. Negri Institute is somehow atypical, as it comprises a series of groups working within and outside the Laboratory of Clinical Pharmacology.

The M. Negri Institute does not have clinical facilities, nor academic affiliations: therefore, there is no formal teaching commitment, nor the possibility of providing University titles.

The Clinical Pharmacology group provides post-doctoral research opportunities, through stages which are tailored to the individuals who apply and who are requested to participate in the research programmes of the group for an appropriate period of time. The main fields of interest include: the cardiovascular area (from molecular biology, to animal models, to the full range of clinical trials, to general and clinical epidemiology); mother and child health (with specific focus on epidemiology of vaccination, perinatal care, drugs in pregnancy, paediatric general practice); health and drug information (with highly developed knowledge on drugs in pregnancy with orientation also to the public at large); the rational use of drug and development of controlled research methodology in general practice.

A general characteristics of the groups working under the responsibility of M. Bonati, D. Coen, R. Latini has been the development of hospital and general practice based networks, which include now several hundreds of clinical departments in various disciplines and several hundred general practitioners. A close and productive collaboration has been established with the Italian Society of Hospital Pharmacists (SIFO), mainly in the areas of pharmaco-epidemiology and human experimentation.

Because of the wide scope of the groups, a 'representative' selection of references would be difficult. They are available on request.

Napoli
University Federico II

Our Unit of Clinical Pharmacology is devoted to the following activities
- Therapeutic drug monitoring in biological fluids: antibiotics, antiepileptics, immunosuppressants, antineoplastics, antiarrythmics, bronchodilators, drugs of abuse and biogenic amines. The following methodologies for measurement of mentioned drugs and substances are used: high performance liquid chromatography, column chromatography, radioimmunoassay, fluorescence polarization immunoassay, microparticle enzyme immunoassay, thin dry film multilayer immunoassay.
- Drug surveillance.
- Drug epidemiology.
- Elaboration and update of the Hospital Drug Formulary.
- Guidelines for prophylactic antibiotics in surgical procedures.

The staff consists of several professors of pharmacology and medical doctors with experience in the field of clinical pharmacology.
The Unit of Clinical Pharmacology is affiliated to the Section of Pharmacology, Department of Neurosciences, School of Medicine, 'Federico II University' of Naples, where a postgraduate school of Pharmacology with a special training programme in clinical pharmacology exists. The training lasts for 4 years. The school follows an EU indication and it will issue a title recognized by the EU.

Currently, the main researches of our Unit of Clinical Pharmacology are devoted to the following objectives:
a. Study of the pharmacokinetics of the immunosuppressant agents (cyclosporine and FK 506) in organ transplanted patients.
b. Evaluation of potential pharmacokinetic and pharmacodynamic interference between cyclosporine and other coadministered drugs (azathioprine, steroids, lipid lowering drugs, antibiotics) in organ transplanted patients.
c. Study of the pharmacokinetics of metotrexate in rheumatoid arthritis.
d. Therapeutic monitoring of aminoglycosides in premature newborns.

References

Capone D, De Marino V, Pisanti N, De Marino V (1994) A new dry chemistry immunoassay: comparison with a fluorescence polarization system. Eur Rev Med Pharmacol Sci 16: 9194

Capone D, Gentile A, Stanziale P, Imperatore P, D'Alessandro R, D'Alto V, Basile V (1996a) Drug interaction between cyclosporine and josamycin in a kidney transplanted patient. Fundamen Clin Pharmacol 10: 172

Capone D, Aiello C, Santoro GA, Gentile A, Stanziale P, D'Alessandro R, Imperatore P, Basile V (1996b) Drug interaction between cyclosporine and two antimicorbial agents, josamycin and rifampicin, in organ transplanted patients. Int J Clin Pharm Res 26: 7376

Capone D, Gentile A, Vajro P, De Vincenzo A, Brengola C, Guerriero S, De Silva C, Basile V(1997a) Therapeutic monitoring of tacrolimus. Role of the trough level. Pharmacol Res 35S: 105

Capone D, Gentile A, Guerriero S, Basile V (1997b) Possible interference of digoxin like immunoreactive substances with digoxin serum assay in subgroups of patients. Pharmacol Res 35S: 105

Capone D, De Marino V, Fontana R, Notaro R, De Marino V, Pisanti N (1997a) Effects of different routes of cyclosporin A administration on blood levels in patients undergoing bone marrow transplantation. Bone Marrow Transplant 19: 369372

Capone D, Imperatore P, Gentile A, Stanziale P, Sabbatini M, Basile V (1997b) Usefulness of therapeutic monitoring of tacrolimus in kidney transplanted recipients. Nephrol Dial Transplant, in press

Pisanti N, Stanziale P, Imperatore F, D'Alessandro R, De Marino V, Capone D, De Marino V (1997) Lack of effect of gemfibrozil on cyclosporine blood concentrations in kidney transplanted patients. Am J Nephrol, in press

Padova

The Cardiovascular Clinical Pharmacology Unit of the University of Padua Medical School offers the following research and training programme

- Pharmacokinetic-pharmacodynamic correlations in patients treated with antiarrhytmic drugs. Evaluation of the ECG effects during combined treatment with Class Ib and Class III.
- In vitro effects of inotripic agents evaluated in diseased human myocardial strips.
- Search for ECG markers to evaluate the risk of proarrhythmic effects.

Clinical and research facilities
HPLC, clinical electrophysiological devices, library, etc.

References

Padrini R, Piovan D, Busa M, Al-Bunni M, Maiolino P, Ferrari M (1993a) Pharmacodynamic variability of flecainide assessed by QRS changes. Clin Pharmacol Ther 53: 59-64

Padrini R, Piovan D, Javarnaro A, Cucchini F, Ferrari M (1993b) Pharmacokinetics and electrophysiological effects of i.v. ajmaline. Clin Pharmacokinet 25: 1-8

Padrini R, Butrous G, Camm AJ, Malik M (1995) Algebraic decomposition of the TU-wave morphology patterns. PACE 18: 2209-2215

Piovan D, Padrini R, Svaluto Morelo G, Magnolfi G, Zordan R, Pellegrino PA, Ferrari M (1995) Verapamil and norverapamil plasma levels in infants and children during chronic oral treatment. Ther Drug Monit 17: 60-67

Yang Q, Padrini R, Bova S, Piovan D, Magnolfi G (1995) Electrophysiological interactions between pinacidil, a potassium channel opener, and class I antiarrhytmic agents in guinea-pig perfused heart. Br J Pharmacol 114: 1745-1749

Yang Q, Padrini R, Piovan D, Ferrari M (1997) Cardiac effects of quinidine on isolated perfused guinea pig hearts after in vivo quinidine pretreatment. Br J Pharmacol 122: 7-12

Zeppellini R, Bolognesi R, Javernaro A, De Domenico R, Libardoni M, Tsialtas D, Piovan D, Padrini R, Cuchini F (1993) Effect of dobutamine on left ventricular relaxation and filling phase in patients with ischemic heart disease and preserved systolic function. Cardiovasc Drug Ther 7: 325-331

Zordan R, Padrini R, Bernini V, Piovan D, Ferrari M (1993) Influence of age and gender on the 'in vitro' serum protein binding of flecainide. Pharmacol Res 28: 259-264

Pisa

University of Pisa

The research and training programme of the postgraduate school of Pharmacology, subspeciality of clinical Pharmacology, is performed within the Division of Pharmacology and Chemotherapy of the Department of Oncology, School of Medicine and Dentistry of the University of Pisa. Trainees are involved in full-time activity on the theory and application to the clinical setting of drug monitoring, pharmacokinetics and toxicology of drugs, in particular chemotherapeutic and immunosuppressant agents, within phase I-II clinical studies. A substantial research activity is also devoted to the clinical pharmacology of drugs acting on cardiovascular, gastrointestinal and central nervous systems as well as on agents for the treatment of endocrinological disorders.

The postgraduate School of Pharmacology offers a research facility in the Division of Pharmacology and Chemotherapy of the Department of Oncology; the clinical facility is within the Pisa University Hospital.

The teaching staff of the postgraduate school of Pharmacology, subspeciality of clinical pharmacology, includes a full professor of pharmacology (Professor Mario Del Tacca) and a number of associate and assistant professors of pharmacology and related disciplines covering various aspects of human pathology and treatment.

Applicants with a valid MD degree who wish to apply for the postgraduate School of Pharmacology may send their application to the University of Pisa. The deadline for submission of applications may vary in October; please contact in advance the Head of the School for deadline information. Two positions are available each year; the selection of applicants is based on the scientific value of their MD thesis, publications and a written and oral selection based on general knowledge of pharmacology, human pathology, biochemistry and clinical medicine.

References

Campa M, Zolfino I, Senesi S, Bernardini N, Danesi R, Ducci M, Oleggini M, Di Stefano R, Mosca F, Lazzarini A, Del Tacca M (1990) The penetration of roxithromycin into human skin. J Antimicrob Chemother 26: 87-90

Conte PF, Baldini E, Gennari A, Michelotti A, Salvadori B, Tibaldi C, Danesi R, Innocenti F, Gentile A, Dell'Anna R, Biadi O, Mariani M, Del Tacca M (1997) Dose-finding study and pharmacokinetics of epirubicin and paclitaxel over 3 hours: a regimen with high activity and low cardiotoxicity in advanced breast cancer. J Clin Oncol 15: 2510-2517

Danesi R, La Rocca RV, Cooper MR, Ricciardi MP, Pellegrini A, Kragel PJ, Paparelli A, Del Tacca M, Myers CE (1996) Clinical and experimental evidence of inhibition of testosterone production by suramin. J Clin Endocrinol Metabol 81: 2221-2230

Danesi R, Falcone A, Conte PF, Del Tacca M (1997) Pharmacokinetic optimisation of the treatment of cancer with high-dose zidovudine. Clin Pharmacokinet 11: 456-462

Del Tacca M, Danesi R, Blandizzi C, Zolfino I, Senesi S, Panattoni E, Gabriele M, Marcucci M, Favini P, Campa M (1993) Periodontal tissue distribution and efficacy of cefpodoxime proxetil in acute odontogenic infections. Drug Invest 5: 313-319

Falcone A, Pfanner E, Cianci C, Danesi R, Bertuccelli M, Brunetti I, Del Tacca M, Conte PF (1995) Suramin in metastatic colorectal cancer patients pretreated with fluoropyrimidine-based chemotherapy: a phase II study. Cancer 75: 440-443

Falcone A, Danesi R, Dargenio F, Pfanner E, Brunetti I, Del Tacca M, Nethersell ABW, Conte PF (1996) Intravenous azidothymidine with 5-fluorouracil and l-leucovorin: a phase I-II study in previously untreated metastatic colorectal cancer patients. J Clin Oncol 14: 729-736

Innocenti F, Danesi R, Di Paolo A, Loru B, Favre C, Nardi M, Bocci G, Nardini D, Macchia P, Del Tacca M (1996) Clinical and experimental pharmacokinetic interaction between 6-mercaptopurine and methotrexate. Cancer Chemother Pharmacol 37: 409-414

Macchiarini P, Danesi R, Mariotti R, Marchetti A, Fazzi P, Bevilacqua G, Mariani M, Giuntini C, Del Tacca M, Angeletti CA (1990) Phase II study of high-dose epirubicin in untreated patients with small cell lung cancer. Am J Clin Oncol 13: 302-307

Zolfino I, Senesi S, Campa M, Di Vito A, Mosca F, Favini P, Ducci M, Danesi R, Del Tacca M (1992) Human skin disposition of cefpodoxime after oral administration of its proxetil ester. J Antimicrob Chemother 30: 731-733

Udine
University of Udine

Research And Training Programme: established in 1991, the Institute of Clinical Pharmacology and Toxicology of University of Udine is continually developing improved analytical methods for therapeutic drug monitoring (TDM) and pharmacokinetics/dynamics in order to individualize and optimize specific therapies according to physicians' queries (mainly concerning antimicrobial, antineoplastic, anticonvulsant, antiparkinsonian, antiasthmatic, antitubercular, cardioactive and immunosuppressive drugs). Current research activities include: optimal monitoring strategies for pharmacokinetic studies, clinical trials and patient care; improved methods for population pharmacokinetic modeling; pharmacoepidemiology and pharmacoeconomy.

The Institute is particularly interested in the postgraduate medical education (meetings and congresses on Pediatric Clinical Pharmacology and Clinical Neuropsycopharmacology in Geriatrics). Recently (September 16-18, 1992), the Institute organized in Grado (Italy) the 1st European Congress on Clinical Pharmacology and Toxicology Services devoted to the various aspects of our discipline (from research to health care).

Clinical and research facilities: multiuser database shared on the local area network; a liquid-mass spectrometer, HPLCs, capillary electrophoreses and ultracentrifuges are among the many resources available. Software is available for use in pharmacokinetic research applications. Current computer programmes include: WINNONLIN, Abbott Pharmacokinetic System (PKS), P-PHARM.

The University: the institute is linked to the Chair of Pharmacology,

Faculty of Medicine, University of Udine. Clinical pharmacology is taught to undergraduate students during the 5th year at medical school by means of seminars and practical interactive computer-aided exercises on pharmacokinetics emphasizing its main role in optimizing therapy in patients with various physiopathological conditions.

Staff: Physicians: Professor Mario Furlanut (Director), Dr Massimo Baraldo, Dr Federico Pea, Dr Donatella Poz, Dr Guang Wu (fellowship) Biologist: Dr Loretta Franceschi

Chemist: Dr Maria Teresa Feruglio, Technicians: Riccardo Ciofuli, Lucia Dose.

Application procedures: at present no positions available
Inquiries: Dr Federico Pea, phone: +39 432 559830.

References

Baraldo M, Furlanut M, Puricelli C (1994) No effect of clodronate on cyclosporine A blood levels in heart transplanted patients simultaneously treated with diltiazem and azathioprine. Ther Drug Monit 16: 435

Benetello P, Furlanut M, Zara G, Baraldo M, Hassan E (1993) Plasma levels of levodopa and its main metabolites in parkinsonian patients after conventional and controlled-release levodopa-carbidopa associations. Eur Neurol 33: 69-73

Benetello P, Furlanut M, Fortunato M, Pea F, Baraldo M (in press) Levodopa and 3-O-methyldopa in cerebrospinal fluid after levodopa-carbidopa association. Pharmacol Res

Benetello P, Furlanut M, Fortunato M, Baraldo M, Pea F, Tognon A, Testa G (in press) Oral gabapentin disposition in epileptic patients after high-protein meal. Epilepsia

Damiani D, Michieli M, Michelutti A, Pea F, Baraldo M, Fanin R, Russo D, Furlanut M, Baccarani M (1995) P170-related multidrug resistance. Enhancement of idarubicin content in leukemic cells with cyclosporine in vivo: a report of two cases. Leukemia 9: 1792-1795

Furlanut M, Benetello P, Spina E (1993) Pharmacokinetic optimisation of tricyclic antidepressant therapy. Clin Pharmacokinet 24 (4): 301-318

Furlanut M, Baraldo M, Pea F, Albanese MC, Albertini A, Puricelli C (1994) Effect of fluctuations of blood cyclosporine concentrations on renal function. Transplant Proc 26: 2574-2575

Furlanut M, Baraldo F, Pea V, Marzocchi V, Croattino L, Galla F (1996a) Blood concentrations and clinical effect of cyclosporin in psoriasis. Ther Drug Monit 18: 544-548

Furlanut M, Baraldo M, Galla F, Marzocchi V, Pea F (1996b) Cyclosporin nephrotoxicity in relation to its metabolism in psoriasis. Pharmacol Res 33: 349-352

Galla F, Marzocchi V, Croattino L, Poz D, Baraldo M, Furlanut M (1995) Oral and intravenous disposition of cyclosporine in psoriatic patients. Ther Drug Monit 17: 302-304

Verona
Borgo Roma University Hospital

The Clinical Pharmacology Unit, Institute of Pharmacology of Verona is located in the Borgo Roma University Hospital, in the south zone of the city. The activities in clinical pharmacology are carried out within the National Health System and in the context of national and international research programmes. They focus on drug safety (special reference to spontaneous reporting system, codifying systems and computerized approach to problems in drug safety), and pharmacokinetics of antitumoral drugs.

The activities are briefly summarized

a Spontaneous reporting system: the Unit is the reference for the adverse drug reaction reports within the Verona region, and gives information on adverse drug reactions to the health care professional. In the attempt to improve the National ADR reporting system, since 1988 ADR reports from physicians and pharmacists in the Veneto Region have been collected and analysed. The analysis of the data have been made interacting with the WHO Collaborating Centre for the International Drug Monitoring (Uppsala, Sweden) using also the database of the Centre where the ADR spontaneous reports from 50 countries are collected (today about 2,000,000). The Unit became recently 'WHO Reference Centre For Education And Communication In International Drug Monitoring';

b Bulletins: since May 1994 the Unit has published quarterly a bulletin on adverse drug reactions, 'Focus'. Since May 1997 Focus is part of the International Society of Drug Bulletins (ISDB).

c Research activities within the 'European Pharmacovigilance Research Group' (BIOMED projects – case control studies on pancreatitis, attitudinal survey of adverse drug reaction reporting by health care professionals, etc.)

d Studies on pharmacokinetics of antitumoral drugs.

The staff is composed of the director, Professor Giampaolo Velo, three research assistants and postgraduate students.

References
Belton KJ, Gram LF, Royer RJ, Feely J, McGettigan P, Velo GP et al. (1997) Attitudinal survey of adverse drug reaction reporting by health care professionals across the European Union. Eur J Clin Pharmacol 52: 423-427

Bonetti A, Franceschi T, Apostoli P, Cetto GL, Recaldin E, Molino A, Leone R (1994) Cisplatin pharmacokinetics in elderly patients. Ther Drug Morit 16: 477-482

Bonetti A, Franceschi T, Apostoli P, Messori A, Sperotto L, Cetto GL, Molino AM, Leone R (1995) Cisplatin pharmacokinetics using a five-day schedule during repeated courses of chemotherapy in germ cell tumors. Therapeutic Drug Monitoring 17: 25-32

Bonetti A, Apostoli P, Zaninelli M, Pavanel F, Colombatti M, Cetto GL, Franceschi T, Sperotto L, Leone R (1996) Inductively coupled plasma mass spectroscopy quantitation of platinum-DNA adducts in peripheral blood leukocytes of patients receiving cisplatin- or carboplatin-based chemotherapy. Clin Cancer Res 2: 1829-1835

Conforti A, Leone R, Moretti U, Guglielmo L, Velo GP (1995) Spontaneous reporting of adverse drug reactions in an Italian region: six years of analysis and observations. Pharmacoepidemiology and Drug Safety, vol 4: 129-135

Franceschi T, Sperotto L, Leone R (1996) Inductively coupled plasma mass spectroscopy quantitation of platinum-DNA adducts in peripheral blood leukocytes of patients receiving cisplatin- or carboplatin-based chemotherapy. Clin Cancer Res 2: 1829-1835

Leone R, Ghiotto E, Conforti A, Velo GP (1999) Potential interaction between ocular chloramphenicol. Ann Pharmacoter (in press)

Leone R, Conforti R, Ghiotto E, Moretti U, Valvo E, Velo GP (1999) Nimesulide and renal impairment. Eur J Clin Pharmacol (in press)

Guglielmo L, Leone R, Moretti U, Conforti A, Spolaor A, Velo GP (1993) Antibiotic prescribing patterns in Italian hospital inpatients with pneumonia, chronic obstructive pulmonary disease and urinary tract infections. Ann Pharmacother 27: 18-22

Guglielmo L, Leone R, Moretti U, Conforti A, Velo GP (1994) Antimicrobial drug utilisation in hospitals in Italy and other european countries. Infections Vol 22 (suppl 3): S176-S181

Leone R, Conforti A, Moretti U, Guglielmo L, Velo GP (1996) Indagine conoscitiva sulle attitudini dei medici italiani nei confronti della segnalazione delle reazioni avverse da farmaci. SIMG 1: 18-21

Guglielmo L, Leone R, Moretti U, Conforti A, Velo GP et al. (1997) Aetiology and therapy of community-acquired pneumonia: hospital study in northern Italy. Eur J Clin Pharmacol 51: 437-443

Glaxo Wellcome Clinical Pharmacology Unit

The Clinical Pharmacology Unit has 12 fully-monitored beds and it is located at Glaxo Wellcome Research site in Verona, Italy. It provides comprehensive facilities for almost all types of clinical pharmacology studies. Various aspects of drug action are assessed including pharmacokinetics, pharmacodynamics, metabolism, safety and tolerabiltiy.

The studies performed at the Unit are on new chemical entities, including first administration to humans as well as on established compounds. Novel formulations or devices are assessed in addition to more routine formulation developments and bioequivalence testing. New methodology to advance drug development is also in progress (methacholine challenge, skin blister, sputum-induced, gastric pH monitoring). The Clinical Pharmacology Unit has also specialized panels of volunteers (e.g. atopic subjects) and the possibility of carrying out studies with subjects suffering from well-established diseases (diabetes, hypertension, etc.).

The Unit personnel consists of five staff members. These being two research physicians of which one is head of the Unit, one junior research physician, one clinical research nurse and one administrative assistant. A specially recruited bank of nurses appropriately qualified and trained plus physicians from the Emergency Department of the local Hospital provide additional staff cover during study periods.

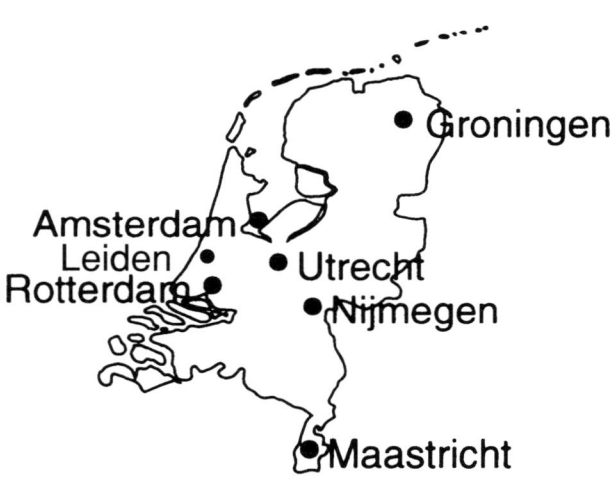

The Netherlands

Clinical pharmacology is not recognized as a separate medical speciality in The Netherlands. However, clinical pharmacology is recognized as an area of interest within the speciality of internal medicine. In this context, clinical pharmacology is defined as research and use of drugs in the treatment of patients as well as drug research carried out in healthy volunteers. In order to become recognized as a clinical pharmacologist, the candidate must be able to demonstrate knowledge of general pharmacology and advanced expertise in one or more of the following fields: adverse effects, intoxication, interpretation of drug concentrations in body fluids, collaboration with either pharmacists or microbiologists, with regard to therapeutic drug monitoring, participation in hospital drug formulary committees and clinical trial methodology, for instance as a member of a review committee.

The training programme for a clinical pharmacologist is as follows

- Basic training: 4 years of training in internal medicine, including cardiology, pulmonology and out-patient care.
- Specific training: (1) Compulsory (12 months): seeing out-patients in clinical pharmacology and follow-up on patients intoxicated by drugs. (2) Facultative (6 months): Three of the following items: a) a pharmacokinetic course, b) practical work at the Dutch Center for Monitoring of Adverse Drug Reactions, c) practical work at the National Center for Intoxication, d) practical work in a hospital pharmacy. e) a course in planning and execution of clinical trials.
- Science: The trainee must participate in a research project leading to at least one publication and one presentation in a well recognized meeting.

The Dutch Society of Clinical Pharmacology and Biopharmaceutics was founded in 1979. The task of the Society is to promote and improve the training and research in clinical pharmacology in The Netherlands. At the moment, the Society has about 240 members.

Twice a year, the Society organizes meetings where both scientific papers and organizational matters are presented. In the past, joint meetings have been organized together with the Dutch Society of Pharmacology, the Dutch Society of Pharmacy as well as with the Flemish and German Societies of Clinical Pharmacology.

Leopold Meyler was appointed the first professor in clinical pharmacology in 1968 at the State University of Groningen. At present, there are five professors of clinical pharmacology in The Netherlands (part- or full-time) and two extraordinary professors of pharmacotherapy granted by the Foundation for Medical Pharmaceutical Research. All seven professors are active participants in the undergraduate teaching in basic pharmacology (together with the professors of this discipline), clinical pharmacology and pharmacotherapy. The professors are also active in the postgraduate training of specialists in internal medicine and hospital pharmacists.

The Minister for Health, Welfare and Sports as well as the Minister for Science and Education are politically responsible for clinical pharmacology in The Netherlands.

There is no formal relationship between the Dutch Society of Clinical Pharmacology and Biopharmaceutics, the pharmaceutical industry and the Dutch Drug Regulatory Agency. However, the Foundation for Medical Pharmaceutical Research is funded by the pharmaceutical companies in The Netherlands, and in this way they contribute to teaching and research in clinical pharmacology.

Addresses

Amsterdam
Professor CJ van Boxtel
Academisch Medisch Centrum
Department of Clinical Pharmacology
Meibergdreef 9
1105 AZ Amsterdam
Phone: +31 20 566 5298
Fax: +31 20 696 5976
E-mail: CvanBoxtel@xs4all.nl

Dr JHM Schellens
Netherlands Cancer Institute
Department of Medical Oncology
1066 CX Amsterdam
Phone: +31 20 512 2569/9111
Fax: +31 20 512 2572
E-mail: JHM@nki.nl

Groningen
Professor D de Zeeuw
Department of Clinical Pharmacology
Faculty of Med. Sciences
University of Groningen
Anthonius Deusinglaan 1
9713 AV Groningen
Phone: +31 050 363 2810

Fax: +31 050 363 2812
E-mail: d.de.zeeuw@med.rug.nl

Leiden
Professor AF Cohen
Centre for Human Drug Research
Zernikedreef 10
2333 CL Leiden
Phone: +31 71 524 6400
Fax: +31 71 524 6499

Professor H Mattie
Academisch Ziekenhuis Leiden
Department of Infectious Diseases, C5-P
Albinusdreef 2
Postbus 9600
2300 RC Leiden
Phone: +31 71 526 2290
Fax: +31 71 526 6758
Email:mattie@rullf2.medfac.leide-nuniv.nl

Maastricht
Dr LMAB Van Bortel
Division of Clinical Pharmacology
Department of Pharmacology
Maastricht University
P.O. Box 616
6200 MD Maastricht
Phone: +31 43 383 1343 or 1417
Fax: +31 43 367 0940
E-mail: l.vanbortel@farmaco.uni maas.nl

Nijmegen
Professor PABM Smits
Sint Radboudziekenhuis
233 Pharmacology
P.O. Box 9101
6500 HB Nijmegen
Phone: +31 24 361 3691
Fax: +31 24 361 4214

Utrecht
Professor JMA Sitsen
Department of Clinical Pharmacology
Rudolf Magnus Instituut
Universiteitsweg 100
3584 CG Utrecht

Training Centres in The Netherlands

Amsterdam
Academisch Medisch Centrum
Research and training in Clinical Pharmacology is supported by the Department of Clinical Pharmacology & Pharmacotherapy, chaired by the Professor of Clinical Pharmacology, and the Department of Medicine, respectively, of the University of Amsterdam and the University Hospital of Amsterdam. The University of Amsterdam was founded in 1632 and the origins of its Medical School can be traced back to 1669. Since 1984 this Medical School with all its disciplines has been housed in the AMC on the outskirts of Amsterdam. The University Hospital of Amsterdam is a facility with all medical specialities and over 800 beds. Clinical pharmacology teaching to some 200 new medical students each year and to clinical staff is the responsibility of the Department of Clinical Pharmacology & Pharmaco-therapy.

The programme provides broad training in clinical pharmacology, including early concentration response studies in man, phase III studies, participation in ADR monitoring and TDM in collaboration with the hospital pharmacy. Trainees will be offered the opportunity to improve their knowledge in the fields of statistics, epidemiology and pharmacological techniques as the need arises. Through the involvement of the Department of Clinical Pharmacology & Pharmacotherapy in, among others, the Hospital Formulary Committee and the Ethics Review Board trainees can be exposed to such activities.

Among the major clinical areas of interest are immunopharmacology, pulmonary pharmacology, drug safety, genetic polymorphism and the pharmacology of drugs for tropical diseases. Clinical facilities include all the clinical and clinical research services of the AMC. The Laboratory for Clinical Pharmacology is fully equipped for the determination of a wide range of drugs. Computer facilities for PK-PD modelling and for analysis of population kinetics are available.

The Laboratory of Clinical Pharmacology is currently staffed with five faculty members, two of them holding joint appointments in the Department of Medicine. At the moment, there are two graduate students and two other trainees in the programme, both of which are specialists in Internal Medicine. Recently, a specialist in tropical medicine from Vietnam finished a 1-year training in the programme. The Laboratory has its own secretarial support and employs two full-time technicians.

Those interested in the programme should write to the director, Professor CJ van Boxtel, stating their career goals and specifics about their formal training. Fellowship training can be made available for candidates with the MD degree and preferably with clinical training in internal medicine or paediatrics.

Candidates will be assisted in seeking foundation support. Supplementation of grants which falling below needed levels might be made from locally available funds.

References

Butter JJ, van den Berg BTJ, Portier JG, Kaiser G, van Boxtel CJ (1996) Determination by HPLC with electrochemical detection of formoterol RR and SS enantiomers in urine. J Liquid Chromatogr (Clin Appl) 19: 993-1005

Jonkers RE, Braat MCP, Koopmans RP, van Boxtel CJ (1995a) Pharmacodynamic modelling of the drug induced down regulation of a beta(2)-adrenoceptor mediated response and the lack of restoration of receptor function after a single high dose of prednisone. Eur J Clin Pharmacol 49: 37-44

Jonkers RE, Braat MCP, Koopmans RP, van Boxtel CJ (1995b) Pharmacodynamic modelling of the drug induced down regulation of a beta(2)-adrenoceptor mediated response and the lack of restoration of receptor function after a single high dose of prednisone. Eur J Clin Pharmacol 49: 37-44

Koopmans R-P, Jonkers RE, Braat MCP, van Boxtel CJ (1995) Pharmacokinetic-pharmacodynamic modelling as applied to bronchial asthma. Clin Pharmacokinet 29: 213-220

Tran Khac Dien, de Vries PJ, Nguyen Xuan Khanh, Koopmans R-P, Le Nguyen Binh, van Boxtel CJ, Dao Dinh Duc, Kager PA (1997) Effect of food intake on pharmacokinetics of oral artemisinin in healthy Vietnamese subjects. Antimicrob Agents Chemother 41: 1069-1072

van Boxtel CJ (1993) Strategies for PMS of new drugs in the EC. Pharmacoepidemiol Drug Safety 2: S7-S10

van den Berg BTJ, Portier EJG, van den Berg M, van Boxtel CJ (1994) First high-performance liquid chromatography assay of formoterol concentrations in the low pg/ml range. Ther Drug Monit 16: 196-199

van den Berg BTJ, Smeets JJ, van Boxtel CJ, Maesen FPV (1995) Evaluation of different doses of formoterol from a newly developed powder inhalation device in asthmatic patients. Fundam Clin Pharmacol 9: 593-603

The Netherlands Cancer Institute-Antoni van Leeuwenhoek Hospital
The training in Clinical Pharmacology is certified by the Dutch Society for Clinical Pharmacology and Biopharmacy. The Netherlands Cancer Institute is a specialized oncology center with approximately 200 beds and a large outpatient clinic for solid tumor as well as hematologic malignancies. There is strong interest in early clinical and pharmacologic studies with anticancer agents, which studies are actively supported by bioanalysis and pharmacokinetics in the Pharmacy Department. There are close links with the other more fundamental research divisions of the institute, such as the division of Experimental Therapy, focused on translational research, and the division of Molecular Biology.

Training takes place in the clinic, under the supervision of Professor Jan H.M. Schellens, MD PhD and in the laboratory of the Pharmacy department, which is headed by Professor Jos H. Beijnen, PhD.

Main research interests are clinical pharmacology, bioanalysis, pharmacokinetics, pharmacodynamics, population pharmacokinetics and -dynamics, drug formulation and biotransformation *in vitro* and *in vivo*.

There are close links with the Slotervaart Hospital which is a medium size regional hospital. There is a research network for early clinical studies initiated by the Netherlands Cancer Institute, which consists of the Netherlands Cancer Institute, the University Hospital Utrecht and the Medical Spectrum Twente, which is a large regional hospital.

There are close links with the Faculty of Pharmacy of the University Utrecht, where JH Beijnen and JHM Schellens both hold a professorship.

Leiden
The clinical pharmacology department at Leiden University Centre is part of the Leiden Amsterdam Center for Drug Research, a multidisciplinary academic institute and is integrated in CHDR, a non-profit drug research unit in Leiden.

Training in all aspects of clinical pharmacology can be provided. The department is not registered as an official training site by the Dutch Society for Clinical Pharmacology but an application for this is pending.

The research programme involves cardiocascular and CNS human pharmacology with healthy volunteers and patients as subjects.

The research facilities for human studies are custom built in 1994 and offer full possibilities for pharmacokinetic and dynamic research in man. Collaborations with numerous clinical departments of the Leiden University Medical Center are in existence for studies in patients.

Leiden University has the full range of faculties, including all science subjects and all medical subjects. The Leiden Amsterdam Centre for Drug research integrates the preclinical disciplines involved in drug research and human clinical pharmacological research, and teaching is co-ordinated by the Centre for Human Drug Research (CHDR).

The staff consists of physicians, specialized nursing staff, pharmacological scientists, a statistician-pharmacokineticist, a computer system analyst and secretarial staff. The department is headed by Professor AF Cohen, MD, PhD, FFPM. Senior staff members are Dr J van Gerven MD PhD, senior lecturer and dr K Burggraaf MD, PhD, lecturer.

Enquiries: please contact Professor AF Cohen or Dr J van Gerven.

References

Boer Ad, Kluft C, Gerloff J, Dooyewaard G, Gunzler WA, Beier H, Meer FJMv, Cohen AF (1993) Pharmacokinetics of saruplase, a recombinant unglycosylated human single-chain urokinase-type plasminogen activator and its effects on fibrinolytic and haemostatic parameters in healthy male subjects. Thromb Haemostas 70 (2): 320-325

Cohen AF, Kroon JM, Schoemaker HC, Breimer DD, Vliet-Verbeek Av, Brandenburg HC (1993) The bioavailability of digoxin from three oral formulations measured by a specific HPLC assay. Br J Clin Pharmacol 35: 136-142

Gerven JMAv, Schoemaker HC, Jacobs L-D, Reint A, Ouwersloot-v.d.Meij MJ, Hoedemaker HGJ, Cohen AF (1996) Self-medication of a single headache episode with ketoprofen, ibuprofen or placebo, home-monitored with an electronic patient diary. Br J Clin Pharmacol 42: 475-481

Griensven JMTv, Jusko WJ, Lemkes HHPJ, Kroon JM, Verhorst CJ, Chiang ST, Cohen AF (1995) Tolrestat pharmacokinetics and pharmacodynamic effects on red blood cell sorbitol in normal volunteers and insulin-dependent diabetics. Clin Pharmacol Ther 58: 631-640

Griensven JMTv, Huisman L, Stuurman T, Dooijewaard G, Kroon JM, Schoemaker HC, Kluft C, Cohen AF (1996) Effects of increased liver blood flow on the kinetics and dynamics of recombinant tissue-type plasminogen activator. Clin Pharmacol Ther 60: 504-511

Hollander AAMJ, Rooij Jv, Lentjes EGWM, Arbouw F, Bree Jv, Schoemaker HC, Es LAv, Woude FJv, Cohen AF (1995) The effect of grapefruit juice on cyclosporine metabolism in transplant patients. Clin Pharmacol Ther 57: 318-324

Koster RW, Cohen AF, Hopkins G, Beier H, Gunzler WA, Wouw PAv (1994) Pharmacokinetics and pharmacodynamics of saruplase, an unglycosylated single-chain urokinase-type plasminogen activator, in patients with acute myocardial infarction. Thromb Haemostas 71(5): 740-744

Rooij Jv, Stegen GHDv, Schoemaker HC, Kroon C, Burggraaf J, Hollaar L, Vroon TFFP, Smelt AHM, Cohen AF (1995) A placebo controlled parallel study on the effect of two types of coffee oil on serum-lipids and -transaminases: identification of chemical substances involved in the cholesterol-raising effect of coffee. Am J Clin Nutr 61: 1277-1283

Schoemaker HC, Houwelingen HCv (1994) Repeated measures for two within-subject factors; analysis and missing data solutions. J Biopharmac Stat 4: 173-188

Stevenick ALv, Schoemaker HC, Hartigh Jd, Rijnkels JM, Pieters MSM, Breimer DD, Cohen AF (1994) Effects of intravenous temazepam. I. Saccadic eye movements and electroencephalogram after fast and slow infusion to pseudo steady state. Clin Pharmacol Ther 55: 535-545

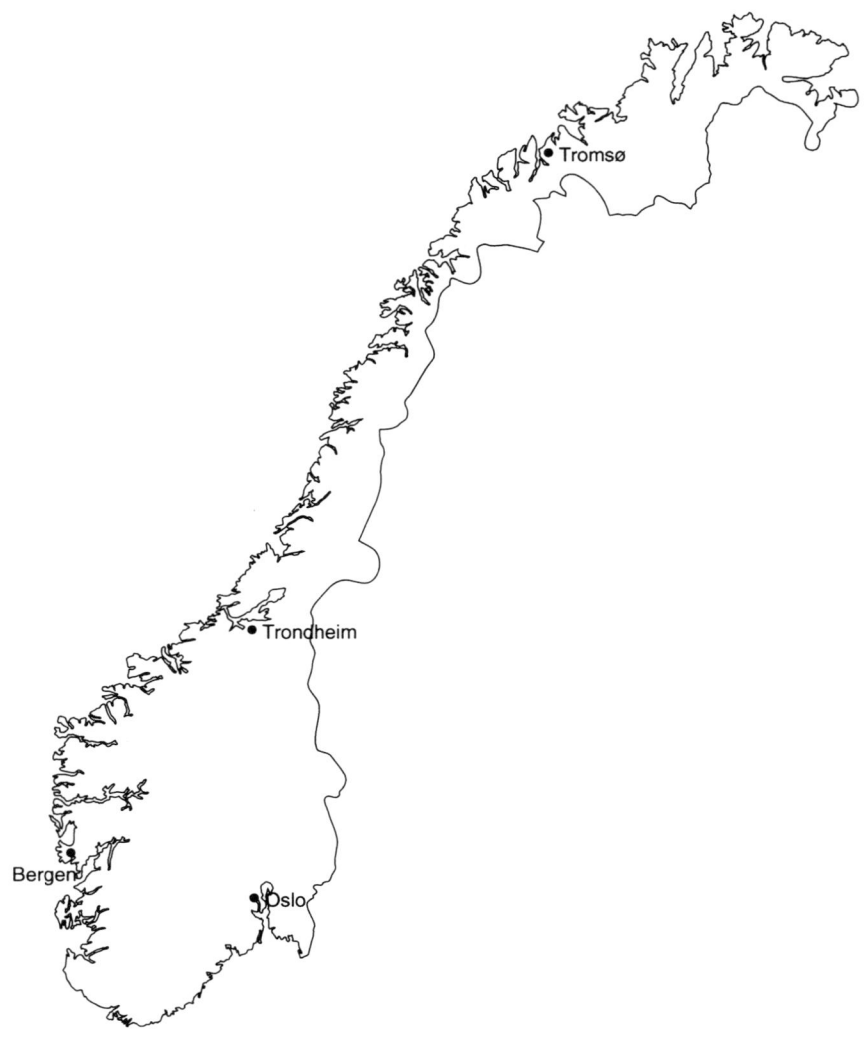

Norway

Clinical pharmacology is formally recognized as a medical speciality. The training lasts 5 years after graduation as an MD. One year must be spent in clinical medicine, and the remainder 4 years in a recognized department of clinical pharmacology. However, up to 2 of the 4 years may be spent at a department or an institute of basic pharmacology. During the training, the trainee follows intensive courses in basic pharmacology, clinical pharmaco-dynamics and clinical pharmacokinetics, clinical trial, pharmacoepidemiology and forensic toxicology. [A detailed training programme (in Norwegian) is available on request at the Norwegian delegate to the council].

The Norwegian Society of Clinical Pharmacology was formally recognized by the Norwegian Medical Association in 1989. In 1995, the total number of members was 40. The tasks of the Society are mainly the same as those of the EACPT, just at the national level. The first department in pharmacotherapy was established in Oslo in 1964. Units or departments in clinical pharmacology were established at all the five university hospitals, including Tromsø, Trondheim, Bergen and two in Oslo during the years 1972-76. More recently, positions in clinical pharmacology have been established at the National Institute of Forensic Toxicology, at the National Cancer Hospital in Oslo and at the Psychiatric Clinic, Vinderen in Oslo.

The course in pharmacology for medical students consists of 70-90 lectures. Teaching in clinical pharmacology is included to a variable extent during the clinical courses. All units or departments in clinical pharmacology are active in the postgraduate training in the subject.

There is no formal relationship between clinical pharmacology and the pharmaceutical industry in Norway. However, through the Norwegian Medical Association, the Society of Clinical Pharmacology receives invitations to participate in relevant committees and propositions. Individual members of the Society may also be members in the different committees of the Drug Regulation Agency.

Addresses

Bergen
Professor P M Ueland
Institute of Pharmacology and
Toxicology
Haukeland Hospital
N-5021 Bergen
Norway

Oslo
Professor O Brørs
Section of Clinical Pharmacology and
Toxicology
Clinical Chemistry Department
Ullevål Hospital
N-0407 Oslo

Professor J Mørland
National Institute of Forensic
Toxicology
P.O. Box 495 Sentrum
N-0105 Oslo
Phone: +47 2204 2700
Fax: +47 2238 3233

Professor H Olsen
Central Laboratory
National Cancer Hospital
Montebello
N-0310 Oslo
Phone: +47 2293 4000
Fax: +47 2273 0725

Professor HE Rugstad
Department of Clinical Pharmacology
Rikshospitalet
N-0027 Oslo

Tromsø
Professor J Aarbakke
Department of Clinical Pharmacology
Regional Hospital in Tromsø
N-9038 Tromsø

Trondheim
Dr T Aamo
Institute of Pharmacology and Toxicology
Medical Technical Centre
Olav Kyrres gate 3
N-7006 Trondheim

Dr T Rygnestad
Institute of Pharmacology and Toxicology
Medical Technical Centre
Olav Kyrres gate 3
N-7006 Trondheim
Phone: +47 7355 0165
Fax: +47 7355 0166
E-mail: Tarjei.Rygnestad@relis.rit.no

Dr O Spigset
Institute of Pharmacology and Toxicology
Medical Technical Centre
Olav Kyrres gate 3
N-7006 Trondheim
Phone: +47 7355 0163
E-mail: olav.spigset@relis.rit.no

Training Centres in Norway

Trondheim

The Section of Clinical Pharmacology at the Regional and University Hospital in Trondheim, Norway is a part of the Department for Pharmacology and Pharmacy, which in addition to Clinical Pharmacology includes the Hospital Pharmacy and the Section for Education, Information and Regional Centre for Registration of Adverse Drug Effects. The Section is staffed with 12 persons, including three physicians (two consultants and one resident), six bioengineers, one technical engineer, one secretary and one laboratory assistant.

At our laboratory, we perform a wide variety of clinical pharmacological analyses, both in TDM, drugs of abuse (screening and verification) and detection and quantification of poisons. At present, we are doing approximately 120 different analyses on a regular basis and our annual total is approximately 55000 analyses (1997).

Our department is recognized as a training institution in clinical pharmacology by the Norwegian Medical Association. To be able to enter the training programme, one has to be recognized as a medical doctor in Norway.

Academic posts at the Section for clinical pharmacology are held at the Institute of Pharmacology and Toxicology at the medical faculty, The Norwegian university of Science and Technology, which was established in 1975. The Faculty admits 90 students annually. At present, there are two persons attached as senior lectures; one in clinical toxicology and one in psychopharmacology. The research activities are focused on SSRIs and clinical toxicological problems.

The department also participates in post-marketing surveillance programmes concerning new psychoactive drugs. The aim is to pick up analytical methods of new drugs in order to participate in the evaluation of the role of TDM in the use of these drugs.

The section will be able to accommodate one trainee or research fellow in clinical pharmacology. Applications can be addressed to the head of department. Applications or plans for funding must be included.

Inquiries to: Dr T Rygnestad

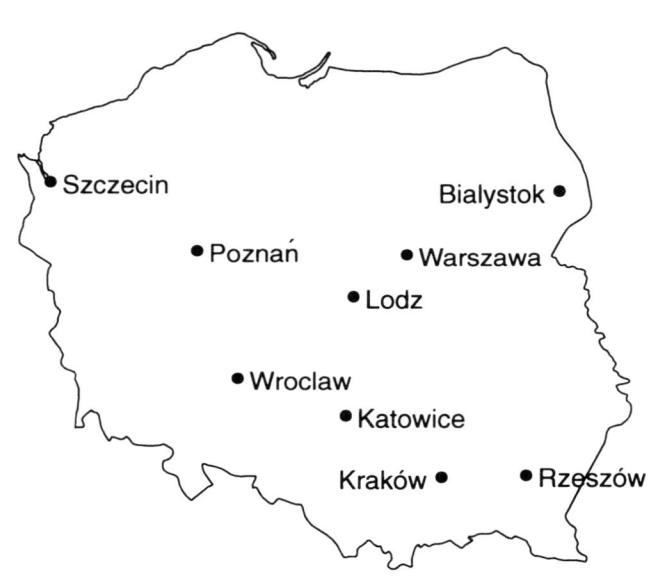

Poland

Clinical pharmacology is an official medical speciality in Poland. To become a specialist in clinical pharmacology, the trainee must initially obtain a first degree specialization in internal medicine, paediatrics, surgery or another clinical speciality. It takes 36 months to become a specialist in clinical pharmacology and this includes 6 weeks spent at an intensive care unit and 6 weeks spent at a therapeutic drug monitoring unit. The training ends with an exam in the following topics: (1) therapy of heart failure, (2) therapy of coronary heart diseases, (3) therapy of hypertension, (4) the clinical pharmacology of the autonomic nervous system, (5) psychotropic drugs, (6) therapy of gastrointestinal diseases, (7) therapy of haematological diseases, (8) anaesthetic drugs, (9) chemotherapy, (10) cronopharmacology

The Section of Clinical Pharmacology in the Polish Society of Pharmacology was established in 1981, and the total number of members was about 40. The Polish Society of Clinical Pharmacology and Therapeutics was established as an independent society in 1996. The Society is presently being organized and new members are being recruited.

There are 12 departments of clinical pharmacology in Poland. Clinical pharmacology is taught to medical students and to students of stomatology during their fifth and fourth year of training, respectively. The course consists of 15 lectures. In addition, clinical pharmacologists in Poland each year organize a series of lectures on selected topics in clinical pharmacology.

The Minister of Health and Social Welfare is responsible for clinical pharmacology. Clinical pharmacology has no formal relationship to the Drug Regulation Agency. Clinical pharmacologists collaborate with the pharmaceutical industry with regard to pharmacokinetic studies.

Addresses

Bialystok
Professor J Braszko
Department of Clinical Pharmacology
ul. Mickiewicza 2c
PL-15-222 Bialystok
Phone: +48 85 22975

Katowice
Professor ZS Herman
Departments of Pharmacology and
Clinical Pharmacology
Silesian Univesity School of Medicine
ul. Medyków 18
PL-40-752 Katowice
Phone: +48 32 2523902

Krakow
Professor E Kostka-Trabka
Department of Clincal Pharmacology
ul. Grzegorzecka 16
PL-31-531 Krakow
Phone: +48 12 211168

Professor J Szymura-Oleksiak
Department of Clinical Pharmacology
ul. Medyczna 9
PL-30-688 Krakow
Phone: +48 12 554021

Lodz
Professor H Adamska-Dyniewska
Department of Clinical Pharmacology
ul. Kniaziewicza 1/5
PL-91-347 Lodz
Phone: +48 42 511059

Professor J Drzewoski
Department of Clinical Pharmacology
ul. Kopcinskiego 22
PL-90-153 Lodz
Phone: +48 42 783172

Poznań
Professor A Mrozikieicz
Department of Clinical Pharmacology
Karol Marcinkowski University of
Medical Sciences
ul. Dluga 1/2
PL-61848 Poznań
Phone: +48 61 521021
Fax: +48 61 529472

Rzeszów
Professor J Splawinski
Department of Clinical Pharmacology
District Hospital no. 2
ul. Lwowska 60
PL-35-301 Rzeszów

Szczecin
Professor J Wójcicki
Department of Clinical Pharmacology
ul. Al. Powstanców Wlkp. 72
PL-70-111 Szczecin
Phone: +48 91 820863

Warszawa
Professor A Czlonkowski
Department of Clinical Pharmacology
ul. Krakowskie Przedmieście 26/28
PL-00-927 Warszawa
Phone: +48 22 262116

Professor A Mazurek
Professor A Czarnecki
Professor J Splawinski
Department of Clinical Pharmacology
ul. Chelmska 30/34
Instytut Lekow
PL-00-725 Warszawa
Phone: +48 22 412940

Wroclaw
Professor K Orzechowska-Juzwenko
Chair of Clinical Pharmacology
ul. Mikulicza – Radeckiego 2
PL-50-368 Wroclaw
Phone: +48 71 216182

Training Centres in Poland

Katowice
Silesian University School of Medicine

The Department of Clinical Pharmacology carries out investigations of the influence of the treatment by neuroleptics and antidepressants in patients (with schizophrenia or depressive illness, respectively) on the activity of macrophages natural killer cells and the level of cytokines in plasma. The release of cytokines by cultured macrophages from hyperlipidaemic or hypertensive patients before, during, after the treatment by hypolipaemic or antihypertensive drugs, respectively.

Enkephalin and neuropeptide level in cerbrospinal fluid of patients after head trauma.

Teaching
The obligations are carried out in practical classes 30 h/semester during 5th year of the medical study. Discussion of individual clinical cases and their pharmacotherapy.

Lectures, 15 h/semester, topics: chemotherapy of infections, selected problems of pharmacotherapy of cardiovascular, gastrointestinal and respiratory diseases, geriatric clinical pharmacology and therapeutics, therapeutic drug monitoring, psychotropic drugs in the hands of the general practitioner, clinically important drug interactions.

The facilities of the department consists of 10 beds in the clinic of internal medicine, equipment for radioimmunoassays, HPLC, equipment for investigations on tissue cultures, molecular biology methods (Southern, Northern blotting), TDx, six computers.

The staff consists of one professor MD, PhD, one professor PhD, one associate professor MD, four doctors MD, three doctors PhD, four technicians and one secretary.

The clinical activities are devoted to drug monitoring, controlled clinical trials, consultations in clinics of University hospitals mainly: internal medicine, surgery, neurosurgery and intensive care.

References
Brunier DP, Herman ZS, Nahler GR (1996) Conducting clinical trials in Poland. Applied Clinical Trials (5): 40-44

Gil D, Hartleb J, Gonciarz Z, Michalski A and Herman Z (1993) Circadian rhythm of human alfa atrial natriuretic peptide in chronic active hepatitis. Arch Gastroenterohepatol 12 (3-4): 150-153.

Golba KS, Deja M, Woś S, Bachowski R, Szalanski, Mrozek R, Herman ZS (1995) Reactivity of isolated human right atria to norepinephrine in various disease states. J Physiol Pharmacol 46 (3): 323-328

Herman ZS (1996) Neuropeptide Y (NPY) and its mRNA in discrete brain areas after subchronic administration of neuroleptics. Acta Neurobiol Exp 56: 55-61

Herman ZS (1997) Minireview: Carbon monoxide: a novel neural messenger or putative neurotransmitter? Pol J Pharmacol 49: 1-4

Herman ZS (1997) Minireview: Agmatine – a novel endogenous ligand of imidazoline receptors. Pol J Pharmacol 49: 85-88

Kowalski J (1997) Effect of enkephalins and endorphins on cytotoxic activity of natural killer cells and macrophages/monocytes in mice. Eur J Pharmacol 326: 251-255

Stachura Z, Kowalski J, Obuchowicz E, Huzarska M, Herman ZS (1997a) Concentration of enkephalins in cerebrospinal fluid of patients after severe head injury. Neuropeptides 31 (1): 78-81

Stachura Z, Obuchowicz E, Herman ZS (1997b) Neuropeptide Y-like immunoreactivity in lumbar cerebrospinal fluid of patients after severe head trauma. Neuropeptides 31 (1): 12-14

Rzeszów

Basic research on antiplatelet drugs. Three lines of research: (1) evaluation of mechanism of antiplatelet drugs, including search for a new thromboxane synthase/receptor inhibitor; (2) synergism of antiplatelet drugs used in clinics; and (3) bioavailability studies. Clinical facilities: outpatient clinic and four clinical beds. Methods: whole blood platelet aggregation, other methods of platelet aggregation, isolation of platelets – human blood, ex vivo and in vitro studies.

Bioavailability of various generics of domestic and foreign origin. Staff: two MDs and two PhDs, one technical help and nurses employed according to needs. Training offered: (1) research on activity of drugs on human platelets, (2) active participation in bioavailability and bioequivalence (based on pharmacodynamics) studies, including (in details): protocol, basic statistics, and measurements of plasma levels. Food ($ 10/day), accommodation ($20/day) at the hospital. Apply to Professor J. Splawinski, District Hospital no. 2.

Wroclaw

Wroclaw University of Medicine

The scientific and teaching staff of the department consists of three physicians (two are specialists of internal diseases, one of them is a specialist of anaesthesiology), four pharmacists [two (PhDs) are specialists of II degree of clinical pharmacy], one biologist.

Chair and Department of Clinical Pharmacology consists of three main laboratories
- Laboratory of pharmacogenetics.
- Laboratory of clinical pharmacokinetics.
- Laboratory of therapeutic drug monitoring.

The department carries out clinical-pharmacological studies primarily concerning problems of individualization and hence the optimalization of pharmacotherapy. Studies on pharmacogenetics, pharmacokinetics, patopharmacokinetics, especially drug biotransformation problems, therapeutic drug monitoring, monitoring of drug unwanted effects, liver and kidney function during pharmacotherapy and effects of drug interactions.

In more detail, the scientific activity of the Department consists of
a Pharmacogenetic studies on the genetically determined drug oxidation and acetylation polymorphism in a Polish population, in neoplastic and allergic diseases in psychiatric and neurological pathological syndromes, during antiarrhythmic and psychotropic drug treatment.
b Studies on phenazone kinetics as a marker of metabolic efficiency of the liver in neoplastic diseases, under the influence of the environmental factors, in endocrinopathies, in hepatic and renal insufficiency before and after pharmacotherapy, monitoring of liver and kidney function during antineoplastic and cardiac drug treatment.
c Studies on practical aspects of therapeutic drug concentration monitoring of such drugs as methotrexate, antiepileptic drug (especially in children), digoxin, aminoglycosides, theophylline, cyclosporine.
d Studies on angiotensin converting enzyme inhibitors interactions.

The Department co-operates very closely with the hematological, oncological, nephrological, urological, endocrinological, cardiological, psychiatric, neurological, internal, paediatric and allergological, anaesthesiological and intensive care clinics and various hospital wards in the region of Wrocaw regarding research and the provision of information and health service.

The Department is involved in lectures, seminars, classes for sixth year medical and fifth year pharmacy students are carried out and postgraduate courses, lectures, round table conferences, seminars in clinical pharmacology are organized for physicians of different specialities and for pharmacists.

The main training topics
- Practical aspects on pharmacokinetics.
- Individualization of pharmacotherapy/pharmacotherapy in the elderly, in children, in pregnant and lactating women, in hepatic and renal insufficiency, clinical significance of drug interactions, of pharmacogenetic, chronopharmacology, therapeutic drug monitoring.
- Drug side effects.
- Clinical trials on new drugs according to GCP and their ethical aspects.

References

Orzechowska-Juzwenko K (1997) Basis of Clinical Pharmacology. Volumed, Wrocaw

Orzechowska-Juzwenko K, Pawlik J, Niewinski P, Milejski P, Dembowski J, Turek J, Godzik A, Swiebodcki L, Hora Z (1994a) Genetically determined sparteine oxidation polymorphism in a polish population. Eur J Clin Pharmacol 5(46): 481

Orzechowska-Juzwenko K, Niewiski P, Pawlik J, Milejski P, Dembowski J, Swiebodcki L, Lorenz J (1994b) Genetically determined sparteine oxidation and sulfadimidine acetylation polymorphism in patients with non occupational urinary bladder cancer. Materia Medicina Polona 26: 145

Orzechowska-Juzwenko K, Jawiska-Tarnawska E, Niewinski P, Loboz-Grudzie K, Rzemisawska Z, Dmochowska-Perz M, Sawin J (1995) Evaluation of the influence of oxidation phenotype serum concentration of propafenone and its metabolite on antiarrhythmic efficacy in patients with atrial fibrillation in long term therapy: Eur J Clin Pharmacol 49: A159

Orzechowska-Juzwenko K, Niewinski P, Cieliski P, Milejski P, Hudziec P, Ziemba B, Pajk K, Hurkacz M, Rzemisawska Z (1997a) Evaluation of genetically determined sparteine oxidation and sulfadimidine acetylation polymorphism in women with breast cancer. The Breast 6: 38

Orzechowska-Juzwenko K, Jawiska-Tarnawska E, Hurkacz M, Loboz-Grudzie K (1997b) Monitorowanie czynnoci nerek u chorych na samoistne nadcinienie ttnicze leczonych enalaprylem. Pol Arch Med Wewn 1: 15-21

Wiela-Hojeska A, Orzechowska-Juzwenko K, Sociak M, Unolt J, Hurkacz M, Bogusawska-Jaworska J (1995) High dose methotrexate treatment in children with osteogeneic sarcoma. Ther Drug Monit 17: 403

Wiela-Hojeska A, Sociak M, Orzechowksa-Juzwenko K, Bogusawska-Jaworska J, Unolt J, Adamska M (1996) Leczenie rednio duymi i duymi dawkami metotreksatu u dzieci z chorobami nowotworowymi ukadu krwiotworczego. Acta Haematologica Polona 27: 309

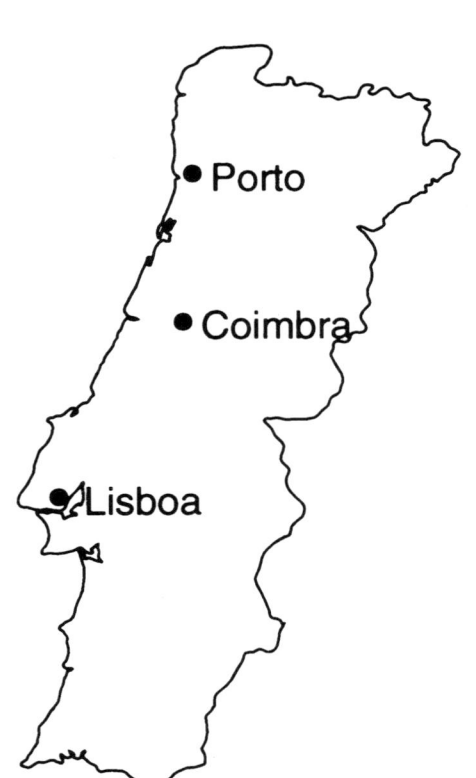

Portugal

Clinical pharmacology became an official medical speciality in Portugal in 1993. The first requirement is to spend 2 years in basic pharmacology at the Department of Pharmacology of the Medical Faculty. After that, the trainee must follow a training programme of 2 years in various clinical disciplines, including internal medicine, cardiology and paediatrics.

In addition to a chair in pharmacology and therapeutics, a separate chair in clinical pharmacology has been established at the University of Coimbra, where clinical pharmacology is taught to the medical students during their final year. Recently, a new Department of Clinical Pharmacology has been established at the Medical Faculty of the University of Oporto. Postgraduate training in clinical pharmacology is also given to both physicians working in hospitals and in the pharmaceutical industry.

The Portuguese Association of Clinical Pharmacology (PACP) is composed of 52 clinical pharmacologists and physicians working in the pharmaceutical industry. The Association held its first two national meetings in 1996, and on this occasion both scientific and administrative matters were discussed. There is a protocol describing the collaboration between the Portuguese Association of Clinical Pharmacology and the Portuguese Pharmacological Society.

Addresses

Coimbra
Professor Frederico Teixeira
Institute of Pharmacology and Experimental Therapeutics
Faculty of Medicine
University of Coimbra
3000 Coimbra
Phone: +351 39 37708
Fax: +351 39 36200

Lisboa
Dr Miguel APC Vigeant Gomes
R. Alfonso Albuquerque, 6
2765 Estoril

Porto
Professor Jorge Polónia
Institute of Pharmacology and Therapeutics
Faculty of Medicine
University of Porto
4200 Porto

REPUBLIC OF IRELAND

Clinical Pharmacology and Therapeutics in the Republic of Ireland has for many years been regulated by the Joint Committee on Higher Medical Training comprising the three Royal Colleges of Physicians in the United Kingdom and the Royal College of Physicians of Ireland. The criteria for entry into training and curriculum and structure are therefore similar to those of the United Kingdom and are described in that section.

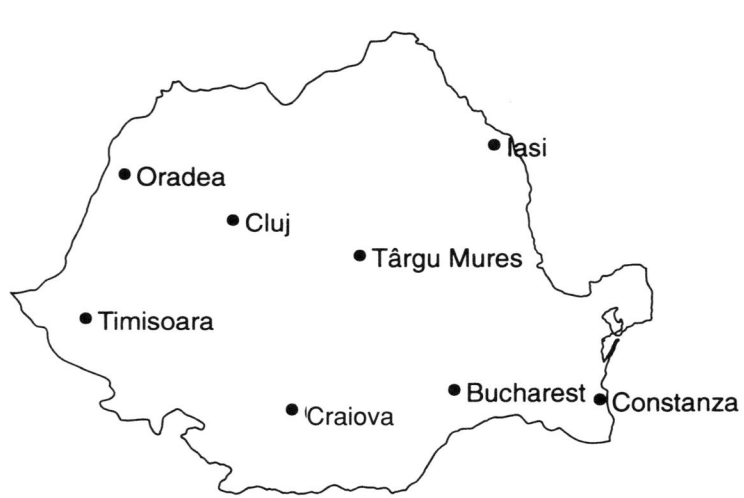

Romania

Clinical pharmacology is not recognized as an independent speciality in Romania, but rather as an area of expertise for physicians who are specialists in one of 23 clinical specialities such as internal medicine, surgery and paediatrics. To become an expert in clinical pharmacology requires an additional training for 6 months. The training programme in clinical pharmacology consists of lectures, workshops and daily clinical practice.

In 1980, the Romanian Society of Pharmacology and Therapeutics emerged from the Society of Physiology and Pharmacology, but last year this society was transformed to the Romanian Society of Pharmacology, Therapeutics and Toxicology. The members are pharmacologists, clinical toxicologists and clinicians with a main interest in therapeutics. The total number of members is around 100, and the Society is affiliated to the Romanian Medical Association. The Society organizes scientific activities in the field of experimental pharmacology, clinical pharmacology, therapeutics and clinical toxicology. Another important task is to be responsible for the postgraduate training in clinical pharmacology. There are bonds to several other scientific societies under the Romanian Medical Association.

There are chairs in pharmacology but no separate chairs in clinical pharmacology at the medical faculties in Bucarest, Cluj, Iasi, Timisoara, Târgu Mures, Oradea and Constanza. The undergraduate teaching of medical students comprises both experimental and clinical pharmacology. However, before 1985, the teaching did not include clinical pharmacology. This was changed so that now 120 lectures in basic pharmacology are given in the third year of the medical study while a series of 20-30 lectures in clinical pharmacology is given in the fourth year. The teaching in clinical pharmacology is integrated in the various modules of internal medicine. The programme for the undergraduate training in clinical pharmacology shows some variability among the different chairs. Clinical pharmacology is also offered to physicians during their postgraduate training.

The Romanian Minister of Education is resposnsible for the undergraduate teaching in clinical pharmacology, and the Minister of Health is responsible for the postgraduate training in the discipline. All of the chairs in pharmacology have direct connections to the Pharmaceutical Direction of the Health Minister, the Institute of Drug Control, the Drug Commission and the pharmaceutical industry in Romania.

Addresses

Bucharest
Professor V Stoescu
Universitatea de Medicina Si Farmacie
Bucharest
Facultatea de Medicina, Catera de Farmacologie
Bd. Eroii Sanitari nr. 8
76241 Bucharest
Phone: +40 1 638 3010/167
Fax: +40 1 311 0984
E-mail: ifulga@univermed-cdgm.ro

Professor E Manolescu
Universitatea de Midicinä si Farmacie
Bucaresti
Facultatea de Medicina, Catedra de Farmacologie
Bd. Eroii Sanitari nr. 8
76241 Bucharest

Professor V Voicu
Universitatea de Medicina Si Farmacie
Bucaresti
Facultatea de Medicina
Clinical de Toxicologie
Spitalul de Urgenta
Calea Floreasca nr. 8
Bucharest
Phone: +40 1 212 0107/219
Fax: +40 1 311 2993
E-mail: ifulga@univermed-cdgm.ro

Cluj
Conf Dr V Sandor
Universitatea de Medicina Si Farmacie
Cluj
Catedra de Farmacologie
Str. E. Grigorescu nr. 2-4
Cluj
Phone: +40 6442 0552
Fax: +40 6442 0552

Constanza
Conf Dr St Surdulescu
Universitatea Ovidius Constanza
Facultatea de Medicina
Catedra de Farmacologie
St. Ion Voda nr. 58
Constanza
Phone: +40 4163 5800/14

Craiova
Conf Dr Valentin Cârlig
Universitatea de Medicina si Farmacie
Craiova
Catedra de Farmacologie
Str. Petru Rares nr. 4
Craiova

Iasi
Professor O Mungiu
Universitatea de Medicina Si Farmacie
Iasi

Catedra de Farmacologie
Str. Universitazii nr. 19
Iasi
Phone: +40 3211 6104
Fax: +40 3221 1820

Oradea
Professor B Cuparencu
Universitatea de Medicina Si Farmacie
Oradea
Catedra de Farmacologie
Str. Vaida Voievod nr. 5
Oradea
Phone: +40 5942 7350

Timisoara
Professor I Gligor
Institutul de Medicina Timisoara
Catedra de Farmacologie
Piaza Eftimie Murgu nr. 2
Timisoara
Phone: +40 5613 7612

Târgu Mures
Conf Dr M Monea
Universitatea de Medicina Si Farmacie
Târgu Mures
Catedra de Farmacologie
Str. Gh. Marinescu nr. 38
Târgu Mures
Phone: +40 6513 2813

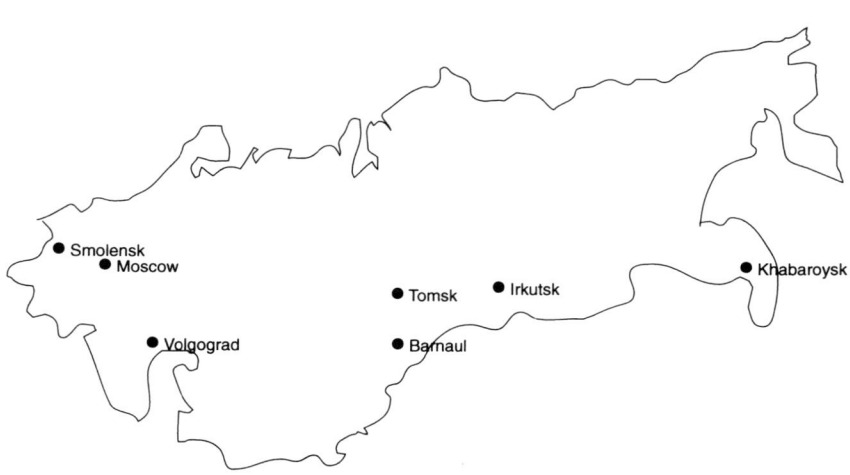

Russia

Clinical pharmacology was officially recognized as an independent medical speciality in 1982. Trainees need 3 years of clinical training after they have obtained their MD degree. Besides, they must have followed a series of separate courses in clinical pharmacology. Once the candidate has performed a series of postgraduate studies in clinical pharmacology and has defended a candidate thesis, he or she is recognized as a scientist in the area. However, the highest scientific level in clinical pharmacology is achieved through a doctoral thesis. In 1984, a Section of Clinical pharmacology was established within the Russian Pharmacological Society. The chairman of the Section is vice chairman of the Society. In 1995, an independent Society of Pharmacology and Therapeutics was established.

Clinical pharmacology is taught at 44 medical schools, several universities and at all the institutes of pharmacology. Research in clinical pharmacology is carried out both at the majority of the research institutes of the Russian Academy of Medical Sciences as well as by the Russian Health Ministry.

A course consisting of 54 lectures in clinical pharmacology is given during the fifth year of the medical study. Clinical pharmacology is also a separate course of 92 lectures during the fourth year in the schools of pharmacy. During the course in clinical pharmacology at the medical schools, the following items are reviewed

- The general principles of clinical pharmacology
- Adverse drug reactions and drug-drug interactions
- Pharmacodynamics and pharmacokinetics.

The course aims at teaching the students how to select the most effective and safe drug in the right dose for the treatment of a particular disorder and to carry out dose adjustment in accordance with either the pharmacological effects or the pharmacokinetic parameters of the drug. The mechanism of action, indications and contra-indications, dosage and dose adjustment of the individual classes of drugs are taught during the course in internal medicine. Since 1982, a commission within the Ministry of Health has evaluated the quality of the teaching in clinical pharmacology. Every second year, there is a conference dealing with new methods of teaching and development in the subject.

Most of the medical schools in Russia also organize postgraduate courses in clinical pharmacology and therapeutics that typically last 3-6 weeks.

Addresses

Barnaul
Professor N Sidorenskova
Altaisky State Medical University
pr. Lenina 40
656099 Barnaul
Phone: +7 3852 225913
Fax: +7 3852 244792
E-mail: capital@barrt.ru

Irkutsk
Dr L Muller
Irkutsky Medical Institute
st Krasnogo vosstaniya 1
664003 Irkutsk
Phone: +7 246777

Khabarovsk
S Suleimanov
Chabarovsky Medical Institute
st K. marksa 35
680000 Khabarovsk

Moscow
Professor VG Kukes
Russian Associations of Pharmacologists
Department of Clinical Pharmacology
Moscow Medical Academy
Petrovsky Blvd., 8
103051 Moscow
Phone: +7 95 200 2791
Fax: +7 95 209 6858
E-mail: nii_tml@mail.sitek.ru

Professor LI Olbinskaya
Department of Clinical Pharmacology and Pharmacotherapy
Moscow Medical Sechenov Academy
Bolshaya Pirogovskaya 2/6
119881 Moscow – Russia
Phone: +7 957 248 75 44
Fax: +7 957 239 25 53
E-mail: gofman@gofman.com

Smolensk
Professor L Stratchounsky
Smolensk State Medical Academy
Department of Clinical Pharmacology and Antimicrobial Chemotherapy
P.O. Box 5
Smolensk 19
214019 Russia
Phone: +7 812 553401 or 552327
Fax: +7 812 550624
E-mail: cliph@iph.smolensk.rospack.ru

Tomsk
Dr E Goldberg
Tomsky Institute of Pharmacology
pr. Lenina 3
634028 Tomsk
Phone: +7 418379

Volgograd
V.I. Petrov
Department of Clinical Pharmacology
Square of Pavshikh Borcov 1
400 066 Volgograd
Russia
Fax: + 7 (-) 33 68 00

Training Centres in Russia

Moscow
Moscow Medical Academy
Training school for doctors and research pharmacodynamics programme. Three hundred clinic beds, pharmacodynamic laboratory, ECG, ultrasound, bicycle exercise testing, Holter and ambulatory blood pressure monitoring devices.

The staff consists of five MD professors, five docents, eight assistants, postgraduates, doctors.

Training in general questions of pharmacokinetics, pharmacodynamics; pharmacokinetic and pharmacodynamic of cardiovascular drugs, pulmonary drugs, gastrointestinal drugs.

Application procedures: directly contact with Professor VG Kukes.

References
Olbinskaya LI (1993) Influence of benazepril and captopril on blood pressure, glucocorticoides and progesterone in essential hypertensives. J Human Hypertension 7: 603-606
Olbinskaya LI (1994) Influence of smoking and coffee on 24-h blood pressure and its variability in essential hypertensives. J Ambualtory Monitoring 7 (2): 143
Olbinskaya LI (1995a) Neurohormonal activity and electrolyte balance in essential hypertension with and without heart failure. J Heart Failure 2 (1): 487
Olbinskaya LI (1995b) Heart failure: kidney kinines mechanism of management. J Heart Failure 2 (1): 1143
Olbinskaya LI (1995c) Has captopril the antiischemic effects? In: New trends in atherosclerosis, vascular diseases and cardiovascular therapy, Monte Carlo p. 127
Olbinskaya LI (1997) Indapamide as one of the modern diuretics in the treatment of hypertension. J Hypertension 15 (Suppl. 4): 175

Smolensk

Research programme
- clinical pharmacology of antibiotics
- pharmacoepidemiology of antibacterials
  pharmacoeconomics of antibacterials
  epidemiology and antibiotic resistance of respiratory pathogens
  epidemiology and resistance of gram-negative nosocomial bacteria

Training programme: clinical pharmacology – general course
Clinical and research facilities: the department is situated at Smolensk Regional Clinical Hospital (1400 beds) and has close working relationships with other hospitals of our city.

The laboratory of the Hospital for routine biochemistry, haematology and urine analysis, is certified by Russian and International external Quality Assurance – NEQAS (UK), INSTAND (Germany).

The laboratory is a well-equipped facility for HPLC, EMIT, clinical microbiology, analytical gel electrophoresis, PCR.

The university: Smolensk State Medical Academy was founded in 1924. More than 3,000 students study in four faculties (General, Paediatric, Dentologist and Postgraduate).

Staff: Clinical Research Group, Clinical Microbiology Research Group, Molecular Biology and Pharmacokinetics Laboratory.

Application procedure: directly or through Local Healthcare Authorities, inquiries to Professor Leonid S. Stratchounski, MD, PhD.

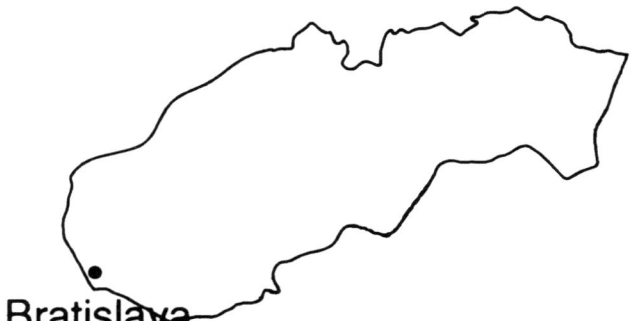

Slovakia

Clinical pharmacology has been an independent medical speciality since 1979. The recognition was given by the Ministry of Health. The training in clinical pharmacology lasts 5 years. After having obtained their MD degree, the trainees must first work for 3 years in either internal medicine or paediatrics. This is followed by 3 years of specialized training in clinical pharmacology organized by the Subchair of Clinical Pharmacology at the Postgraduate School of Medicine in Bratislava. The theoretical part of the specialized training consists of both lectures and courses in clinical pharmacology, and the practical part consists of active participation in the service at one of the recognized departments of clinical pharmacology in Bratislava. The 2 years also comprises a short stay in the Department of Pharmacology at the University. The training is ended by a board examination.

The Slovak Society of Clinical Pharmacology was established in 1990 through the efforts of several members from the Pharmacological as well as Internal Medicine Societies. The Society presently has about 180 members. The Society organizes an annual conference, the seminar 'Medicamenta Nova' and one or two meetings where actual problems of drug policy is discussed. The main tasks of the Society is to stimulate research in drug development and evaluation, research in outcome measures but also promote the input of clinical pharmacology in the health care delivery In order to meet these challenges, the Slovak Society of Clinical Pharmacology has established a close collaboration with its sister societies of pharmacology and of internal medicine. There is a very strong need to improve the collaboration with primary health care physicians. The health care system in Slovakia is presently undergoing big changes, and the Society of Clinical Pharmacology together with the Ministry of Health and the Drug Regulation Agency is very active in the formulating of a drug policy.

The first subchair in clinical pharmacology was established at the Postgraduate Medical School in Bratislava in 1979. The next subchair in clinical pharmacology was established in 1990 at the School of

Medicine at the Comenius University in 1990. Teaching in clinical pharmacology is provided during the fifth year of the medical study, and the course consists of 24 lectures. A similar course is provided at the School of Pharmacy.

There is one in-patient department of clinical pharmacology at the Institute of Preventive and Clinical Medicine in Bratislava. The department houses the chair in clinical pharmacology at the Postgraduate school of Medicine. The department is involved in phase I-III trials. In addition to the in-patient department, there are four out-patient departments in Bratislava and five out-patient departments in the regional hospitals.

The Minister of Health is responsible for the further development of the discipline, but clinical pharmacology is only supported with small grants from the Slovak government. The Society of Clinical Pharmacology collaborates with the State Institute for Drug Control, which serves as the national drug regulation agency. The collaboration with the pharmaceutical industry is expanding in these years.

Addresses

Bratislava
Assistant Professor L Boňeková
Department of Clinical Pharmacology
Faculty of Medicine
Comenius University
Sasinkova 4
813 76 Bratislava
Slovak Republic
Phone: +421 7 5357 232
Fax: +421 7 5357 508

Professor Dzúrik
Department of Clinical Pharmacology
Institute Preventive and Clinical Medicine
Limbová 14
833 01 Bratislava
Slovak Republic
Phone: +421 7 4379 411
Fax: +421 7 3739 06

Assistant Professor J Holomán
Chair of Clinical Pharmacology
Postgraduate Medical School
Limbová 12
833 03 Bratislava
Slovakia
Phone: +421 7 378 9245
Fax: +421 7 373906, 373739
E-mail: HOLOMAN@UPKM.SANET.SK

Professor M Kriska
Division of Clinical Pharmacology
Institute of Pharmacology
School of Medicine
Comenius University
Sasinkova 4
813 76 Bratislava
Phone: +421 7 5357 232
Fax: +421 7 5358 508
E-mail: kriska@fmed.uniba.sk

Training Centres in Slovakia

Bratislava
Comenius University – School of Medicine
The Division of Clinical Pharmacology constitutes a part of the Institute of Pharmacology, School of Medicine, Comenius University. The division fulfils the educational, scientific and expert requirements of the University and of the Ministry of Health. The main fields of its activity are education and research.

The basic educational programme of the division is pregraduate teaching of clinical pharmacology. It consists of lectures, seminars and courses provided not only for pregraduate but also for postgraduate education. The main priority of the research activity is drug risk evaluation, pharmacogenetics and certain problems of pharmacokinetics. The research and training programme leads to PhD and DSc degrees as well as to specialization in clinical pharmacology.

The core staff consists of one professor, one associate professor, one chemical analyst and one technical assistant.

An important component of the decision is presented by National Drug Information Centre designed for providing drug information to all parts of Slovakia.

References
Brandsteterová E, Romanová D, Králiková D, Boñeková L, Kriska M (1994a) Possibilities of SPE-HPLC for clinical important compounds and in pharmacokinetics. Intern Symposium on Instrumental Analysis, Düsseldorf

Brandsteterová E, Kubalec P, Králiková D, Boñeková L, Kriska M (1994b) On-line SPE-HPLC in Pharmacology. ISPP 94, Heidelberg, Germany

Brandsteterová E, Kubalec P, Králiková D, Boñeková L, Kriska M (1994c) Automatic SPE and PHLC of quinidine in plasma. J Chromatogr A 665: 101-104

Kriska M, Boñeková L, P. Gibala (1993) The problem of risk evaluation in antimicrobial drug usage. Abstracts from 6th Interscience symposium on chemotherapy of infection is compromised Host. An official satellite of 18-IOC Stockholm, Smolenice Júl s. 14

Kriska M, Boñeková L, HolomáÁ J, Gibala P (1995) Drug risk evaluation – the role of teaching centres. Thérapie, Suppl. Abstracts of EACPT 1995/1st Congress of the European Association for Clinical Pharmacology and Therapeutics/Paris, France 27-30 Sept. 1995, 140

Chair of Clinical Pharmacology of the Postgraduate Medical School (CCP PMS)
The Subchair is involved in clinical trials (phase I-III), studies on fibrogenesis in chronic liver diseases and hepatopharmacology
The training programme consists of the following items
- Postgraduate education and training in clinical pharmacology (speciality degree in clinical pharmacology).
- Clinical pharmacokinetics.
- Specialized intensive courses in clinical pharmacology and pharmacotherapy.
- Good Clinical Practice – with special regard to applications in hepatology, gastroenterology, nephrology and cardiovascular diseases.

Our clinical and research facilities are confined to the Clinic of Pharmacotherapy of the Institute of Preventive and Clinical Medicine (IPCM) (in- and out-patient) and we are also collaborating with the laboratories of IPCM

Our core staff is made Subchair of Clinical Pharmacology and one associate Professor (medicine – clinical pharmacology) and one second assistant professor (medicine – clinical pharmacology).

We collaborate with researchers and experts from the following institutions: Clinic of Pharmacotherapy (IPCM), Institute of Preventive and Clinical Medicine, Institute of Pharmacology, Faculty of Medicine CU, Slovak Academy of Sciences, National Institute for Drug Control, Ministry of Health and the pharmaceutical industry.

Procedures for applications about training opportunities: the Head of the Department, Assistant Professor J HolomáÁ, should be contacted.

References
Glasa J, Holomán J, Klepanec J, Šoltés L (1996a) Ethics committees and achievment of good clinical practice. Thérapie, 51: s. 269-372

Glasa J, Kaščák M, Holomán J (1996b) Nová klasifikácia chronickej hepatitídy./New classification of chronic hepatitis. Lek. Obzor (Bratislava), 3: p. 71-75

Holomán J (1994) Good Clinical Practice in Hepatology. 1st International Symposium 'Liver and Drugs', Bratislava, Nov. 24-26, GS4, Book of Abstracts

Holomán J (1995) Alcoholism and Alcoholic Liver Injury – Worldwide Problem. EASL Joint International Postgraduate Course in Hepatology, Stará Lesná (Vysoké Tatry), 25-26 May. Course Book and Book of Abstracts

Holomán J, Glasa J (1995) Teaching clinical pharmacology – Postgraduate or continuous education: Missed opportunity? Thérapie, suplément (Abstracts of AECPT), 208

Holomán J, Glasa J (eds), Bechtel PR, Tiribelli C (guest eds.)(1995) Liver and Drugs '94, Progress in Hepato – Pharmacology, Vol. 1, 333 pp, Liver and Drug Fdn., Bratislava

Holomán J, Glasa J (eds), Gangl A, Fehér J (guest eds) (1997a) Liver and Drugs '96 – Cholestatic Liver Diseases, Progress in Hepato-Pharmacology, Vol. 2, 125 pp., Liver and Drug Federation, Bratislava

Holomán J, Glasa J, Veningerová M, Prachár V, Trnovec T (1997b) Genetic polymorphism of sparteine oxidation – occurrence in healthy volunteers in Slovakia. Bratisl. Lek. Listy, 98: p. 89-90

Institute of Preventive and Clinical Medicine

Department of Clinical Pharmacology constitutes a part of the Institute of Preventive and Clinical Medicine (IPCM), which belongs to the Ministry or Health of the Slovak republic and fulfils the scientific, educational and expert requirements of the Ministry of Health on the basis of grants. The department performs the ambulatory and counselling activity, and it also shares a 24-bed ward participating in curative, educational and research activity. The department is also a site of the Subchair of Clinical Pharmacology at the Postgraduate School of Medicine.

The research and training programme of internal members leads to a PhD and DSc degree as well as specialization in clinical pharmacology. The external members stay at the department during the courses, and in addition to signing lectures and seminars they also participate in the visits and the daily life of the department. The training/educational programme is defined by the law and precised by the Postgraduate Medical School.

The IPCM does not belong to any university. However, the members give lectures at the Comenius University in Bratislava, University in Trnava and Medical School in Martin.

The staff consists of one professor, one associate professor, three fully qualified clinical pharmacologists and five residents in clinical pharmacology. Moreover, a biochemical laboratory which is a part of the Department performs not only standard and non-standard clinical biochemistry and clinical pharmacology analyses but also experiments on experimental animals. The preclinical studies are performed primarily to elucidate unexpected findings in the clinical phase of drug development. All four phases of clinical trials are performed with full respect to GCP and GLP criteria and under the auspices of Institutional Review Board.

References

Dubovská D et al. (1995) Pharmacokinetics of acetylsalicylic acid and its metabolites at low doses: A compartmental modeling. Meth Find Exp Clin Pharmacol 17: 67-77

Dzúrik R (1994) Drug registration procedures in Slovakia. Eur J Clin Res 6: 358-363

Dzúrik R, Trnovec T (eds) (1997) Standard Therapeutic Procedures (guidelines, in Slovak) pp 974

Dzúrik R et al. (1995) The prevalence of insulin resistance in kidney diseases. Nephron, 69: 281-285

Okša A et al. (1994) Effects of angiotensin-converting enzyme inhibitors on glucose and lipid metabolism in essential hypertension. J Cardiovasc Pharmacol 23: 79-86

Šebeková K et al. (1996a) Inhibition of glucose uptake by 5-hydroxyindolacetic acid in the isolated rat soleus muscle. Int Urol Nephrol 28: 123-131

Šebeková K et al. (1996b) 31P NMR spectroscopy investigation of free magnesium concentration and intracellular pH in skeletal muscle of patients with essential hypertension with or without insulin resistance. In Halpern MJ (ed). Current Research in Magnesium. Libbey & Co, London, pp. 21-23

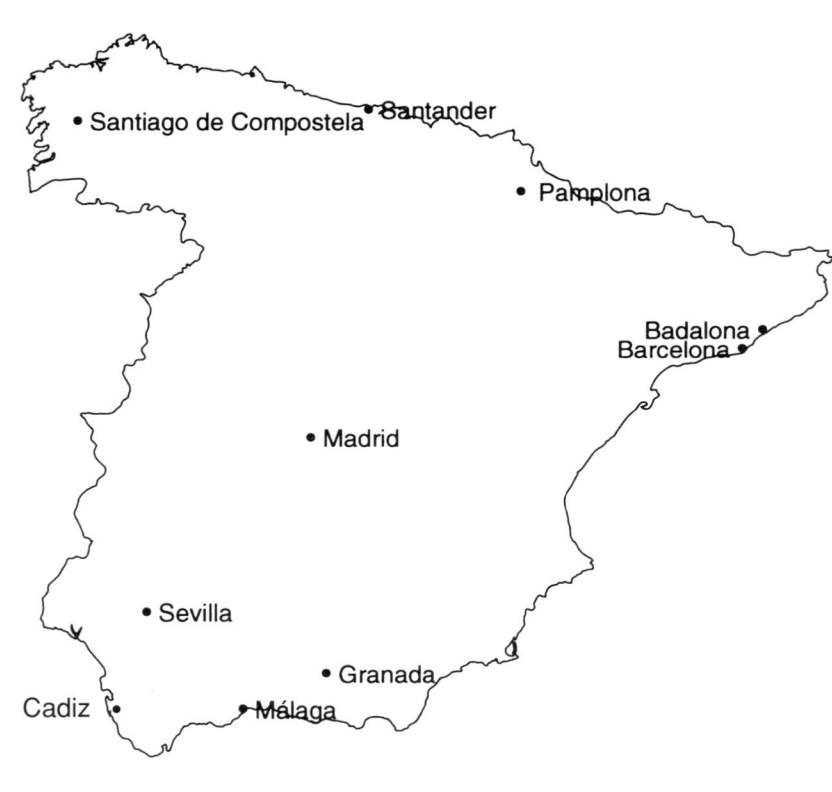

Spain

Clinical pharmacology is an official medical speciality in Spain. Each medical speciality has its own separate training programme. Admission to the 4-year training programme in clinical pharmacology is obtained after the successful passing of a national examination on general medicine which allows entering the residence programme. The speciality and the centre are chosen by rank order. Each medical speciality has a limited training capacity, and presently there are 20 new trainees per year in clinical pharmacology in all of Spain. Eighteen to 24 months in general internal medicine or paediatrics is compulsory. The remaining 24-30 months take place in various compulsory subjects: laboratory (TDM and pharmacokinetics), drug utilization, clinical trial (including preparation and review of protocols and participation in ethics committee meetings), pharmacovigilance and pharmacoepidemiology, drug selection, drug information (e.g. bulletins), therapeutic consultations and primary health care.

The Sociedad Española de Farmacología Clínica [The Spanish Society of Clinical Pharmacology (SEFC)] started its activities in 1981, and it became officially established in 1983. The SEFC meets every year, since 1995, on the pair years, and on the odds it meets during the EACPT Congress. The SEFC has organized several multicentre studies including a clinical trial and several drug utilization studies.

According to the General University Law, clinical pharmacology is not registered as an independent area in the Spanish universities. The undergraduate teaching in pharmaco-therapeutics is somewhat different at each university. Teaching in pharmacology now takes place during the third year in the preclinical part, and during the fourth to sixth year during the clinical part of the medical curriculum.

The Ministry of Health and the Ministry of Education are both responsible for the National Commission on Clinical Pharmacology. The Commission is legally responsible for defining the training programme in clinical pharmacology, and on the accreditation of the units and departments that could serve as training centres.

Addresses

Barcelona
Professor JR Laporte
Hospital Vall d'Hebron
P Vall d'Hebron 119-129
E-08035 Barcelona
Phone: +34 3 428 3029
Fax: +34 3 489 4109
E-mail: JRL@icf.uab.es

Professor J Cami Morell
Institut Municipal d'Assistèucia Sanitària
Hospital Ntra. Sra. del Mar
Department of Pharmacology and Toxicology
Dr Aiguader 80
E-08003 Barcelona
Phone: +34 3221 1009
Fax: +34 3221 3237
E-mail: JCami@imin.es

Professor F Jané
Department of Clinical Pharmacology
Hospital de la Santa Creu i Sant Pau
Av Sant Antoni Maria Claret, 167
E-08025 Barcelona
Phone: +34 3 291 9018
Fax: +34 3 291 9178
E-mail: fjane@santpau.es

Professor P Salvá
Hospital Universitari 'Germans Trias i Pujol'
Crta. de Canyet, s/n
E-08916 Badalona
Phone: +34 3 395 0611
Fax: +34 3 395 4206
E-mail: pausalva@ns.hugtip.scs.es

Cadiz
Professor J Galiana
Department of Clinical Pharmacology
Hospital Universitario de Puerto Real
Crta. Nacional IV, Km. 665
E-11510 Puerto Real. Cádiz
Phone: +34 956 470 356
Fax: +34 956 470 163
E-mail: javier.galiana@uca.es

Granada
Professor M García Morillas
Hospital San Cecilio
Av del Doctor Olariz, 16
E-18005 Granada

Madrid
Professor A Moreno González
Servicio de Farmacología Clínica
Hospital Universitario San Carlos
E-28040 Madrid
Professor P Sánchez García
Hospital 'La Paz'
P° de la Castellana, 261
E-28046 Madrid

Malaga
Professor F Sánchez de la Cuesta
Hospital Clinico Universitario Virgen de la Victoria
Campus Universitario de Teatinos, s/n
E-29070 Málaga
Phone: +34 345 213 1567/72
Fax: +34 345 213 1568

Pamplona
Professor J Honorato Pérez
Clínica Universitaria de Navarra
Av Pío XII, 36
E-31080 Pamplona

Santander
Professor JA Armijo
Hospital Universario Marqués de Valdecilla
Servicio de Farmacologia Clinica
Av De Valdecilla, s/n

E-39008 Santander
Fax: +34 4234 7411

Santiago de Compostela
Professor F Tato Herrero
Hospital General de Galicia

Galeras, s/n
E-15705 La Coruña

Sevilla
Professor J Serrano Molina
Hospital Virgen de la Macarena
Av Doctor Fedriani, 3
E-41071 Sevilla

Training Centres in Spain

Badalona
University Hospital Germans Trial i Pujol
In the Clinical Pharmacology Department, two clinical pharmacologists and one nurse are employed as staff members, further eight persons are employed as granted medicals, chemists and secretaries.

The activities cover different fields, including hospital activities, clinical trials, technical assessment to Institutional Review Board and teaching. Hospital: drug utilization studies, drug information and therapeutic consultation, drug selection, therapeutic drug monitoring laboratory, pharmacovigilance and activities to promote a rational use of drugs. The department participates in all hospital committees related to drug and therapeutics (pharmacy, policy of antibiotics, thromboembolism). We are now performing multi-centre pharmacoepidemiological studies focused on AIDS and heart failure. The executive management and technical assessment of the Institutional Review Board is also a part of our responsibility.

Clinical trials: our department has a phase I-II unit where clinical pharmacokinetic-pharmacodynamic trials are performed, including those of bioequivalence. We have two wards with six beds each (12 in total) to perform studies in healthy subjects. During 1996 and 1997 we have performed nine studies.

I.R.B.: Executive management and technical assessment of 235 investigation projects.

Teaching: we do under- and postgraduate teaching of clinical pharmacology and therapeutics at the Autonomous University of Barcelona. We develop teaching activities on subjects related to pharmacology or therapeutics for the personnel of the Hospital itself and other health areas. Our department has an accredited teaching capacity of one resident per year, and given that the duration of the training programme in our country is 4 years, there are a total of four residents. There are also persons who are carrying out research projects that will be presented as doctoral theses.

Barcelona
Universitat Autonoma de Barcelona (UAB), Institut Català de Farmacologia

The Institute Català de Farmacologia (ICF) is a non-profit Foundation under the patronage of the Department of Health of the local Catalan government, Institut Català de la Salut (which is the public sector provider of health care) and the Autonomous University of Barcelona. It includes the Service of Clinical Pharmacology of Hospitals Vall d'Hebron (which is the main reference hospital of the health system in Catalonia), the Unit of the Department of Pharmacology and Therapeutics of the UAB, and the former ICF, a non-profit civil society. More than 50 professionals work at the ICF, of which 23 have a doctoral degree, 16 are training fellows in clinical pharmacology (in a 4-year training programme), 10 to 15 are foreign fellows, and six are administrative and support personnel. ICF is a WHO Collaboration Centre for Research and Training in Pharmacoepidemiology, and a member of the European Pharmacovigilance Research Group. Its activities are organized in different working areas, as follows:

- Clinical trials – evaluation and follow up of protocols for the Hospital Ethics Committee. Approximately 100 new protocols are evaluated each year, and each year more than 2,000 patients enter clinical trials at the hospital.
- Clinical trials, unit for design, methods, development, and analysis, for external clients.
- Pharmacovigilance, voluntary reporting – in 1982 the ICF pioneered the Spanish system of Pharmacovigilance (Sistema Español de Farmacovigilancia, SEFV). In 1992, the National Coordinating Centre of the SEFV was transferred to the Ministry of Health, and our centre became a regional centre for Catalonia.

Institut Municipal d'Assistència Sanitària (IMIM – Hospital del Mar)
Training programme: 18 months in Internal Medicine (15 months in

General Internal Medicine and 3 months in Intensive Care Unit), 30 months in Pharmacology Unit (pharmacokinetics and TDM, clinical trials, pharmacovigilance, therapeutic consultation, drug information) Research programme: clinical pharmacology of drug abuse (human pharmacology, chemical analysis of drugs of abuse and psychoactive drugs, doping control)

The facilities of the Department of Pharmacology and Toxicology are divided in two areas: clinical (different experimental rooms used to carry-out clinical trial with human volunteers), and analytical laboratory (different section devoted to chemical analysis using HPLC, GC/MS, GC).

The centre is affiliated to the Universitat Autònoma de Barcelona (School of Medicine).

Staff: There are two senior clinical pharmacologists, two chemists, and one pharmacist. There are also auxiliary persons (nurses, technicians), and fellows (three in the clinical pharmacology section) and one resident (training programme in clinical pharmacology).

Anyone interested could write to the address of the Department to obtain information about training programme and fellowships.

References:
Farré M, de la Torre R, Llorente M, Lamas X, Ugena B, Segura J, Camí J (1993) Alcohol and cocaine interactions in humans. J Pharmacol Exp Ther 266: 1364-1373

Boobis AR, Lynch AM, Murray S, de la Torre R, Solans A, Farré M, Segura J, Goodergam NJ, Davies DS (1994) Dietary heterocyclic amines are predominantly converted to their proximate carcinogens by CYPIA2 in humans. Cancer Res 54: 89-94

Lamas X, Farré M, Camí J (1994) Acute effects of pentazocine, naloxone and morphine in opioid-dependent volunteers. J Pharmacol Exp Ther 268: 1485-1492

Lamas X, Farré M, Llorente M, Camí J (1994) Spanish version of the 49-item short form of the Addiction Research Center Inventory (ARCI). Drug Alcohol Depend 35: 203-209

Lamas X, Farré M, Moreno V, Camí J (1994) Effects of morphine in nondependent humans: A meta-analysis. Drug Alcohol Depend 36: 147-152

de la Torre R, Ortuño J, González ML, Farré M, Camí J, Segura J (1995) Determination of cocaine and its metabolites in human urine by gas chromatography/mass spectrometry after simultaneous use of cocaine and ethanol. J Pharmaceut Biomed Anal 13: 305-312

Farré M, Lamas X, Camí J (1995) Sensation seeking amongst healthy volunteers participating in phase I clinical trials. Br J Clin Pharmacol 39: 405-409

Farré M, Terán MT, Camí J (1996) A comparison of the acute behavioral effects of flunitrazepam and triazolam in healthy volunteers. Psychopharmacology (Berlin) 125: 1-12

de la Torre R, Badía R, González G, García M, Pretel J, Farré M, Segura J (1996) Biological cross-reactivity of stimulants screened for in sports drug testing by two fluorescence polarization inmunoassays. J Anal Toxicol 20: 165-170

Farré M, de la Torre R, González ML, Terán MT, Roset PN, Menoyo E, Camí J (1997) Cocaine and alcohol interactions in humans: neuroendocrine effects and cocaethylene metabolism. J Pharmacol Exp Ther 283: 164-176

St Pau Hospital

In the Clinical Pharmacology Department of St Pau Hospital, eight clinical pharmacologists, two neurologists, one psychologist, two statisticians and four nurses are employed as staff members. Furthermore, between granted medical doctors, pharmacists, technicians and secretaries, 16 more persons work with us.

Our activities cover different fields, being hospital activities, clinical trials and teaching the three more relevant ones.

Hospital: drug utilization studies, drug information and pharmacovigilance, and in general all those activities directed to promote rational use of drugs. Our department participates in all hospital committees related with drugs and therapeutics (Pharmacy and Therapeutics; Antibiotics). We are now performing multicentre pharmacoepidemiological studies focused on AIDS and heart failure. The executive management and technical assessment of the Institutional Review Board is also a part of our responsibility.

Clinical trials: our department has a phase I-II unit where clinical pharmacokinetic-pharmacodynamic trials are performed, including those of bioequivalence. We have one ward with 14 beds to perform studies in healthy subjects. There are two more wards, one of them for carrying out studies with patients, and the other one specifically dedicated to evaluate the effect of drugs on CNS. During 1996, we have performed several studies.

Teaching: we do undergraduate and postgraduate teaching of clinical pharmacology and therapeutics at the Autonomous University of Barcelona. Furthermore, we organize a two-year course on Pharmaceutical Industry Medicine, and next year we introduce a Master on European Regulatory Affairs. We also participate in the teaching of pharmacology and statistics in two nurses' schools.

Inquiries to Professor F. Jané.

Cadiz

Research: drug utilization studies, pharmacokinetics of methadone, consequences of the retinoid therapy.

Training programme: according to national regulations.

Madrid
Servicio de Farmacologia Clinica

Our service has an accredited teaching capacity of two residents per year, and given that the duration of the training programme in our country is 4 years, there are a total of eight residents. There are also persons who are carrying out research projects that will be presented as doctoral theses (basically from the Complutense University of Madrid) and/or mini-theses for the Master's programme from different teaching organisms (fundamentally public health and management schools).

The medical staff is made up of a chief of service and three medical specialists. There are also two nurses and two administrative secretaries assigned to the service. The medical personnel carry out pre- and post-graduate teaching activities in the area of clinical pharmacology in Medical and Nursing career studies. Furthermore, they collaborate in developing and organizing teaching activities on subjects related to pharmacotherapy for the personnel of the hospital itself and other health areas. The principal areas of investigation are situated in the 'Studies of Drug Usage' and 'Pharmacovigilance'. However, a 'Phase I Unit' has been functioning during the last 3 months.

References

Bañares A, Jover JA, Fernandez B, Benitez JM, Garcia J, Vargas E, Hernandez C (1997) Patterns of uveitis as a guide in making rheumatologic and immunologic diagnoses. Arthr Rheum 40: 358-370

Cubo E, Sanz R, García-Urra D, Barquero S, Vargas E (1997) Acute cerebellopathy as a probable toxic effect of flucytosine. Eur J Clin Pharmacol 51: 505-506

García Mateos M, Vargas E (1995) Dihidropiridinas. Medicina y función hospitalaria 239-243

Laredo L, Vargas E, García M, Portolés A, Ambit MI, Moreno A (1996) Reacciones adversas a medicamentos en medicina interna. Farm Clin 13: 586-594

Portolés A, Vargas E (1995) Verapamilo: Aspectos farmacológicos y clínicos. Medicina y Función Hospitalaria 1: 164-176

Vargas E (1995) Racionalización en el uso de somatostatina: implicaciones terapéuticas y económicas. Farm Clin 12: 477-482

Vargas E, Portolés A (1995) Fármacos de acción cardiovascular en el paciente anciano. Rev Esp Cardiol 48(s3): 81-88

Vargas E, García-Arenillas M, Laredo L, Martinez M, Portolés A, Moreno A (1996) Adverse drug reactions in a cardiology department. Cause of admission or appearance during hospitalization. Clin Drug Invest 12: 46-52

Vargas E, Puerro M, Portolés A, García M, Ambit MI, Moreno A(1997a) Use of intravenous omeprazole in a university hospital. J Pharm Technol 13: 32-35

Vargas E, Navarro MI, Laredo L, García M, García M, Moreno A (1997b) Effects of drug-drug interactions on the development of adverse drugs reactions. Clin Drug Invest 13: 282-289

Vargas E, Miguel V, Portolés A, Avendaño C, Ambit MI, Torralba A, Moreno A (1997c) Use of albumin in two Spanish university hospitals. Eur J Clin Pharmacol 52: 465-470

Malaga

Teaching activity

Undergraduate: pharmacology: 3rd year at the medical school. 5.5 credits for theory and 5.5 credits for practice; clinical pharmacology: 6th year at the medical school. Total credits: 6. Clinical Pharmacology for nurses: total credits 8.5. Pharmacology at physiotherapists: total credits 6.0

Postgraduate: doctorate courses in basic and clinical pharmacology.

Other courses leading to a Master's degree. Full collaboration with the Medical College Association for update courses.

There is a service of clinical pharmacology in the hospital accredited by the National Commission in Clinical Pharmacology for the official 4-year postgraduate training in clinical pharmacology. Capacity: one resident per year.

Three members of the faculty staff are trained in clinical pharmacology.

The activities developed at the service are mainly: therapeutic drug monitoring, clinical trials, drug selection, utilization and information. Participation in local commissions: policy of antibiotics, pharmacy, ethics committee, pharmacovigilance, and at the national level: National Commission of Drug Evaluation and Rational use and The National Commission on Clinical Pharmacology.

Clinical epidemiology and controlled clinical trials in the field of: hypertension, respiratory disease, hepatology, diabetes, infectious diseases, geriatrics. Pharmacoeconomic studies.

Co-ordination of a multicentric, multidisciplinary (hepatologist and clinical pharmacologist) network for the register of hepatotoxic adverse drug reactions. A project of vigilance with methodology case control is a substudy to establish a possible association between acute hepatic injury and drug consumption.

Drug metabolism. Studies on cytochrome P450 and related enzymatic activities.

Antithrombotic pharmacology. Free radicals and lipid peroxidation.

Radioligand binding studies at muscarinic and serotonergic receptors. Main collaboration with other institutions: 'Mario Negri' Institute di Recerche Farmacologiche (Italy), National Institute for Medical Research (London)

Santander

University of Cantabria School of Medicine, 'M. de Valdecilla' University Hospital

Training programme in clinical pharmacology: our service has two residents per year with a total of eight residents of clinical pharmacology. The training programme in our service includes 20 months in clinical practice, 4 months in our laboratory, and 24 months in clinical pharmacology.

During the 2 years of clinical practice our residents are trained in internal medicine (about 12 months), and other specialities such as infectious diseases, intensive medicine, neurology, haematology or paediatrics (8 months).

The 4 months in our laboratory include the training in drug assay laboratory techniques (we perform more than 20.000 determinations of drugs in our laboratory), clinical pharmacokinetics and statistical procedures and computer software). The remaining 24 months are dedicated to clinical pharmacology activities, mainly therapeutic drug monitoring (we elaborate more than 4000 informs on TDM) and drug information activities, but also drug utilization (Pharmacy and Therapeutics Committee and Infections Committee meetings), clinical trials (Ethics Committee meetings) and pharmacovigilance (we collaborate with the Centre of Pharmacovigilance of Cantabria). Along the 4 years, our residents make part of the emergency team of our hospital both at the Admission Service and at the Internal Medicine Service with a frequency of 5-8 days/month, and participate in the training sessions of our Service (two by week) and in the general training activities of our hospital

Research fields: the main research fields of our service are TDM and antiepileptic drugs, but we are also concerned in anti-infectious and immunosuppressive agents.

Teaching activities: most people in our service are enrolled in the teaching team of the Department of Physiology and Pharmacology of the University of Cantabria. We teach clinical pharmacology at the Faculty of Medicine and at the Nurse School, and we participate in the programme of Doctorate of the Department of Physiology and Pharmacology.

Staff: one Head of Service (physician), three consultants in clinical pharmacology (physicians), eight residents in clinical pharmacology (physicians), two nurses, two laboratory technicians, one laboratory technician assistant and two administrative assistants.

Application procedures: Admission to our training programme is obtained after an examination on medicine contents. This exam has a national character, and applications should be addressed to the IN-SALUD in Madrid.

Inquiries: Professor Juan A Armijo.

References

Armijo JA, De Cos MA (1994) Parent cyclosporine in whole blood by FPIA and EMIT after kidney, heart and liver transplantation. Clin Biochem 6: 488-501

Armijo JA, Cuadrado A, Bravo, Arteaga R (1997) Vigabatrin serum concentration to dosage ratio: influence of age and associated antiepileptic drugs. Ther Drug Monit 491-498

Arteaga R, Herranz JL, Armijo JA (1993) Platelet GABA-transaminase in epileptic children: Influence of epilepsy and anticonvulsants. Epilepsy Res 14: 73-85

Arteaga R, Herranz JL, Armijo JA (1996) Add-on vigabatrin in children with refractory epilepsy: a 4-year follow-up study. Clin Drug Invest 12: 287-297

Calvo-Alén J, De Cos MA, Rodriguez Vlaverde V, Escanllada R, Flórez J, Arias M (1994) Subclinical renal toxicity in rheumatic patients receiving longterm treatment with nonsteroidal antiinflammatory drugs. J Rheumatol 21: 1742-1747.

Castrillón JL, Mediavilla A, Méndez MA, Cavada E, Carrascosa M, Valle R (1993) Syndrome of inappropriate antidiuretic hormone secretion (SIADH) and enalapril. J Int Med 233: 89-91

González-Ruiz M, De Cos MA, Casafont F (1996) Cholestasis-related cyclosporin malabsorption overcome by administration of Sandimmun Neural: dase-report and review of the literature. Clin Drug Invest 11: 60-64

Herranz JL, Artega R, Armijo JA (1996) Three-year efficacy and tolerabliity of add-on lamotrigine in treatment-resistant epileptic children. Clin Drug Invest 11: 214-223

Sacristán JA, Soto JA, De Cos MA (1993a) Erythromycin-induced hypoacusis: 11 new cases and literature review. Ann Pharmacother 27: 950-955

Sacristán JA. De Cos MA, Soto J, Zurbano F, Pascual J, Tasis A. Valle R, De Pablos C (1993b) Ototoxicity of erythromycin in man: electrophysiologic approach. Am J Otol 14: 186-188

Sanchez BM, De Cos MA, Peralta FG, Arribas C, Armijo JA (1996) syva-EMIT 2000 and Roche 'on-line' subject to less interference by digoxin-like factors than Abbott Tdx FPIA i newborns and pregnant women. Clin Chem 42: 974-976

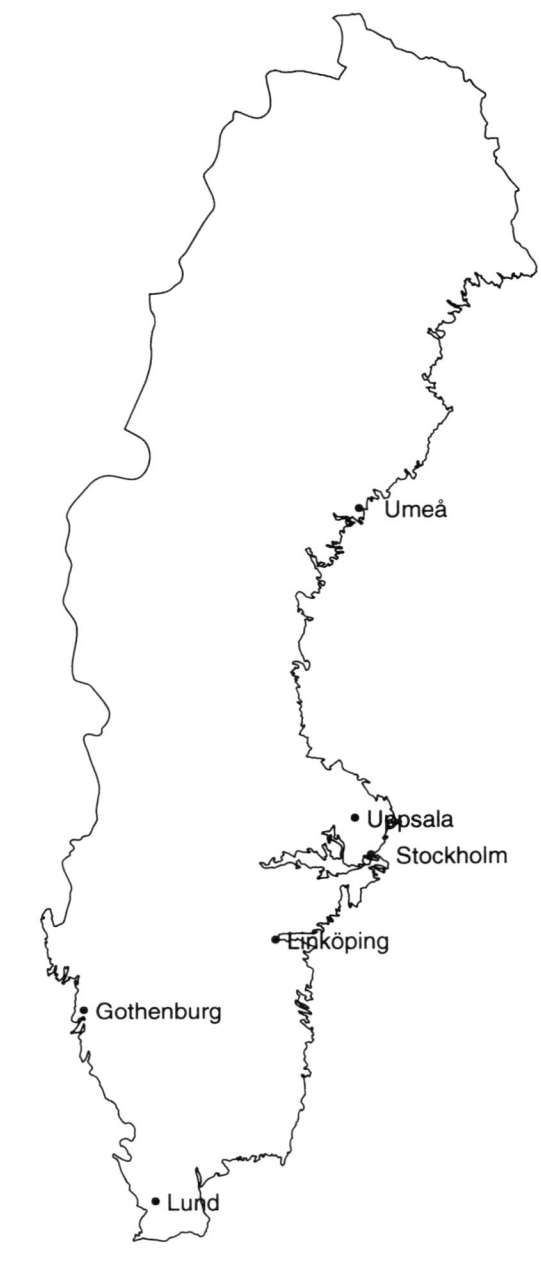

Sweden

Clinical pharmacology is a well established medical speciality in Sweden with chairs in the discipline at all the six medical faculties. The national requirements for becoming a specialist in clinical pharmacology includes the basic medical degree (5 years), 2 years of internship (rotating in medicine, surgery, psychiatry, primary health care) and 5 years of residency. Of these 5 years, one has to be spent in a pharmacotherapeutically oriented clinical discipline and 4 years fulfilled in a clinical pharmacology unit. Of the latter, 1 year may be spent in preclinical pharmacology or in the drug regulatory agency.

The training programme should cover all aspects of the role of clinical pharmacology in health care delivery and a specific research project leading to a PhD (minimally 4 years) in clinical pharmacology. The research areas in the Swedish departments include drug evaluation and clinical trial methodology, assessment of drug effects in man, drug metabolism and clinical pharmacokinetics, pharmacogenetics, PK/PD modelling, pharmacoepidemiology, pharmacovigilance and drug information.

The health care obligations include consultations to regional and local drug committees, the provision of drug problem-oriented information to prescribers as well as patient consultations. The regional drug information centres collaborate and a common database, Drugline, has been created. This database consists of evaluated case stories of patients with pharmacotherapeutic problems and is being produced in collaboration between physicians and pharmacists specializing in drug information. The services also include therapeutic drug monitoring as well as analysis of drugs in drug toxicology and drug abuse. All departments are also involved in clinical drug evaluation during all its phases including post marketing surveillance. Most departments also provide services in drug utilization and pharmacoepidemiology.

A national society was formally created and statutes agreed upon in 1980. An informal society was created some 10 years earlier. The society is consulted in important national pharmacopolitical issues through the Swedish Medical Association.

The number of members is approximately 120, representing hospitals, faculties, the drug regulatory agency and the pharmaceutical industry.

The tasks of the society are to develop the discipline, to catalyse training courses, to arrange scientific meetings together with the Section on Drugs of the Swedish Medical Society and to provide expert knowledge in pending drug issues at national and regional levels. The Society has continuous collaboration with the Swedish Medical Society and the Swedish Medical Association. Further information can be obtained from the chairman: Professor Anders Rane, see below.

Swedish clinical pharmacology began in 1956 with the successive establishment of reader-ships in all medical schools. In 1965, these positions were combined with part-time consultancies to various clinical departments such as internal medicine, psychiatry and paediatrics. The first chair in clinical pharmacology (combined with a position as head physician) was created in 1970 at the new medical school in Linköping. The second chair was founded in 1972 at the Karolinska Institute and based at its new research and teaching hospital in Huddinge in southern Stockholm. Chairs were subsequently established at the universities of Lund in 1975, Gothenburg in 1978, Umeå in 1989 and Uppsala in 1990. There are now about 15 professorial positions in clinical pharmacology in Sweden, including three at the Swedish Medical Products Agency (the national drug control agency). There are six academic departments with from ten to more than 50 staff members and annual budgets of up to SEK 20 million.

All academic units provide undergraduate teaching in clinical pharmacology. Medical students receive in average 2 weeks of instruction during their clinical years. Postgraduate courses for licensed doctors emphasize drug use in different specialities including primary health care and are held at regular intervals. National courses in clinical drug evaluation and clinical trials are arranged annually. All units provide short-term training (1-2 years) to foreign fellows with an interest in clinical pharmacology.

Most departments provide expert knowledge to the Swedish Medical Products Agency (SMPA) in questions related to drug evaluation and drug safety.

Since 1993, the university departments officially collaborate with SMPA in the monitoring of adverse drug reactions. A network in pharmacovigilance co-ordinated from SMPA has been created. Research collaboration with the pharmaceutical industry is encouraged but academic members of the National Society of Clinical Pharmacology are not supposed to be consultants to individual drug firms.

Addresses

Göteborg
Professor Thomas Hedner
Department of Clinical Pharmacology
Sahlgrenska University Hospital
S-413 45 Göteborg
Phone: +46 3160 2983 or 3160 2974
Fax: +46 3182 6723
E-mail: Thomas.Hedner@pharm.gu.se

Linköping
Professor Curt Petersson
Department of Clinical Pharmacology
University Hospital
S-581 85 Linköping
Phone: +46 1322 1745
Fax: +46 1310 4195
E-mail: curt.petersson@far.liu.se

Lund
Professor Karl-Erik Andersson
Department of Clinical Pharmacology
Lund University Hospital
S-221 85 Lund
Phone: +46 46 173350
Fax: +46 46 211 1987
E-mail: Karl-Erik.Andersson@klinfarm.lu.se
Homep: www.klinfarm.lu.se

Stockholm
Professor Paul Hjemdahl
Department of Laboratory Medicine
Division of Clinical Pharmacology
Karolinska Hospital
S-171 76 Stockholm
Phone: +46 8 5177 5293 (office)
   +46 8 5177 5292 (secretary)
Fax: +46 8 308 529
E-mail: Paul.Hjemdahl@mb.ks.se

Professor Anders Rane
Department of Medical Laboratory Sciences and Technology
Division of Clinical Pharmacology
Huddinge University Hospital
S-141 86 Huddinge
Phone: +46 8 585 81068
Fax: +46 8 585 81070

Professor Folke Sjöqvist
Department of Medical Laboratory Sciences and Technology
Division of Clinical Pharmacology
Huddinge University Hospital
S-141 86 Huddinge
Phone: +46 8 585 81068
Fax: +46 8 585 81070
E-mail: folke.sjoqvist@pharmlab.hs.sll.se

Umeå
Professor Rune Dahlqvist
Division of Clinical Pharmacology
Umeå University
S-901 85 Umeå
Phone: +46 90 103 742
Fax: +46 90 120 430
E-mail: Rune.Dahlqvist@clpharm.umu.se

Uppsala
Vacant after 1. March 1999
Uppsala University
Department of Clinical Laboratory Sciences

Division of Clinical Pharmacology
University Hospital
S-751 85 Uppsala
Phone: +46 18 664 261 or 664 260
Fax: +46 18 519 237

Training Centres in Sweden

Göteborg

Sahlgrenska University Hospital
Research and training programme: education in clinical pharmacology for medical and postgraduate students. Main interests of research include cardiovascular, pharmacology, respiratory pharmacology in particular sleep apnoea, gastrointestinal pharmacology and pain mechanisms.

Clinical and research facilities: the activities in clinical pharmacology include therapeutic drug monitoring (TDM) in clinical routine as well as in association with research on pharmacological compounds undergoing clinical development and registration. The problem oriented service covers undertakings in regulatory issues, educational issues and expert consultations in the field of clinical pharmacology. Such activities cover local to regional levels as well as national and international activities.

The analytic service covers plasma and tissue monitoring of drugs using HPLC, gas chromatography, RIA, ELISA and spectrophotometric methods. The routine analytical activity includes therapeutic drug monitoring after referrals from the Sahlgrenska University Hospital or regional hospitals. Additional assays of interest are also performed within the frame of different research and development projects.

Staff: Thomas Hedner, professor and senior clinician; Jan Hedner, Associate professor, senior clinician and specialist in clinical pharmacology; Nils Svedmyr, professor emeritus; Anders Pettersson, MD, PhD and senior clinician; Anders Himmelmann, associate professor, specialist in internal medicine and clinical pharmacology; Jan Lötvall, associate professor and specialist in clinical pharmacology; Bernt Everts, MD, specialist in internal medicine and gastroenterology, Eva Johnsson, MD, PhD; Holger Kraiczi, MD, Anders Mellén, MD.

Application procedures: general application procedures are used.

References

Brandsson S, Rydgren B, Hedner T, Eriksson BI, Lundin O, Sward L, Karlsson J (1996) Postoperative analgesic effects of an external cooling system and intra-articular bupivacaine/ morphine after arthroscopic cruciate ligament surgery. Knee Surg Sports Traumatol Arthrosc 4 (4): 200-205

Carlson JT, Hedner JA, Sellgren J, Elam M, Wallin BG (1996) Depressed baroreflex sensitivity in patients with obstructive sleep apnea. Am J Respir Crit Care Med 154(5): 1490-1496

Everts B, Karlson BW, Herlitz J, Abdon NJ, Hedner T (1997) Effects and pharmacokinetics of high dose metoprolol on chest pain in patients with suspected or definite acute myocardial infarction. Eur J Clin Pharmacol 53 (1): 23-31

Hedner J, Svedmyr N, Lunde H, Mandahl A (1997) The lack of respiratory effects of the ocular hypotensive drug latanoprost in patients with moderate-steroid treated asthma. Surv Ophthalmol

Himmelmann A, Hedner T, Snoeck E, Lundgren B, Hedner J (1996) Haemodynamic effects and pharmacokinetics of oral d- and l-nebivolol in hypertensive patients. Eur J Clin Pharmacol 51(3-4): 259-264

Lindholm LH, Hansson L, Dahlof B, Ekbom T, Hedner T, De FU, Schersten B, Webster PO (1996) The Swedish Trial in old patients with hypertension-2 (STOP-hypertension-2): a progress report. Blood Press 5(5): 300-304

Malmberg AB, Hedner T, Fallgren B, Calcutt NA (1997) The effect of alpha-trinositol (D-myo-inositol 1,2,6-triphosphate) on formalin-evoked spinal amino acid and prostaglandin E2 levels. Brain Res 747(1): 160-164

Stenlof K, Grunstein R, Hedner J, Sjostrom L (1996) Energy expenditure in obstructive sleep apnea: effects of treatment with continuous positive airway pressure. Am J Physiol. 271 (6) E1036-43

Wallen R, Landahl S, Hedner T, Saito Y, Masuda I, Nakao K (1997) Brain natriuretic peptide in an elderly population. J Int Med 242 (4): 307-311

Zhao XH, Sun XY, Edvinsson L, Hedner T (1997) Does the neuropeptide Y Y1 receptor contribute to blood pressure control in the spontaneously hypertensive rat? J Hypertens 15: 19-27

Linköping

Oncological clinical pharmacology: the aim of our studies is to improve cancer chemotherapy by individualizing the treatment based on pharmacokinetic and pharmacodynamic variability. At present, we are focused on changes in drug transport across cell membranes as a resistance mechanism, both detection in clinical samples and the possibilities to reverse such resistance. We are also studying the possibilities to target cancer chemotherapy to malignant cells by linking toxic but non-selective drugs to macromolecular carriers. In addition, we are interested in ameliorating side effects of cancer chemotherapy, in particular the optimal use of novel antiemetics.

Enantioselective chromatography: the analytical work is focused on chiral chromatographic methods based on liquid as well as gas chromatographic techniques. Validated methods are available for amlodipine, citalopram including demethylated metabolites, salbutamol and arabinitol. Enantioselective chromatography has been developed for other substances such as other calciumblockers, terbutaline, venlafaxine, lactic and ketamine.

Physician-patient communication: several projects concerning communication between caregivers and patients are conducted together with the Department of Communication Studies at the University of Linköping. These studies include evaluation of patients' knowledge of their disease and their medication, especially in hypertension, as well as their assessments of risk with the disease and risk reduction with treatment.

Lund
Lund University Hospital
Research and training programme: ongoing research programmes are in the fields of fundamental pharmacology and physiology, pharmacokinetics and pharmacodynamics in humans, adverse reactions, and therapeutic drug monitoring. Especially prominent are the research areas of the lower urinary and genital tracts, and vascular reactivity. Training programmes for residents include clinical trials, therapeutic drug monitoring, drug information, pharmacovigilance and extensive lecturing for medical students and clinical colleagues.

Clinical and research facilities: the newly renovated, 900 square meter Department of Clinical Pharmacology includes an in vitro laboratory (organ baths, electrophysiology, a DNA lab, a cell culture lab, etc.), an analytical routine lab, a drug analysis development lab, animal housekeeping, an eight-bed in-hospital ward for phase I-II clinical trials, a regional drug information centre, and a pharmacovigilance unit.

Lund University and Lund University Hospital: the department is located at the University Hospital in the centre of the old university town of Lund, in the southern part of Sweden. The 300 year old University is a full university with all classical faculties including medicine, odontology, and natural sciences. The town of Lund has about 100,000 inhabitants, and the University has enrolled approximately 30,000 students. The University Hospital is the second biggest hospital in Sweden.

Staff: the department is staffed with 11 physicians, 20 research and technical personnel, five administrative personnel, and more than 10 full time PhD students.

Application Procedure: applications for student advanced courses, PhD programmes, post doc programmes, doctoral training in clinical pharmacology, etc. should be sent to Professor Karl-Erik Andersson.

References

Alm P, Larsson B, Ekblad E, Sundler F, Andersson K-E (1993) Immunohistochemical localization of peripheral nitric oxide synthase-containing nerves using antibodies raised against synthesized C- and N-terminal fragments of a cloned enzyme from rat brain. Acta Physiol Scand 148: 421-429

Andersson K-E, Wagner G (1995) Physiology of penile erection. Physiol Rev 75: 191-236

Bergqvist PBF, Wikell C, Hjorth S, Apelqvist G, Bengtsson F (1997) Effect of citalopram on brain serotonin release in experimental hepatic encephalopathy implications for thymoleptic drug safety in liver insufficiency. Clin Neuropharmacol 20: 511-522

Eriksson T, Björkman S, Roth B, Fyge Å, Höglund P (1995) Stereospecific determination, chiral inversion in vitro and pharmacokinetics in humans of the enantiomers of thalidomide. Chirality 7: 44-52

Ishizuka O, Persson K, Mattiasson A, Naylor A, Wyllie M, Andersson K-E (1996) Micturition in conscious rats with and without outlet obstruction: role of spinal a1-adrenoceptors. Br J Pharmacol 117: 962-966

Johnsson A, Höglund P, Grubb A, Cavallin-Ståhl E (1996) Cisplatin pharmacokinetics and pharmacodynamics in patients with squamous cell carcinoma in the head/neck or oesophagus. Cancer Chemother Pharmacol 39: 25-33

Persson K, Johansson K, Alm P, Larsson B, Andersson K-E (1997) Morphological and functional evidence against a sympathetic or sensory origin of nitric oxide synthase containing nerves in the rat lower urinary tract. Neuroscience 77: 271-281

Vinge E, Nergelius G, Nilsson L-G, Lidgren L (1997) Pharmacokinetics of cloxacillin in patients undergoing hip or knee replacement. Eur J Clin Pharmacol 52: 407-411

Zygmunt PM, Edwards G, Weston AH, Davis CS, Högestätt ED (1996) Effects of cytochrome P450 inhibitors on EDHF-mediated relaxation in the rat hepatic artery. Br J Pharmacol 118: 1147-1152

Zygmunt PM, Edwards G, Weston AH, Larsson B, Högestätt ED (1997) Involvement of voltage-dependent potassium channels in the EDHF-mediated relaxation of rat hepatic artery. Br J Pharmacol 121: 141-150

Stockholm

Huddinge University Hospital

Our main research interests include: (1) interindividual differences in pharmacokinetics and drug metabolism in man, in particular research on pharmacogenetics, interethnic differences in drug metabolism, drug interactions and active drug metabolites; (2) population pharmacokinetics, antipsychotics, immunosuppressants, protease inhibitors; (3) clinical pharmacology of drugs used in tropical diseases; (4) clinical pharmacology of analgesics, particularly opiates; (5) Pharmacoepidemiology: Studies of drug utilisation, prescription monitoring studies, case control studies of severe adverse drug reactions (together with the Section of Adverse Drug Reactions, Swedish Medical Products Agency, Uppsala).

The hospital staff has the following main functions in health care services: (a) to serve in the pharmacokinetic and drug analytical service laboratory with emphasis on consultative interplay with different clinical departments; (b) to participate in our drug educational programmes and in the drug information centre; (c) to offer other drug problem oriented services to prescribers and seeing particular patient groups; (d) to give advice on matters related to clinical drug evaluation; (e) to serve in drug formulary committees.

Our teaching obligations include: (a) teaching of medical students from their third year throughout the medical school, approx. 70 hours/student; (b) postgraduate courses for licensed physicians with special emphasis on rational drug use; (c) advanced teaching of MD, PhD-students in clinical pharmacological research.

Clinical and research facilities: Our space is now about 1400 m^2. There are six distinct activities in the department: the pharmacokinetic and drug analytical service laboratory, the IOC (International Olympic Committee) accredited doping analysis laboratory, the human pharmacology laboratory, the drug information centre, the pharmacoepidemiological section and three new research laboratories including one in molecular pharmacogenetics. We also have access to laboratories for animal work.

The university: the Karolinska Institute is a university entirely focused on education and research in the health care sciences (medicine, dentistry, nursing, physiotherapy, etc.). It is one of the most prestigious medical schools in the world and its Nobel faculty is responsible for awarding the Nobel price in medicine.

The staff: the department has three professorial positions, one adjunct professor, one senior lecturer and four assistant professors. We collaborate with outstanding clinicians in internal medicine, infectious diseases, gastroenterology, transplantation surgery, neurology, psychiatry and primary health care. The total staff comprises about 70 persons and includes engineers, lab technicians, nurses and secretaries.

Application procedures: applications for short (minimum 3 months) or longer (1-2 years) training should be sent to the head of the department.

References

Aden Abdi Y, Gustafsson LL, Erichsson Ö, Hellgren U (1995) Handbook of Drugs for Tropical Parasitic Infections, 2nd edition. Taylor & Francis Publ, London

Bertilsson L, Dahl M-L, Ingelman-Sundberg M, Johansson I and Sjöqvist F (1995) Interindividual and interethnic differences in polymorphic drug oxidation. Implications for drug therapy with focus on psychoactive drugs. In: Advances in Drug metabolism in Man. Pacifici GM and Fracchia GN, pp 85-136, European Commission, Brussels

Chang M, Tybring G, Dahl M-L, Götharson E, Sagar M, Seensalu R, Bertilsson L (1995) Interphenotype differences in disposition and effect on gastrin levels of omeprazole-suitability of omeprazole as a probe for CYP2D19. Br J Clin Pharmacol 39: 511-515

Isacsson G, Wasserman D, Bergman U (1995) Self-poisonings with antidepressants and other psychotropics in an urban area of Sweden. Ann Clin Psychiatry 7: 113-118

Isacsson G, Bergman U, Rich C (1996) Epidemiological data suggest antidepressants reduce suicide risk among depressives. J Affect Disord 41: 1-8

Jerling M, Dahl ML, Åberg-Wistedt A, Liljenberg B, Landell NE, Bertilsson L, Sjöqvist F (1996) The CYP2D6 genotype predicts the oral clearance of the neuroleptic agents perphenazine and zuclopenthixol. Clin Pharmacol Ther 59:423-428

Marandi T, Dahl M-T, Rägo L, Kivet RA, Sjöqvist F (1997) Debrisoquin and S-mephenytoin hydroxylation polymorphisms in a Russian population living in Estonia. Eur J Clin Pharmacol 53: 257-260

Sjöqvist F, Borgå O, Dahl M-L, Orme ML (1997) Fundamentals of clinical pharmacology. In Avery's Drug Treatment. Principles and Practice of Clinical Pharmacology and Therapeutics. 4th ed. Speight TM, pp 1-73. Adis Press, Auckland

Ståhle L, Alm C, Ekquist B, Lundquist B, Tomson T (1996) Monitoring free extracellular valproic acid by microdialysis in epileptic patients. Ther Drug Monit 18: 14-18

Wakelkamp M, Alván G, Gabrielsson J, Paintaud G (1996) Pharmacodynamic modeling of furosemide tolerance after multiple intravenous administration. Clin Pharmacol Ther 60: 75-88

Yue QY, Svensson JO, Säwe J, Bertilsson L (1995) Codeine metabolism in three Oriental populations : a pilot study in Chinese, Japanese and Koreans. Pharmacogenetics 5: 173-177

Karolinska Hospital
The main research areas of Clinical Pharmacology at the Karolinska Hospital are cardiovascular and oncological pharmacology and drugs of abuse. The cardiovascular group has special expertise in haemostasis, especially platelet function in vivo, and sympatho-adrenal mechanisms. The pathophysiological and therapeutic importance of stress mechanisms in cardiovascular disease is investigated. The largest collaborative project so far is the Angina Prognosis Study In Stockholm (APSIS), which evaluates treatment effects in, and pathophysiological aspects of stable angina pectoris. The main interests of the oncological group are: multiple drug resistance and its mechanisms, possibilities of targeting cytostatic drugs to cancer cells by means of carrier molecules, cellular cholesterol metabolism, the therapeutic development of nucleoside analogs for cancer treatment, and the treatment and prevention of nausea during cytostatic drug treatment. The drugs of abuse programme focuses on further developments of biochemical diagnosis and monitoring of abstinence, and on the improvement of methadone treatment in opiate abusers. The department has a staff of 50, of whom two-thirds are employed by the Hospital and one-third by the Karolinska Institute. Inquiries may be directed to Paul Hjemdahl.

References

Gruber A, Areström I, Albertioni F, Björkholm M, Peterson C, Vitols S (1995) Mdr1 gene expression in peripheral blasts from patients with acute leukemia only rarely increases during disease progression after combination chemotherapy. Leukemia and Lymphoma 18: 435-442

Helander A, Beck O, Jones W (1996) Laboratory tests for recent alcohol consumption: comparison of ethanol, methanol, and 5-hydroxotryptophol. Clin Chem 42: 618-624

Held C, Hjemdahl P, Rehnqvist N, Wallén NH, Björkander I, Eriksson SV, Forslund L, Wiman B (1997) Prognostic implications of fibrinolytic variables in patients with stable angina pectoris treated with verapamil or metoprolol. Results from the APSIS study. Circulation 95: 2380-2386

Hiltunen AJ, Lafolie P, Martel J, Ottoson E-C, Boréus L-O, Beck O, Borg S, Hjemdahl P (1995) Subjective and objective symptoms in relation to plasma methadone concentrations in methadone patients. Psychopharmacology 118: 122-126

Hjemdahl P, Chronos N, Wilson D, Bouloux P, Goodall A (1994) Epinephrine sensitizes human platelets in vivo and in vitro as studied by fibrinogen binding and P-selectin expression. Arterioscl Thromb 14: 77-84

Larsson PT, Wallén NH, Hjemdahl P (1994) Norepinephrine-induced human platelet activation in vivo is only partly counteracted by aspirin. Circulation 89: 1951-1957

Lindqvist M, Kahan T, Melcher A, Hjemdahl P (1994) Acute and chronic calcium antagonist treatment elevates sympathetic activity in primary hypertension. Hypertension 24: 287-296

Rehnqvist N, Hjemdahl P, Billing E, Björkander I, Eriksson SV, Forslund L. Held C, Näsman P, Wallén NH (1996) Effects of metoprolol versus verapamil in patients with stable angina pectoris B the Angina Prognosis Study In Stockholm (APSIS). Eur Heart J 17: 76-81

Skoglund K, Söderhäll S, Beck O, Peterson C, Wennberg M, Hayder S, Björk O (1994) Plasma and urinary levels of methotrexate and 7-hydroxy-methotrexate in children with ALL during maintenance therapy with weekly oral methotrexate. Med Pediat Oncol 22: 187-193

Vitols S, Norgren S, Juliusson G, Tatidis L, Luthman H (1994) Multilevel regulation of low density lipoprotein receptor and 3-hydroxy-3-methylglutaryl coenzyme A reductase gene expression in normal and leukemic cells. Blood 84: 2689-2698

Umeå
Norrland University Hospital

The research areas of the Department are: (1) genetic and environmental factors controlling variability in drug disposition; (2) clinical pharmacology of antidepressants and neuroleptics; (3) serotonin receptors as markers for disease and treatment response; (4) clinical pharmacokinetics of anticancer drugs – an analytical platform and use of microdialysis; (5) adverse drug reactions drug epidemiology

The Department is active in: (1) teaching of medical students from their third year and throughout altogether around 30 hours per student; (2) postgraduate teaching for physicians and other health service personnel about rational drug use, potential problems with drugs and about new drugs and treatment recommendations, and (3) training of MDs for specialist competence within clinical pharmacology and training of PhD students to doctoral thesis in clinical pharmacology.

The area for clinical pharmacology is around 450 m². It is located within the University Hospital, which is situated a few yards from the University campus. Clinical pharmacology and its closest neighbour basic pharmacology form a common department with two separate sections but also share some common resources.

The clinical pharmacology unit is made up of five units: the TDM and drugs of abuse service laboratory (HPLC and GCMS), the human pharmacology laboratory, the research laboratory

(HPLC), the drug information centre, and the adverse drug reaction unit. Apart from that, the senior clinical pharmacologists are much involved in local and regional drug formulary committee work. The cover area for medical service within clinical pharmacology is the northern half of Sweden, housing just below 1 million people. Among other activities our unit houses the co-ordinating editor and editorial office for the European Journal of Clinical Pharmacology.

Umeå University is a young (from the 1960s) enthusiastic and rapidly growing full university situated in Umeå in northern Sweden. The number of students presently is 23,000 and the medical faculty accepts 122 students annually.

The clinical pharmacology staff is presently 19 persons including physicians, nurses, secretaries, chemists, laboratory technicians and pharmacists. The staff includes one full professor and two assistant professors.

Applications for both shorter visits and longer (12 years) training periods should be submitted to the head of clinical pharmacology.

References

Hedenmalm K, Sundgren M, Granberg K, Spigset O, Dahlqvist R (1997) Metabolism of codeine and ethylmorphine and their metabolites in urine in relation to CYP2D6 phenotypes. Ther Drug Monit 19: 643-649

Hägg S, Joelsson L, Mjörndal T, Spigset O, Oja G, Dahlqvist R (In press) Prevalence of diabetes/hyperglycemia in clozapine treated patients and patients treated with depot neuroleptics. J Clin Psychiatry

Smedh K, Spigset O, Allard P, Mjörndal T, Adolfsson R (In press) Platelet 3Hparoxetine and 3HLSD binding in seasonal affective disorder and the effect of light treatment. Biol Psychiat

Spigset O, Adielsson G (1997) Combined serotonin syndrome and hyponatraemia caused by a citaloprambuspirone interaction. Int Clin Psychopharmacol 12: 6163

Spigset O, Hägg S (1998) Excretion of psychotropic drugs into breast milk. Pharmacokinetic overview and therapeutic implications. CNS Drugs 9: 11134.

Spigset O, Mjörndal T (1997) Serotonin 5HT2A receptor binding in platelets from healthy subjects as studied by (3H)lysergic acid diethylamide (3HLSD): intraand interindividual variability. Neuropsychopharmacology 16: 285-293

Spigset O, Hedenmalm K, Dahl ML, Wiholm BE, Dahlqvist R (1997a) Seizures and myoclonus associated with antidepressant treatment: assessment of potential risk factors, including CYP2D6 and CYP2C19 polymorphisms and treatment with CYP2D6 inhibitors. Acta Psychiatr Scand 96: 379-384

Spigset O, Granberg K, Hägg S, Norström Å, Dahlqvist R (1997b) Relationship between fluvoxamine pharmacokinetics and CYP2D6/CYP2C19 phenotype polymorphisms. Eur J Clin Pharmacol 52: 129-133

Spigset O, Granberg K, Hägg S, Söderström E, Dahlqvist R (1998) Nonlinear fluvoxamine disposition. Br J Clin Pharmaccl 45: 257-263

Sundgren M, Hedenmalm K, Spigset O (In press) Simultaneous analysis of nine benzodiazepine compounds in urine by GC/MS and solidphase extraction. Analytical Pharmacology

More reading clinical service as well as teaching and research activities within the department is available on http.//server.pharm.umu.se/rutor.htm

Uppsala
Uppsala University

Areas of competence: specialist consultations in clinical pharmacology, problem-oriented as well as patient-related questions, including adverse drug reactions. Therapeutic drug monitoring (drug analyses). Drug analyses in evaluations of intoxications and adverse drug reaction. Pharmacogenetic counselling in therapeutics; pharmacogenetic tests (genotyping and phenotyping). Clinical drug trials, pharmacokinetics, drug information service, assessment of drug metabolism in man, in vitro as well as in vivo. Chemotherapeutic drug resistance in tumour cell-lines and in isolated tumour cells from patients with malignancies for prediction of tumour response. Metabolism, kinetics and effects of opioids in patients.

Research programme:
- Physiological and endocrine regulation of human drug metabolism. Studies in experimental animals and humans utilising molecular biology techniques for DNA, RNA as well as enzyme protein analyses. Clinical studies in humans using appropriate probe drugs for estimates of fractional clearance representing different enzymatic pathways.
- Developmental pharmacology: in vitro studies of human feal tissues. In vivo studies of development of metabolic capacities in children. Age effects on expression of different phenotypes.
- Pharmacology of the prostate: studies of crucial target enzymes and effects of endocrine intervention in prostate cancer and benign prostate hyperplasia.
- Clinical pharmacology of neuroendocrine intervention with drug metabolism: Focus on monoaminergic intervention by neuroleptic

and opioid agents. Studies of the effects on cytochrome P450 oxidations and glucuronidation reactions.
- Development and application of new tumour models and concepts for preclinical identification of new pharmacological principles for clinical development. This includes the implementation of a drug evaluation programme based on human tumour cell lines and primary cultures ranging from high-capacity screening for anticancer activity and mechanical classification to 'phase II trials in vitro' and in vivo evaluation in animal tumour models.
- Evaluation of new pharmacokinetic and pharmacodynamic methods for guiding phase I/II anticancer drug development. This programme involves the study of predictive methods for optimal use of preclinical information to assist in selection of suitable diagnoses and patients, optimal starting dose and escalation procedure for phase I and early phase II trials of novel anticancer agents.
- Application of laboratory methods for prediction of clinical cytotoxic drug resistance. Optimising the clinical application of a flurometric microculture toxicity assay (FMCA) of primary human tumor cells from patients with malignant tumours, in combination with estimates of plasma drug exposure and tumour cell regrowth after chemotherapy, is a major goal of this project.

Clinical duties of the department
- Drug analytical and pharmacokinetic advice. The hospital division analyses some 15-20 drugs for therapeutic monitoring. Pharmacokinetic advice is based on conventional and population-based pharmacokinetics.
- Drug information service. Collaboration between clinical pharmacologists and pharmacists from the hospital pharmacy.
- Problem-oriented clinical pharmacology service. Drug formulary committee of the hospital and of the country council.

Teaching
- Medical students in the second through fourth year of the curriculum. Seminars, lectures, therapy, conferences, group teaching, etc.
- Post-graduate international course in Clinical Drug Development. A 20-week full-time course (30 EC points). The course is given in English and aimed at graduates with background from medical,

pharmaceutical, or natural sciences education.
- Post-graduate teaching for groups of specialists in different clinical disciplines. Tutorial teaching of MD, PhD students and introductory courses for research.

Equipment and methods: immunoassay drug analytical facilities, HPLC drug analyses, DNA sequencing, Taqman machine for real-time PCR detection (ABI prismTM 7700).

PCR: cytosensor equipment, automatic ELISA, microtitre well-based fluorimetry, immunocyto-chemistry.

Department localization in hospital: The Section of Clinical Pharmacology is located centrally in the hospital and occupies about 300m^2 (to be expanded within the next few years). Laboratory for drug analyses. Laboratory for genotyping. Separate laboratories for RNA and protein work. Animal experiment facilities adjacent to laboratory. Human clinical pharmacology laboratory.

Uppsala University is the oldest university in Sweden and was inaugurated in the late 15th century. It includes all faculties, except dentistry. Adjacent and partially co-located are a multitude of departments at the Swedish agricultural university.

A Centre for Drugs is to be created through informal collaboration and exchange programmes between the faculties of Medicine, Pharmacy and Veterinary Medicine, the medical Products Agency, Pharmacia & Upjohn, and different departments in the Faculty of Natural Sciences, and the Positron Emission Tomography Centre. Several projects are performed through collaboration with different sections within Departments of Medicine, Neurology, Oncology, Pathology, clinical Genetics, Paediatrics, Paediatric Surgery, Psychiatry, etc.

Staff: the Section of Clinical Pharmacology has one professor, one senior lecturer, and three post-doc positions. The total staff is about 30 persons including six or seven physicians, pharmacists, two engineers, technicians, secretaries and nurses. Currently, there are 14 PhD student positions.

Application for short or long training in clinical pharmacology are to be submitted to the Section Head.

References

Dhar S, Nygren P, Botling J, Csóka K, Nilsson K, Larsson R (1996) Anticancer drug characterization using a human tumor cell line panel representing different forms of drug resistance. Br J Cancer 74: 888-896

Fridborg H, Jonsson B, Nybren P, Csóka K, Nilsson K, Öberg G, Kristensen J, Bergh J, Tholander B, Olsen L, Jakobsson Å, Larsson R (1994) Activity of cyclosporins as resistance modifiers in primary cultures of human hematological and solid tumors. Br J Cancer 70: 11-17

Hakkola J, Pasanen M, Purkunen R, Saarikoski S, Pelkonen O, Mäenpää J, Rane A, Raunio H (1994) Expression of xenobiotic metabolizing cytochrome P450 forms in human adult and fetal liver. Biochem Pharmacol 48: 59-64

Jonsson E, Fridborg H, Csóka K, Nygren P, Larsson R (1997) Cytotoxic activity of topotecan in human cell lines and primary cultures of human tumor cell from patients. Br J Cancer 76: 211-19

Ladona MG, Lindström B, Thyr C, Peng D, Rane A (1991) Differential foetal development of the O- and N-demethylation of codeine and dextromethorphan in man. Br J Clin Pharmacol 32: 295-302

Larsson R, Nygren P (1994) Cytotoxic activity of topoisomerase Ii inhibitors in primary cultures of tumor cells from patients with human hematologic and solid tumors. Cancer 74: 2857-2862

Nygren P, Fridborg H, Csóka K, Sundström C, de la Torre M, Kristensen J, Bergh J, Hagberg H, Glimelius B, Rastad J, Tholander B, Larsson R (1994) Detection of tumor specific cytotoxic drug activity in vitro using the fluorometric microculture cytotoxicity assay and primary cultures of tumor cells from patients. Int J Cancer 56: 715-720

Rane A, Liu Z, Henderson C, Wolf CR (1995) Divergent regulation of cytochrome P450 enzymes by morphine and pethidine: a neuroendocrine mechanism? Mol Pharmacol 47: 57-64

Wadelius M, Darj E, Frenne G, Rane A (1997) Induction of CYP2D6 in pregnancy. Clin Pharmacol Ther 62: 400-407

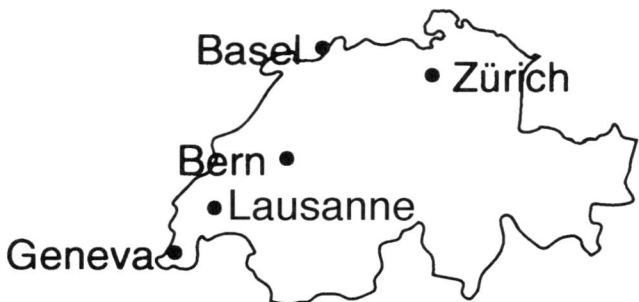

Switzerland

In Switzerland, it is possible to obtain two different specialist titles in clinical pharmacology. The first title is the so-called sub-speciality title (clinical pharmacology FMH) of the Swiss National Board of Physicians (Foederatio Medicorum Helveticorum). The sub-speciality is added to the main speciality (e.g. internal medicine, pediatrics, surgery etc.) at the same level as other sub-specialities such as cardiology, neprology, intensive care etc. The second title is the so-called specialist title (clinical pharmacologists SPC/SKP) given by the Clinical Pharmacology Section (SPC) of the Swiss Society of Pharmacology and Toxicology. This title may be given to physicians, pharmacists or other specialists in biological sciences with appropriate training.

The national requirements to become a specialist depend on the actual title. To become a FMH specialist requires at least 2 years of training after the main speciality training has been completed (usually 5 years out of a total of 7 years). The training aims at providing the candidates with a sound knowledge in the major fields of clinical pharmacology (clinical pharmacokinetics, pharmacodynamics, drug therapy, therapeutic drug monitoring, clinical toxicology, clinical trial methodology, and biometrics, GCP, ethical and legal issues, pharmacoepidemiology and pharmacoeconomy. The candidates must attend postgraduate courses organized by the Swiss Society of Pharmacology and Toxicology and pass an examination. The FMH specialist title can only be granted to candidates with a Swiss medical diploma. The SPC/SKP specialist title given by the Section of Clinical Pharmacology requires at least 6 years of training after graduation, and 4 years must be spent in a training centre of clinical pharmacology. The candidates must be well trained in the different fields of clinical pharmacology (see above). The candidates must obtain a medical degree (MD or PhD) and they must attend at least two courses in clinical pharmacology. Their scientific activity must be documented by at least four publications in the field of clinical pharmacology. The specialist title is available for candidates with a foreign academic degree. Each year, the Section of Clinical Pharmacology organizes two to three courses in clinical pharmacology. Well established courses in clinical pharmacology are organized outside of Switzerland.

The Section of Clinical Pharmacology of the Swiss Society of Pharmacology and Toxicology was founded in Geneva in 1978. Its goals are to develop research in clinical pharmacology in order to improve patient treatment, to encourage the teaching in clinical pharmacology, to sustain the interest of clinical pharmacologists and to maintain ties with sister societies outside Switzerland. The Section presently has 120 members.

The first chairs in clinical pharmacology were established in Berne (1964) and in Basel and Geneva in 1970. Today, there are five academic chairs: Basel, Berne, Geneva, Lausanne and Zürich. They are all active in undergraduate teaching, organizing the official national examination at the end of the medical study and postgraduate teaching of drug therapy in the main medical specialities (internal medicine, psychiatry, geriatric medicine etc.).

Due to the fact that Switzerland is a federation of states (cantons), the centres of clinical pharmacology are under local political administration (Ministry of Health and Welfare and Ministry of Education). At the federal level, the Ministry of Interior Affairs is responsible for both research and teaching.

The clinical pharmacologists of Switzerland are very active in the Swiss-based pharmaceutical industry and at the Office of Drugs Control. Academic clinical pharmacologists are also members of the Swiss board of experts for drug registration and pricing authorities.

Addresses

Basel
Dr Jürgen Drewe
Division of Clinical Pharmacology
Kantonsspital Basel
Petersgraben 4
CH-4031 Basel
Phone: +4161 265 2525
Fax: +4161 265 5401

Bern
Professor B Lauterburg
Professor J Reichen
Institut für Klinische Pharmakologie
Universität Bern
Murtenstrasse 35
CH-3010 Bern
Phone: +4131 632 3191

Fax: +4131 632 4997
E-mail: blauterburg@ik.unibe.ch
reichen@ikp.unibe.ch
Homep: www.cx.unibe.ch/ikp/

Professor S Vozeh
Medical Division
Intercantonal Office for the Control of Medicines
Erlachstrasse 8
CH-3000 Bern 9
Phone: +41 31 322 0345
Fax: +41 31 322 0432
E-mail: iksmed@uniplus.ch

Geneva
Professor P Dayer
Division of Clinical Pharmacology
University Hospital
Rue Michell-du-Crest 24
CH-1211 Geneva 14
Phone: +4122 372 9932
Fax: +4122 372 9940
E-mail: Pierre.Dayer@hcuge.ch

Lausanne
Professor J Biollaz
Division of Clinical Pharmacology
Centre Hospitalier Universitaire Vaudois
Beaumont 06-632
CH-1011 Lausanne CHUV
Phone: +4121 314 4262
Fax: +4121 314 4266

Reinach
Dr E Fröhlich
Drug Safety
Roche Pharma (Schweiz)
Schönmattstrasse 2
CH-4153 Reinach
Phone: +4161 715 4111
Fax: +4161 715 4112

Zürich
Professor PJ Meier
Klinische Pharmacologie und Toxikologie
Universitätsspital
CH-8091 Zürich
Phone: +411 255 2068
Fax: +411 820 3054

Training Centres in Switzerland

Berne

The following research areas are covered: isolation and characterization of copper and iron transporters (Professor M Solioz); pathophysiology and treatment of portal hypertension (Professor J Reichen); molecular mechanisms in cirrhosis (Professor M Solioz and Professor J Reichen); antioxidative defence in alcohol- and drug-induced liver disease (Professor BH Lauterburg); ion transport and signal transduction in the hepatocyte (Dr JF Dufour); carnitine transport and metabolism (PD Dr S Krähenbühl); theory and application (in particular drug analysis) of capillary electrophoresis (Professor W Thormann); clinical pharmacology of anti-infectious agents (Dr B Lee); multicentre trials in the treatment of chronic liver disease (Professor J Reichen).

The department offers doctoral studies in pharmacology/clinical pharmacology and in molecular biology. The programme is open to qualified candidates (diploma in medicine, pharmacy, biology). Clinical training is offered in hepatology (in conjunction with the Division of Gastroenterology) and clinical pharmacology. The department of clinical pharmacology runs an outpatient clinic and is closely affiliated with the university hospital where it offers a consultation service. Members of the department work closely with the department of clinical research so that a critical mass of expertise in all fields of biomedical research is available.

There are about 300 m^2 of research space, superbly equipped with the most modern tools for analytical tasks and work in cell and molecular biology.

The staff consists of seven senior staff members (four MDs, three PhDs), a varying number of doctoral and post-doctoral students, 13 technicians and nine supporting staff. There is an outpatient facility (five day beds) with four research nurses and access to a four-bed clinical investigation unit in the Department of Medicine. Applications should be sent to one of the directors. Further information can be garnered on our homepage at http://www.cx.unibe.ch/ikp

References

Forestier M, Reichen J, Solioz M (1996) Application of mRNA differential display to liver cirrhosis: Reduced fetuin expression in biliary cirrhosis in the rat. Biochem Biophys Res Communications 225: 377-383

Helbling B, Von Overbeck J, Lauterburg BH (1996) Decreased release of glutathione into the systemic circulation of patients with HIV infection. Eur J Clin Invest 26: 38-44

Hufschmid E, Theurillat R, Wilder-Smith CH, Thormann W (1996) Characterization of the genetic polymorphism of dihydrodeine O-demethylation in man via analysis of urinary dihydrocodeine and dihydromorphine by micellar electrokinetic capillary chromatography. J Chromatogr B 678: 43-51

Krähenbühl St, Reichen J (1996) Carnitine metabolism in patients with chronic liver disease. Hepatology 25: 148-153

Küpfer A, Aeschlimann C, Cerny T (1996) Methylene blue and the neurotoxic mechanisms of ifosfamide encephalopathy. Eur J Clin Pharmacol 50: 249-252

Lebbe C, Reichen J, Wartna E, Sägesser H, Poelstra K, Meijer DKF (1997) Targeting naproxen to non-parenchymal liver cells protects against endotoxin induced liver damage. J Drug Targ 4: 303-310

Strausak D, Solioz M (1997) CopY is a copper-inducible repressor of the enterococcus hirae copper ATPases. J Biol Chem 272: 8932-8936

Von Heeren F, Verpoorte E, Manz A, Thormann W (1996) Micellar electrokinetic chromatography separations and analyses of biological samples on a cyclic planar microstructure. Anal Chem 68: 2044-2053

Geneva

The major research in vitro drug biotransformation in vivo/in vitro forecasting of drug metabolism, clinical pharmacokinetics, computer-based predictions of drug interactions, pain pharmacology.

Our division is a hospital-based centre with a laboratory and a clinical investigation unit. Clinical pharmacology service for hospital physicians and general practitioners, multidisciplinary pain clinic. Two specialized clinical pharmacology units affiliated to the division: Unit of Geriatric Clinical Pharmacology (Head Dr N Vogt), and Unit of Clinical Psychopharmacology (Head Dr P Schulz).

The division is affiliated to the Geneva University's Faculty of Medicine.

The division has three permanent positions for fully trained specialists, positions for consultant physicians, trainees physicians, doctoral students (MD and PhD), laboratory and clerical staff, for at total of 20 people.

For applications: contact Professor P Dayer

References

Desmeules J, Gascon MP, Dayer P, Magistris M (1991) Impact of environmental and genetic factors on codeine analgesia. Eur J Clin Pharmacol 41: 23-26

Leemann T, Dayer P (1995) Quantitative prediction of in vivo drug metabolism and interactions from in vitro data. In: Pacifici GM, Gracchia GN Eds, Advances in drug metabolism in man, chapter 22, p. 783-830, Office for Official Publications of the European Communities, Luxembourg

Leemann T, Bonnabry P, Dayer P (1994) Selective inhibition of major drug metabolizing cytochrome P450 isozymes in human liver microsomes by carbon monoxide. Life Sci 54: 951-956

Piletta P, Porchet HC, Dayer P (1991) Central analgesic effect of acetaminophen but not of aspirin. Clin Pharmacol Ther 49: 350-354

Transon C, Leemann T, Vogt N, Dayer P (1995) In vivo inhibition profile of cytochrome p450TB (CYP2C9) by (+/-)-fluvastatin. Clin Pharmacol Ther 58: 412-417

Transson C, Leemann T, Dayer P (1996a) In vitro comparative inhibition profiles of major human drug metabolising cytochrome p450 isozymes (CYP2C9, CYP2D6 and CYP3A4) by HMG-CoA reductase inhibitors. Eur J Clin Pharmacol 50: 209-215

Transson C, Lecoeur S, Leemann T, Beaune Ph, Dayer P (1996b) Interindividual variability in catalytic activity and immunoreactivity of three major human liver cytochrome p450 isozymes. Eur J Clin Pharmacol 51: 79-85

Coquoz D, Porchet HC, Dayer P (1993) Central analgesic effects of desipramine, fluvoxamine, and moclobemide after single oral dosing: A study in healthy volunteers. Clin Pharmacol and Ther 54: 339-344

Desmeules JA, Piguet V, Collart L, Dayer P (1996) Contribution of monoaminergic modulation to the analgesic effect of tramadol. Br J Clin Pharmacol 41: 7-12

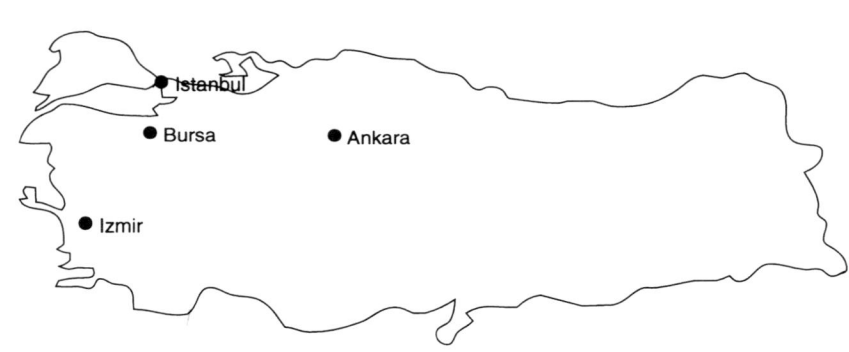

Turkey

Medical pharmacology is an official medical speciality in Turkey although there are some departments which include 'clinical pharmacology' in their title. Clinical pharmacology is not an official speciality yet, but is likely to get official approval in the near future. Since 1993, the Ministry of Health has established guidelines for clinical drug research in accordance with the similar guidelines of the European Union. As a consequence, certain clinics at the medical schools and some of the state training hospitals have participated in international drug trials.

The Turkish Pharmacological Society was founded in 1966 and it has about 400 members. The Society does not have a section of clinical pharmacology, but an independent society of clinical pharmacology was established in 1996, and the Society is still in the making.

There are no chairs in clinical pharmacology in Turkey. However, a doctoral training programme in clinical pharmacology has been developed by the Department of Pharmacology at the Hacettepe University. Although the programme was approved by the Institute for Graduate Studies in Health Sciences, it has been stopped without reason by higher bodies. Turkish pharmacologists are presently fighting to overcome this difficulty. In 1996, a Turkish textbook on clinical pharmacology and regulations was published, and the same year the first unit of clinical pharmacology was opened at the Hacettepe University in Ankara. In some of the Turkish medical schools, a course in clinical pharmacology is part of the curriculum. However, in most cases, the content is pharmacology applied to therapeutics, rather than actual clinical pharmacology. The Ministry of Health is responsible for registration involved in clinical drug trials in Turkey.

Addresses

Ankara
Professor H Ayhan
Department of Pharmacology and
Clinical Pharmacology
Ankara University Medical School
TR-06100 Ankara
Phone: +90 312 310 3010

Professor SO Kayaalp
Ahmet II aşim 95-A/24
Dikmen
TR-06460 Ankara
Phone: +90 312 238 1093
Fax: +90 312 482 1103

Professor FC Tulunay
Department of Pharmacology and Clinical Pharmocology
Medical School of Ankara University
Sihhye, 06100 Ankara
Phone and Fax: +90 312 311 6495
E-mail: tulunay@dialup.ankara.eda.tr

Bursa
Professor BK Kiran
Uludag University Medical School
Department of Pharmacology and
Clinical Pharmacology
Görükle Kampusu
TR-16059 Bursa
Tel: +90 224 442 8316
Fax: +90 224 442 8189
E-mail:
bkkiran@uu20.bim.uludag.edu.tr

Istanbul
Professor H Koyuncuoglu
Istanbul University
Medical School

Department of Pharmacology
Çapa
TR-34390 Istanbul
Fax: +90 212 631 7514

Professor Kemal Berkman
Marmara University Medical School
Department of Pharmacology
Haydarpasa
Istanbul
Phone: +90 216 347 5594

Professor E Eskazan
Istanbul University
Cerrahpasa Medical School
Department of Pharmacology
Cerra pasa/Istanbul
Phone: +90 212 586 1557
              +90 212 587 6878
Fax: +90 212 633 0131
E-mail: eeskazan@istanbul.edu.tr

Izmir
Professor Hülya Güven
Dokuzeylül University Medical School
Department of Pharmaoclogy
Inciralti
TR-35100 Izmir
Phone: +90 232 277 7333
Fax: +90 232 277 7333

Professor A Evinç
Ege University Medical School
Department of Pharmacology
Bornova
TR-35100 Izmir
Tel: +90 232 3882862
Fax: +90 232 3422142
E-mail: evinc@bornova.ege.edu.tr

Training Centres in Turkey

Ankara

Ankara University

The Department of Pharmacology and Clinical Pharmacology of Ankara University Medical School was founded in 1946. The scope of the department has been research, training and service of basic and clinical pharmacology. It has completed its legal institutionalization in Clinical Pharmacology in 1996. There are five full-professors, four associate professors, six research assistants and eight PhD students in the department who are all medical doctors. The training programme of the discipline to medical students has been reorganized in 1987 to cover both basic and clinical pharmacology using a problem-based learning system which has been proved to be effective by all means. The training policy has also been widened to new target populations, clinicians. All kinds of clinical pharmacological service have long been given and are, for the time being, given to whom it is necessary (e.g. Ministry of Health, hospitals, drug industry).

References

Cila E, Alpaslan M, Melli M, Tokgözoglu M (1994) Prostaglandin E2 activity in the synovial like membrane. J Arthroplasty 9 (1): 67-71

Inan S, Soydan C, Tulunay FC (1994a) MMPI profiles of Turkish headache sufferers. Headache 34: 152

Inan L, Tulunay FC, Güvener A, Tokgöz G, Inan N (1994b) Characteristics of headache in migraine without auro and episodic tension type headache in Turkish population to H S classification. Cephalgia 14: 171

Soygür H, Palaoglu Ö, Ekarsu ES, Ayhan H (1994) Diltiazem significantly improves the negative symptoms of chronic schizophrenia: a double blind, placebo controlled clinical study. J Ankara Med School 16 (4)

Soygür H, Palaoglu Ö, Altinörs N, Çorapçioglu D, Erdogan G, Ayhan H (1997) Melperone treatment in an organic delusional syndrome induced by hyperprolactinemia: a case report. Eur Neuropsychopharmacol 7: 161-163

Tulunay M, Demiralp S, Taştan S, Akalin H, Özyurda U, Çorapçioglu T, Akarasu ES (1993) Complement (C3-C4) and C-reactive protein responses to cardiopulmonary bypass and protamine administration. Anesth Intens Care 21: 50-55

Tulunay FC, Onaran O, Uçar A, Ünal N, Usanmaz S, Tulunay M, Erbay E (1994) Pharmacokinetics of Fludex (Indapamid) manufactured in Turkey Medical Network Cardiology 1: 185-188

Tulunay M, Tulunay FC, Alkiş N, Özdemir N, Akat M, Yavuzer Ş (1996) Double blind comparison of ketorolac and metamizol in postthoracotomy pain. Turk J Med Sci 26: 333-338

Hacettepe University

The Department of Pharmacology and Toxicology of Hacettepe University Medical School was founded in 1965. In addition to its relatively heavy involvement in experimental pharmacology in animal subjects including neuropharmacology, cardiovascular pharmacology, pharmacology or serotonin and central autonomic control, it has also been involved in genetic polymorphism of drug metabolizing enzymes in the Turkish population since 1985. Its clinical pharmacology unit was established in 1996. The academic staff consists of five professors and two associate professors. The department offers PhD programmes in pharmacology and toxicology. There are nine PhD students including research assistants as of early 1998. The undergraduate medical education was given in the framework of an integrated system. Inclusion of an applied pharmacology course to medical curriculum is underway. The department has sufficient relevant infrastructure to conduct experimental works.

References

Bozkurt A, Başçi NE, Kalan S, Tuncer M, Kayaalp SO (1990) N-Acetylation phenotyping with sulphadimidine in a Turkish population. Eur J Clin Pharmacol 38: 53-56

Bozkurt A, Başçi NE, Işimer A, Kayaalp SO (1991) Polymorphic debrisoquine metabolism in a Turkish population. Clin Pharmacol Ther 55: 399-401

Başçi NE, Bozkurt A, Kortunay S, Işimer A, Kayaalp SO (1996) Proguanil metabolism in relation to S-mephenytoin oxidation in a Turkish population. Br J Clin Pharmacol 42: 771-773

Bozkurt A, Başçi NE, Işimer A, Sayal A, Kayaalp SO (1996) Metabolic ratios of four probes of CYP2D6 in Turkish subjects: a crossover study. Eur J Drug Metab Pharmacokinet 21: 309-314

Hanioglu-Kargi S, Başçi NE, Soysal H, Bozkurt A, Günsel E, Kayaalp SO (1998) The penetration of ofloxacin into human aqueous humor given by various routes. Eur J Ophthalmol 8: 139-143

Kortunay S, Başçi NE, Bozkurt A, Işimer A, Sayal A, Kayaalp SO (1998, in press) The hydroxylation of omeprazole correlates with S-mephenytoin and proguanil metabolism. Eur J Clin Pharmacol

Bornova/Izmir

Our department was founded in 1958, 3 years after the foundation of the Medical Faculty of Ege University. Besides our experimental studies, our laboratory provides support to the other clinics of the university hospital which is one of the biggest in Europe with a capacity of 2000 beds. The determination of drug concentrations in body fluids by EMIT (Enzyme Multiplied Immune Technology) also provides us data for pharmacokinetic and pharmacodynamic studies.

The academic staff consists of three professors and two associate professors. We have a postgraduate education of 3 years for medical doctors in our department who are selected with an examination, and at the end of the education programme they become pharmacologists. There are five doctors in our department at the moment continuing this programme. Our laboratory is mainly focused on in vitro studies on isolated organ chambers. We are especially interested in sepsis, arthritis, diabetes, renal failure and pharmacology of pain.

Bursa

The research activity of the Department of Pharmacology and Clinical Pharmacology at the Uludag University Medical School is mostly in basic pharmacology. The main subject of interest is documented in the publications. The training is also mainly focused on basic pharmacology. Some training and research in clinical pharmacology have in the recent years mostly been concerning bioequivalence studies.

The Department has very good equipment for classical pharmacological and biochemical pharmacological research. The Department is also responsible for the daily activities of the hospital. We are responsible for the measurements of about 90 biochemical and pharmacological parameters for patients (such as blood levels, some drugs, insulin, noradrenaline, oestrogen, progesteron, etc.). We have no clinical section in the hospital, but beds can be arranged within the department of internal medicine when making bioavailability or bioequivalance studies.

The Uludag University is a new university (25 years old) developing quite fast. It is in a large, green campus with about 10 schools, 15 km from the centre of Bursa.

The department has five full time staff and six assistants. The academic staff members are mostly graduated from medical school. There are also a number of chemists and laboratory technicians.

Any academic person can apply directly to the department head. We can provide them with working facilities, but no salary. An exception is if the applicant comes from a NATO country. Then, the salary problem can be solved through a NATO grant.

References

Büyükuysal L, Ulus IH, Aydin S, Mogol E, Kiran BK (1994) Comparison of relative bioavailability and pharmacokinetic characteristics of three different tablet formulations of amlodipine in healthy volunteers. Uludag Üniv. Typ Fak Derg 1: 70

Büyükuysal RL, Ulus IH, Aydin S, Kiran BK (1995) 3,4Diaminopyridine and choline increase in vivo acetylcholine release in rat striatum. Eur J Pharmacol 281: 179-185

Savci V, Gürün S, Ulus IH, Kiran BK (1996a) Intracerebroventricular injection of choline increases plasma oxytocin levels in conscious rats. Brain Res 709: 97-102

Savci V, Gürün MS, Ulus IH, Kiran BK (1996b) Effect of intracerebroventricularly injected choline on plasma ACTH and bendorphin levels in conscious rats. Eur J Pharmacol 309: 275-280

Ulus IH, Aydin S, Mogol E, Büyükuysal L, Gürün S, Kiran BK (1994a) Bioavailability of sultamicillin in healthy volunteers following oral administration of sulta-micillin base and sultamicillin tosylate. Uludag Üniv. Typ Fak Derg 1: 55

Ulus IH, Büyükuysal L, Aydin S, Mogol E, Gürün S, Kiran Bk (1994b) Comparison of bioavailability of sultamicillin in healthy volunteers following oral administration of two different tablet formulations. Uludag Üniv. Typ Fak Derg 1: 59

Ulus IH, Arslan BY, Savci V, Kiran BK (1995) Restoration of blood pressure by choline treatment in rat made hypotensive by haemorrhage. Br J Pharmacol 116: 19111-917

Istanbul

Cerrahpaşa University Medical School

The Department of Pharmacology of Istanbul University Cerrahpaşa Medical School was established in 1967 when the University of Istanbul, Faculty of Medicine was divided into Cerrahpaşa Faculty of Medicine and Istanbul Faculty of Medicine. Originally, it was a therapy clinic but now it is a research and education centre. It has seven staff members and eight research assistants. In the Department there is also a clinical epilepsy treatment centre. Various drug assays including antiepileptic drugs, cytotoxics, antibiotics are provided for clinical and research purposes. Vasodepressive substances, oxytocin activity and toxicity tests are provided for the pharmaceutical industry.

References

Akkan AG, Mutlu I, Özyazgan S, Gök A, Yigit U, Özüner Z, Ôenses V, Pekel H (1997) Comparative tear concentrations of topically applied ciprofloxacin, ofloxacin and norfloxacin in human eyes. Int J Clin Pharm Ther 35(5): 214-217

Aykaç B, Erolçay H, Dikmen Y, Öz H, Yillar DO (1995) Comparison of intrapleural versus intravenous morphine for postthoracotomy pain management. J Cardiothorac Vasc Anesth 9(5): 538-540

Bozkurt P, Kaya G, Süzer Ö (1996) Diazepam serum concentration-sedative effect relation-ship in patients with liver disease. Middle East J Anesthesiology 13 (4): 405-413

Çetinkale O, Yazici Z (1997) Early postburn fatty acid profile in burn patients. Burns 23: 392-399

Eşkazan E, Aslan S (1992) Antiepileptic therapy and teratogenicity in Turkey. Int J Clin Pharmacol Ther Toxicol 30 (8): 261-264

Süzer A, Süzer Ö, Aykaç Z (1997) Comparison of midazolam and propofol effect on cerebral metabolism during cardiopulmonary bypass. Br J Anaesth 78(2): A52

Süzer A, Süzer Ö, Aykaç Z (1998) Comparison of midazolam, thiopental, propofol and etomidate on the prevention of desaturation during rewarming phase of hypothermic cardiopulmonary bypass. Submitted to Eur J Anaesthesiol

Umut S, Gemicioglu B, Yildirim N, Barlas A, Özüner Z (1992) Effect of theophyline in chronic obstructive lung disease. Int J Clin Pharmacol Ther Toxicol 30(5): 149-152

Yillar DO, Akkan AG, Akcasu A, Özüner Z (1991) The influence of choline ascorbate on the blood levels of ascorbic acid in humans. Int J Clin Pharmacol Ther Toxicol 29(6): 228-230

Çapa, Istanbul

The Department of Pharmacology, Istanbul University Istanbul (Çapa) Medical School was founded in 1967 when the former single Faculty of Medicine was divided into two separate schools. The Department of Pharmacology of the former medical school, which was the oldest in Turkey, had been involved in studies in clinical pharmacology for a long time as a clinic of therapeutic studies. The new Department is carrying out clinical investigations in part in collaboration with the clinical departments of the medical school. A special outpatient unit for research founded in 1976 has been doing investigations in hypertensive patients. The Department increased its capacity in clinical pharmacological studies by commissioning its staff members at clinics and foreign centres involved in clinical pharmacological studies under a clinical pharmacology training programme. Nowadays, one of the associate professors (Dr Yagiz Üresin) is heavily involved in clinical pharmacological studies.

References

Eroglu L, Ôimşek S, Yazici O, Keyer M, Yüksel Ô (1979) A study of the relationship between serum lithium and plasma cortisol levels in manic depressive patients. Br J Clin Pharmacol 8: 89-90

Koyuncuoglu H (1983) The treatment with L-aspartic acid of persons addicted to opiates. Bull Narcot 35: 11-15
Koyuncuoglu H (1995) The combination of tizanidine markedly improves the treatment with dextromethorphan of heroin addicted outpatients. Int J Clin Pharmacol Ther 33: 13-19
Koyuncuoglu H, Saydam B (1990) The treatments of heroin addicts with dextromethorphan: a double-blind comparison of dextromethorphan with chlorpromazine. Int J Clin Pharmacol Ther Toxicol 28: 147-151
Sener AI, Ceylan ME, Koyuncuoglu H (1986) Comparison of the supressive effects of L-aspartic acid and chlorpromazine + diazepam treatments on opiate abstinence syndrome signs in men. Arzneimittelforschung 36: 1684-1686
Yazici O, Gümüşcü K, Esin Y, Kandemir E, Üçok A, Şen D, Eroglu L (1994) Changes in serum calcium and magnesium levels during the early phase of lithium treatment. Prediction of the prophylatic response. Lithium 5: 53-58

Marmara University
Marmara University School of Medicine was founded in 1983 and the Department of Pharmacology started its activities by the end of 1986. The following are the academic staff members of the department: Professor Kemal Berkman, MD and Head of the department; Professor Sule Oktay, MD and PhD; Associate Professor Filiz Onat, MD, PhD. There are five doctoral students.

Basic medical pharmacology
– The main fields of research of the department are (1) autonomic system pharmacology: cholinergic system: muscarinic receptors subtypes (2) central nervous system pharmacology: cholinergic, GABAergic and glutamergic control of blood pressure and epilepsy.
– Teaching activities: (1) graduate teaching: School of Medicine (2nd and 3rd year; in English), Nursing Schools, School for Radiology Technicians, (2) Postgraduate teaching: Masters and PhD programmes in pharmacology.

Clinical pharmacology
– Research: several clinical studies (mainly phase IV) are being conducted in collaboration with the Department of Cardiology.

- Bioequivalence: two bioequivalence studies have been conducted in collaboration with the Internal Medicine Department). We have applied to the Ministry of Health to get an approval for such studies and now developing our unit in collaboration with the Gastro-enterology Institute

Teaching: (1) Clinical pharmacology course for phase IV medical students during their Internal Medicine Clerkship. Problem-based rational pharmacotherapy teaching model is being used. (2) Elective Clinical Pharmacology Clerkship for phase V.

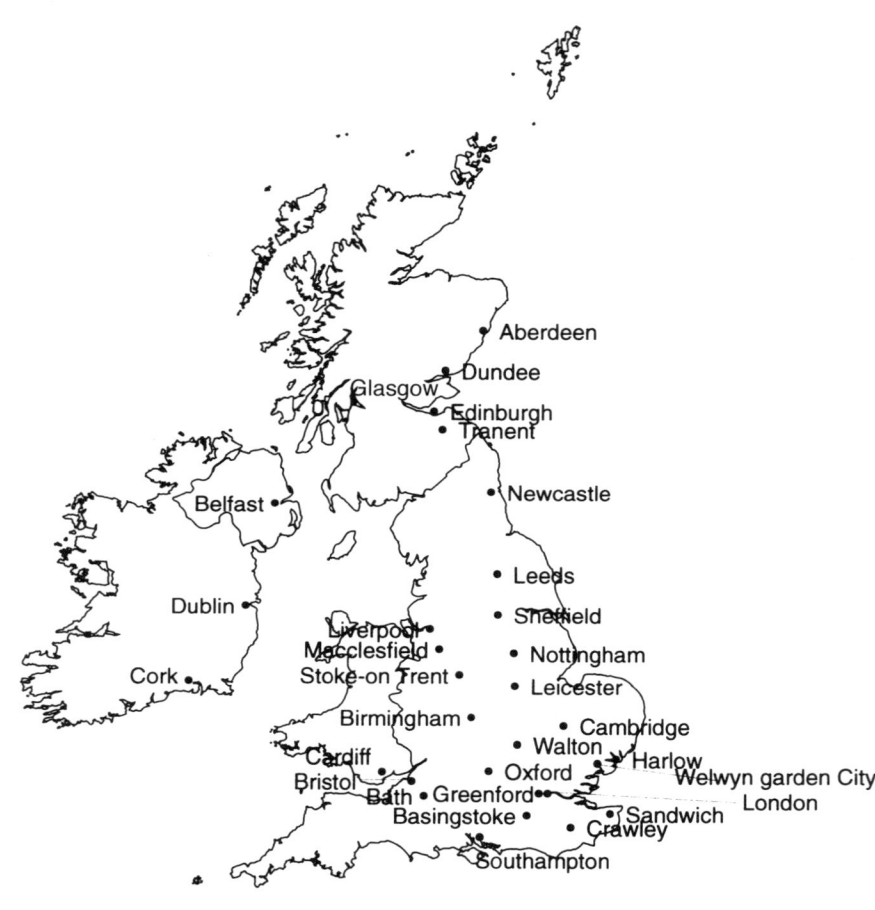

United Kingdom

Clinical Pharmacology and Therapeutics (CPT) is an accepted speciality for clinical training in the UK but most trainees will also be trained in parallel in General Internal Medicine (G(I)M). The training in Clinical Pharmacology and Therapeutics has undergone a substantial change in the last few years as a result of moves to integrate clinical training in the UK with that seen in the body of Europe. The usual pattern of training following registration will be a minimum period of 2 years of general professional training at the Senior House Officer level. After obtaining the diploma of membership of one of the Royal College of Physicians (by examination), the trainee will then usually obtain a Specialist Registrar post that has been approved for Higher Medical Training in CPT and G(I)M. The period of training will normally take 5 years after which time the individual will be able to obtain a certificate of competition of specialist training (National Health Service (CCST)) and will then be able to apply for a consultant post in the National Health Service or a similar post elsewhere in Europe.

The training in G(I)M will equip the trainee to manage a wide variety of general medical problems The CPT training will be available in most of the universities in the UK and at least 16 new posts have been established in association with the pharmaceutical industry. The period of higher Medical Training in CPT allows for up to 2 years spent in acquiring research skills. However, in some cases, trainees will wish to spend longer than this in order to fully understand the discipline. It is expected that many will spend 3 years or so in research enabling them to obtain a doctoral degree. Trainees will be expected to obtain some management training and experience in medical audit. A curriculum has now been established in CPT, including both obligatory and recommended experience. The full curriculum will be available on request. The obligatory experience states that the trainee should have a sound knowledge of:
 – Drug action in man
 – Clinical pharmacokinetics

- The theory and practice of statistics and experimental design
- The evaluation of scientific literature
- The interpretation of preclinical pharmacological and toxicological studies
- The design and conduct of phase I clinical studies of new drugs
- Rational and cost-effective use of medicines
- The role and function of a Drug and Therapeutics Committee (by attendance as a full member)
- The development and management of drug formularies
- The communication and educational skills required to teach medical and professional colleagues concerned with health care.

The recommended experience includes knowledge about phase II and III studies, adverse drug reactions, drug epidemiology, therapeutic drug monitoring, drug overdose, Research Ethics Committees and National regulatory requirements.

Clinical pharmacology is well established as an academic discipline in most universities in the UK. The majority of university medical schools have a department or a division of clinical pharmacology and give the clinical pharmacologist an acute service role. Over the last few years, the subject area has become somewhat less visible in the university setting. This is because of amalgamation of clinical pharmacology with other disciplines (e.g. as physiological sciences or medicine) while in other, cases the success of individual chair holders has led them to take over chairs of medicine or deans of faculties. In London, there has also been a progressive programme of amalgamation of medical schools.

Clinical pharmacologists often have direct responsibility for both inpatient and outpatient care, while in a few cases, they may only be involved in outpatient care or be part of the therapeutic drug monitoring service. The teaching of clinical pharmacology and therapeutics to both medical students and to postgraduates is a major responsibility and all units have an active research programme.

Outside the universities, a number of smaller units, usually with one or two trained clinical pharmacologists, work in the National Health Service. There has been surprisingly little expansion of clinical pharmacology in the National Health Service. This is partly due to the emphasis on the internal marker and generating income and also the difficulty of defining the clinical role for pure clinical pharmacology. In contrast, clinical pharmacology has developed in the pharmaceutical industry, and most research-based companies in the UK have an active clinical pharmacology unit.

The aim is to consolidate the role of clinical pharmacology. Most current posts are clinical academic posts at the senior lecturer, reader or professorial level. It is expected that more posts will be available in the future in the National Health Service, in the pharmaceutical industry and with regulatory bodies.

Most clinical pharmacologists belong to the British Pharmacological Society (BPS) which has over 2500 members. There is an active clinical section which meets twice each year and has 700 members, many of whom come from other European countries. The honorary secretary of the clinical section is: Professor David Webb, Edinburgh.

Addresses

Aberdeen
Professor JC Petrie
Clinical Pharmacology Unit
Department of Medicine and Therapeutics
Polwarth Building
Foresterhill
Aberdeen A25 2ZD
Phone: +441224 681818
Fax: +44 1224 699884

Bath
Dr P Bennett
Clinical Pharmacology Unit
Royal United Hospital
Combe Park
Bath BA1 3NG
Phone: +441225 824536

Belfast
Professor RG Shanks
Department of Therapeutics and Pharmacology
Queens University of Belfast
Whitla Medical Building
97 Lisburn Road
Belfast BT9 7BL
Phone: +44 1232 335770
Fax: +44 1232 438346
E-mail: r.g.shanks@qub.ac.uk

Birmingham
Dr MJ Kendall
Department of Clinical Pharmacology
Queen Elizabeth Hospital
Birmingham B15 2TH
Phone: +44 121 627 2383

Bristol
Dr CJC Roberts
Consultant Senior Lecturer in
Clinical Pharmacology & Therapeutics
Division of Medicine, Level 5
Bristol Royal Infirmary
Bristol BS2 8HW
Phone: +44 117 928 2254

Bucks
Head of Clinical unit
Clinial Pharmacology

Hoechst Marion Roussel Ltd.
Walton Manor
Walton
Milton Keynes
Bucks MK7 7AJ
Phone: +44 1908 201 185
Fax: +44 1908 680 463

Cambridge
Professor MJ Brown
Clinical Pharmacology Unit
Level 2, F and G Block
Box 110
Addenbrooke's Hospital
Hills Road
Cambridge CB2 2QQ
Phone: +44 1223 336743
Fax: +44 1223 216893
E-mail: mjb14@medschl.cam.ac.uk

Cardiff
Professor A Richens
Department of Pharmacology and Therapeutics
University of Wales College of Medicine
Heath Park
Cardiff CF4 4XN
Phone: +44 1222 755944

Cheshire
Dr S Cunningham
Zeneca Pharmaceuticals
Goup Head, Clinical Pharmacology
Mereside, Alderley Park
Macclesfield
Cheshire SK10 4TF
Phone: +44 1625 514892

Dr AJ Williams
Zeneca Pharmaceuticals
Chief Clinical Pharmacologist
Mereside, Alderley Park
Macclesfield
Cheshire SK10 4TF
Phone: +44 1625 514892

Cork
Professor MB Murphy
Pharmacology & Therapeutics Department
University College
Cork
Ireland
Phone: +353 2134 5599
Fax: +353 21343211

Dublin
Professor J Feely
Pharmacology and Therapeutics Department
Trinity College
Dublin 2
Ireland
Phone: +353 1608 1563
Fax: +353 1671 3507
E-mail: jfeely@mail.tcd.ie

Professor D Fitzgerald
Department of Clinical Pharmacology
Royal College of Surgeons in Ireland
123 St. Stephen's Green
Dublin 2
Ireland
Phone: +353 1478 0200
Fax: +353 1478 1200

Dundee
Professor DG McDevitt
Department of Clinical Pharmacology and Therapeutics
Ninewells Hospital and Medical School
Dundee DD1 9SY
Scotland
Phone: +44 1382 632180
Fax: +44 1382 644972
Email: j.l.orr@dundee.ac.uk

Professor J McEwen
Department of Clinical Pharmacology
and Therapeutics
Ninewells Hospital and Medical School
Dundee DD1 9SY
Scotland
Phone: +44 1382 646 317
Fax: +44 1382 645 606

Edinburgh
Professor DJ Webb
Christison Professor of Therapeutics
and Clinical Pharmacology
University Department of Medicine
Western General Hospital
Edinburgh EH4 2XU
Scotland
Phone: +44 31 343 6017
Fax: +44 31 332 1205
E-mail: D.J.Webb@ed.ac.uk

Glasgow
Dr MJ Brodie
Epilepsy Unit
Department of Medicine and Therapeutics
Western Infirmary
Glasgow G11 6NT
Scotland
Phone: +44 141 211 2572

Professor J Reid
Regius Professor of Medicine &
Therapeutics
Department of Medicine and
Therapeutics
Gardiner Institute
Western Infirmary
Glasgow G11 6NT
Scotland
Phone: +44 141 211 2886
Fax: +44 141 339 2800
E-mail: j.l.reid@clinmed.gla.ac.uk

Greenford
Dr N Baber
Glaxo Wellcome Research & Development
Greenford Road
Greenford
Middlesex UB6 0HE
Phone: +44 181 966 3484
Fax: +44 181 869 1017
E-mail: NSB1438@ggr.co.uk

Dr G Rapeport
Head of Clinical Pharmacology Department
Glaxo Wellcome Research & Development
Greenford Road
Greenford
Middlesex UB6 0HE
Phone: +44 181 966 4581
Fax: +44 181 966 2757

Hants
Dr S Wise
Lilly Research Centre
Dextra Court
Chapel Hill
Basingstoke
Hants RG21 5SY

Harlow
Dr DG Scibberas
Merck Sharp & Dohme Research Labs
Clinical Pharmacology Europe
Terlings Park
Eastwick Road
Harlow, Essex CM20 2QR
Phone: +44 1279 440157
Fax: +44 1279 440156

Dr TCG Tasker
Director & Vice President, Clinical
Pharmacology Europe
SmithKline Beecham Pharmaceuticals
New Frontiers Science Park South

Third Avenue
Harlow
Essex CM19 5AW
Phone: +44 1279 644740
Fax: +44 1279 644404
E-mail: TimothyqCqTasker@SBPHRD.COM@INET

Inveresk
Dr W Nimmo
Inveresk Research
Tranent EH 2NE
Scotland
Phone: +44 1875 614 545
Fax: +44 1875 514 555
E-Mail: walter.nimmo@iri.iri.btx400.co.uk

Leeds
Professor H Bird
University of Leeds
Clinical Pharmacology Unit
Chapel Allerton Hospital
Chapeltown Road
Leeds LS7 4SA
Phone: +44 113 292 4721
Fax: +44 113 292 4723

Dr M Feely
Department of Medicine
Martin Wing
Leeds General Infirmary
Leeds LS1 3EX
Phone: +44 1132 432 799

Leicester
Professor D Barnett
Division of Clinical Pharmacology
University of Leicester
Robert Kilpatrick Clinical Sciences Building
Leicester Royal Infirmary
P.O. Box 65
Leicester LE2 7LX
Phone: +44 116 252 3126
Fax: +44 116 252 3108
E-mail: dbbl@le.ac.uk

Leics
Dr GT Dixon
Department of Clinical Pharmacology
Astra Charnwood
Bakewell Road
Loughborough
Leics LE11 5RH
Phone: +44 1509 644000
Fax: +44 1509 645555
E-mail: geoffrey.dixon@charwood.gb.astra.com
Homep: www.astra.com/charnwood

Liverpool
Professor A Breckenridge
Department of Pharmacology and Therapeutics
New Medical School
Ashton Street
Liverpool L69 3BX
Phone: +44 151 794 5542
Fax: +44 151 794 5540

London
Professor PJ Barnes
Department of Thoracic Medicine
National Heart & Lung Institute
Dovehouse Street
London SW3 6LY
Phone: +44 171 351 8174
Fax: +44 171 351 5675
E-mail: p.j.barnes@ic.ac.uk
Homep: www.nhli.ic.ac.uk/tmed.htm

Professor N Benjamin
Department of Clinical Pharmacology
St. Bartholomew's and the Royal London School
of Medicine and Dentistry
Charterhouse Square
London EC1M 6BQ
Phone: +44 171 415 3402

Fax: +44 171 415 3408
E-mail: N.Benjamin@mds.qmw.ac.uk

Dr J Collier
Department of Pharmacology and
Clinical Pharmacology
St George's Hospital Medical School
Cranmer Terrace
London SW17 0RE
Phone   +44 181 725 5607
Fax: +44 181 682 0487
E-mail: jcollier@sghms.ac.uk

Professor D Davies
Department of Clinical Pharmacology
Royal Postgraduate Medical School
Ducane Road
London W12 0HS
Phone: +44 181 740 3220
Fax: +44 181 749 3439
E-mail: dboland@rpms.ac.uk

Dr I James
Department of Medicine
Royal Free Hospital School of Medicine
Clinical Sciences Building
Pond Street
London NW3 2QG
Phone: +44 171 794 0500

Professor M Lader
Clinical Psychopharmacology
Institute of Psychiatry
De Crespigny Park
Denmark Hill
London SE5 8AF
Phone: +44 171 703 5411, Ext. 3372
Fax: +44 171 252 5437

Professor A Lant
Department of Clinical Pharmacology
and Therapeutics
Chelsea and Westminster Hospital
369 Fulham Road
London SW10 9NH

Phone: +44 181 746 8144
Fax: +44 181 746 8887

Professor JM Ritter
Department of Clinical Pharmacology
UMDS Guys & St Thomas's Hospitals
Block 5 South, St Thomas's Hospital
London SE1 7EH
Phone: +44 171 928 9292
Fax: +44 171 401 2242
E-mail: j.ritter@umds.ac.uk

Professor P Sever
Imperial College School of Medicine
Department of Clinical Pharmacology
St Mary's Hospital
Praed Street
London W2 1PG
Phone: +44 171 725 1117
Fax: +44 171 725 6145

Professor C Swift
Department of Health Care of the Elderly
King's College Hospital School of Medicine and Dentistry
King's College Hospital (Dulwich)
East Dulwich Grove
London SE22 8PT
Phone: +44 171 346 6076
Fax: +44 171 346 6476

Professor P Vallance
Centre for Clinical Pharmacology
The Rayne Institute
University College London
5 University Street
London WC1E 6JJ
Phone: +44 171 209 6340
Fax: +44 171 209 6351
E-mail: patrick.vallance@ucl.ac.uk

Newcastle-upon-Tyne
Professor M Rawlins
Department of Clinical Pharmacology

University of Newcastle
Claremont Place
Newcastle-upon-Tyne NE1 7RU
Phone: +44 191 230 5460

Nottingham
Professor P Rubin
Department of Therapeutics
Floor C South Block
Queen's University Medical Centre
Nottingham NG7 2UH
Phone: +44 115 942 0820

Dr IP Hall
Head of Division
Division of Therapeutics
South Block, C Floor
Queen's Medical Centre
Nottingham NG7 2UH
Phone: +44 115 970 9905
Fax: +44 115 942 2232
E-mail: ian.hall@nottingham.ac.uk

Oxford
Professor D Grahame-Smith
University Unit of Clinical Pharmacology
Radcliffe Infirmary
Oxford OX2 6HE
Phone: +44 186 524 1091

Sandwich
Dr MJ Allen
Director, Early Clinical Research Group
Pfizer Central Research
Ramsgate Road
Sandwich, Kent CT13 9NJ
Phone: +44 1304 618532
Fax: +44 1304 618159
E-mail: Michael-Allen@sandwich.pfizer.com.uk

Sheffield
Professor GT Tucker
Section of Clinical Pharmacology & Therapeutics
Floor L
Royal Hallamshire Hospital
Glossop Road
Sheffield S10 2JF
Phone: +44 114 271 3019
Fax: +44 114 272 0275
E-mail: G.T.Tucker@sheffield.ac.uk

Professor LE Ramsay
Section of Clinical Pharmacology & Therapeutics
Floor L
Royal Hallamshire Hospital
Glossop Road
Sheffield S10 2JF
Phone: +44 114 271 3178
Fax: +44 114 272 0275

Southampton
Professor AG Renwick
Clinical Pharmacology Group
Biomedical Sciences Building
Bassett Crescent East
Southampton SO16 7PX
Phone: + 44 1703 594 272
Fax: +44 1703 594 262
E-mail: AGR@soton.ac.uk

Stoke-on-Trent
Dr JC Mucklow
Department of Clinical Pharmacology
North Staffordshire Hospital NHS Trust
Newcastle Road
Stoke-on-Trent
ST4 6QG
Phone: +44 178 255 2917
Fax: +44 178 255 2918

Walton
Dr JTL Smith
Head of Clinical Unit
Clinical Pharmacology

Hoechst Marion Roussel Ltd.
Walton Manor
Walton
Milton Keynes
Bucks MK7 7AJ
Phone: +44 1908 680447
Fax: +44 1908 680463
E-mail: smithj@msmcr.hoechst.com

Roche Products Ltd.
Broadwater Road
Welwyn Garden City
Hertfordshire AL7 3AY
Phone: +44 1707 365934
Fax: +44 1707 365780
E-mail:
Graham.McClelland@roche.com

Welwyn Garden City
Dr GR McClelland
Department of Clinical Pharmacology
Operations

Training Centres in the United Kingdom

Aberdeen

The Clinical Pharmacology Unit, led by Professor JC Petrie, is part of the Department of Medicine and Therapeutics at the University of Aberdeen. The Unit has a long tradition in medicines evaluation and close working links with the pharmaceutical industry.

Our long standing commitment to teaching Clinical Pharmacology is emphasized in the Masters course which has been running in Aberdeen since 1982. This course has attracted students with clinical and scientific backgrounds from all over the world. The course deals with all aspects of clinical pharmacology and aims to provide a multi-disciplinary approach to the study of drug discovery and development; the mechanism of drug action; pre-clinical and clinical trials; regulatory affairs.

Clinical facilities are centred in a 41-bedded general medical unit incorporating a dedicated stroke unit. The NHS and academic units co-operate closely in a wide range of clinical trials using the computer-assisted shared care protocols for the combined follow-up of patients with the General Practitioner. The joint University/NHS Trust sponsored Medicines Assessment Research Unit, directed by Dr D Galloway, is an additional important training resource for Clinical Pharmacologists.

Academic Staff: Professor JC Petrie; Professor GM Hawksworth; Drs D Galloway; JS McLay; JM Rawles; HM Wallace; MJ McLeod; HS Cameron. NHS Staff: Drs J Webster; A Jeffers; L Gates

Application Procedures/Enquiries: All enquiries should, in the first instance, be made to Professor JC Petrie.

References

Chatterjee PK, Weerackody RP, Mistry SK, Hawksworth GM, McLay JS (1997) Selective antagonism of AT1 receptor inhibits angiotensin II stimulated DNA and protein synthesis in primary cultures of human proximal tubular cells. Kidney International 51: in press

Fraser JHE, Helfrich MH, Wallace HM, Ralston SH (1996) Hydrogen peroxide, but no superoxide, stimulates bone resorption in mouse calvaria. Bone 19: 223-226

Harden PN, MacLeod MJ, Roger RSC, Baxter GM, Connell JMC, Doninczak AF, Junor BJR, Briggs JD, Moss JG (1997) Progression of renovascular renal failure is slowed by renal artery stenting. Lancet 349

Hawksworth GM, Tisocki K, Jones GE (1996a) Culture of human renal medullary interstitial Cells. Human Cell Culture Protocols, Human Press, Totowa, New Jersey, 437-445

Hawksworth GM, Murray GI, Eksins S (1996b) Ultrastructural and metabolic effects after vitrification of precision-cut rat-liver slices with antifreeze proteins. Cryo-letters 17: 157-164

MacLeod MJ, Lee WK, Devlin AM, Caslake M, Anderson N, Packard CJ, Dominiczak MH, Reid JL, Dominiczak AF (1997) Sodium-lithium countertransport, sodium-hydrogen exchange and membrane microviscosity in patients with hyperlipidaemias. Clin Sci 92: 237-246

Weerackody RP, Chatterjee PK, Mistry SK, McLaren J, Hawksworth GM, McLay JS (1997) Selective antagonism of the AT1 receptor inhibits the effect of angiotensin II on DNA and protein synthesis of rat proximal tubular cells. Exp Nephrol 5: 253-262

Petrie JC, Donald P, Findlay A, Grimshaw JM, Harper DR, Howard GCW (Eds) (1996) Helicobacter pylori eradication therapy in dyspeptic disease. A clinical guideline developed by a multiprofessional expert group sponsored by The Clinical Resource And Audit Group (CRAG) and recommended for use in Scotland by The Scottish Intercollegiate Guideline Network (Sign). Edinburgh, 1-37

Petrie JC, Anderson A, Barnwell E, Donaldson K, Grimshaw JM, Harper DR, Howard GCW, Pottinger E (Eds) (1996) Prophylaxis of venous thromboembolism. A national clinical guidelines recommended for use in Scotland by The Scottish Intercollegiate Guideline Network (Sign), Edinburgh, 1-42

Rawles J (1996). Magnitude of benefit from earlier thrombolytic treatment in acute myocardial infarction: New evidence from Grampian Region early anistreplase trial (Great). Br Med J 212-216

Wallace HM (1996) Polyamines in human health. Proc Nutr Soc 55: 351-363

Belfast

The Department of Therapeutics and Pharmacology in Belfast has eight permanent members of staff; five clinical and three scientific appointments. The principal research interests are cardiovascular pharmacology (Professor RG Shanks, Dr JG Riddell, Dr B Silke, Dr BJ McDermott and Dr D Bell); neuropharmacology (Professor DJ King) and oncopharmacology (Dr F Van den Berg). The department is part of the Queen's Univeristy of Belfast and has links with the Belfast City Hospital. The department has a long tradition in medicine evaluation and drug epidemiology.

We are responsible for the teaching of clinical pharmacology to 2nd and 3rd year medical students and drug therapeutics to final year students in the Belfast City Hospital. We also run an intercalated Bachelor of Medical Science degree for medical students wishing to expand their knowledge of clinical pharmacology.

Clinical facilities are provided in a 30-bedded acute medical unit which admits patients from the Greater Belfast Area as part of a 1 in 6 rota. Specialist heart failure, angina and hypertension clinics are also available and we have close liaisons with several other groups of clinicians, in particular cardiologists, diabetologists, rheumatologists and chemical pathologists.

References

Bell D, Millar BC, McDermott BJ (1997) Use of D-myoinositol 1,2,6 triphosphate to inhibit contractile function in rat ventricular cardiomyocytes induced by neuropeptide Y and other cardioactive peptides through phospholipase C. Br J Pharmacol 122: 1655-1660

Green JF, King DJ (1996) Cognitive functioning in schizophrenia: effects of drug treatments. CNS Drugs 6: 382-398

Kelso EJ, Geraghty RF, McDermott BJ, Cameron CHS, Nicholls DP, Silke B (1997) Characterization of a cellular model of cardiomyopathy in the rabbit produced by chronic administration of the antracycline, epirubicin. J Mollecular & Cell Cardiol 29: 3385-3397

Lynch G, King DJ, Buth W, Winson-Davis K (1997) The effects of haloperidol on visual search, eye movements and psychomotor performance. Psychopharmacol 133: 233-239

McAuley D, McGurk C, Nugent AG, Hanratty C, Maguire S, Johnston GD (1997) Forearm endothelium-dependent vascular responses and the potassium-ATP channel. Br J Clin Pharmacol 44: 292-294

McDermott BJ, Millar BC, Dolan FM, Bell D, Balasubramaniam A (1997) Evidence of Y1 and Y2 subtypes of neuropeptide Y receptors linked to opposing postjunctional effects observed in cardiac myocytes. Eur J Pharmacol 336: 257-265

McGurk C, Nugent A, McAuley D, Silke B (1997) Sources of inaccuracy in the use of the Hawksley random-zero sphygmomanometer. Hypertension 15 (12): 1379-1384

Mullan DM, Bell D, Kelso EJ, McDermott BJ (1997) Involvements of ETA and ETB receptors in the hypertrophic effects of endothelin-1 in adult rabbit ventricular cardiomyocytes. J Cardiovasc Pharmacol 29: 350-359

Nugent AG, McGurk C, Hayes JR, Johnston GD (1996) Impaired vasoconstriction to endothelin 1 in patients with NIDDM. Diabetes 45: 105-107

Silke B, Guy S, Riddell JG (1997) Effects of b-adrenoceptor agonists and antagonists on heart rate variability in normal subjects assessed using summary statistics and nonlinear procedures. J Cardiovasc Pharmacol 30: 817-823

Birmingham

The clinical pharmacology section of the Department of Medicine is based in the Queen Elizabeth Hospital, immediately next to the Birmingham Medical School and on the new university campus. The section is lead by Dr MJ Kendall and is based in the Clinical Investigation unit which is part of the Clinical Research Institute.

The clinical pharmacology section is responsible for teaching medical undergraduates clinical pharmacology and therapeutics and runs one of the modules of the University's MSc course in Toxicology. It also has good facilities for PhD students and there are plenty of opportunities for collaborative work.

The Consultant staff and the Special Registrar run one of the five general medical firms in the Queen Elizabeth Hospital. Within the Clinical Investigation Unit, there are good facilities for clinical research, a well-equipped laboratory and good office space. The major interest of the Unit is cardiovascular research particularly in relation to lipids, antioxidants, endothelial damage and hypertension. However, there are also links with clinical pharmacy, Sports Science, Elderly Care medicine, diabetes and drug regulatory affairs.

Academic staff: Dr MJ Kendall, Dr U Martin, Dr RE Ferner, Dr O'Mahoney. NHS staff: Dr R Cramb

References

Clark W, Kendall MJ (1996) Therapeutic advances: riluzole for the treatment of motor neurone disease. J Clin Pharmacol Ther 21: 373-376

Eagles CJ, Kendall MJ (1997) The effects of combined treatment with B1 selective receptor antagonists and lipid lowering drugs on fat metabolism and measures of fatigue during moderate intensity exercise. Br J Clin Pharm 43: 291-300

Kendall MJ (1997) Clinical relevance of pharmacokinetic differences between betablockers. Am J Cardiol 80 (9B): 15J-19J

Kendall MJ, Horton R (Eds)(1998) Preventing coronary artery disease. 2nd Ed. Martin Duntz, London

Kendall MJ, Toescu V, Wallace DMA (1996) Quick and early diagnosis. Lancet 348: 528-529

Marvin G, Sharma A, Aston W, Field C, Kendall MJ, Jones DA (1997) The effects of buspirone on perceived exertion and time to fatigue in man. Exp Physiol 32: 1057-1060

Rajman I, Lip GYH, Cramb R, Maxwell SRJ, Sarifs J, Beevers DG, Kendall MJ (1996) Adverse changes in low density lipoprotein subfraction profile with oestrogen only hormone replacement therapy. Q J Med 89: 771-778

Cambridge

The University Department of Medicine is one of 10 constituent departments of the University of Cambridge Clinical School and consists of a number of divisions, each involved in research related to human disease. The Department has a total of around 200 personnel including about 60 graduate students, 15 holders of clinical research training fellowships, and 10 senior clinical and non-clinical fellowships. The Clinical Pharmacology Unit is part of the Department, although geographically separate from its main accommodation and currently has approximately 35 staff. There are exceptional research facilities for both laboratory and clinical studies. The new Clinical Research Building will open in 1998. This includes a Clinical Investigation Ward for research studies, an entire floor of laboratories for the molecular and pharmacological studies of the Clinical Pharmacology and Cardiovascular Units, and a Research Clinic area with six beds and a non-invasive diagnostic suite. The department's clinical staff work in Addenbrooke's Hospital in close association with their NHS colleagues, with whom they are aligned by speciality interest. The Clinical Pharmacology Unit currently has trainees in joint training programmes with Respiratory Medicine and Renal Medicine and is planning programmes with Cardiology and Diabetology/Encrinology.

Application Procedures: in the first instance, please send a Curriculum Vitae to the Head of the Unit, professor Morris Brown.

References

Brown MJ (1996) The causes of essential hypertension. J Clin Pharmacol 42: 21-27

Brown MJ, Castaigne A, Ruilope LM, Mancia G, Rosenthal, de Leeuw PW, Ebner F (1996) INSIGHT: International Nifedipine GITS Study Intervention as a Goal in Hypertension. Treat J Hum Hypertens 10 (Supplement 3): S157-S160

Dickerson JEC, Garratt CJ, Brown MJ (1995) Management of hypertension in general practice: agreements with and variations from the British Hypertension Society Guidelines. J Hum Hypertens 9: 835-839

Ferro A, Longmore J, Hill RG, Brown MJ (1995) A comparison of the contractile effects of 5-hydroxytryptamine, sumatriptan and MK-462 on human coronary artery in vitro. Br J Clin Pharmacol 40: 245-251

Ferro A, Hall JA, Dickerson JEC, Brown MJ (1997) A prospective study of the effects of prolonged timolol therapy on a- and b-adrenoceptor and angiotensin II receptor mediated responses in normal subjects. Br J Clin Pharmacol 43: 301-308

Hingorani AD, Jia H, Stevens PA, Hopper RV, Dickerson JEC, Brown MJ (1995) Renin-angiotensin system gene polymorphisms influence blood pressure and the response to angiotensin converting enzyme inhibition. Hypertension 13: 1602-1609

Hingorani AD, Sharma P, Jia H, Hopper R, Brown MJ (1996) Blood Pressure and the M235T polymorphism of the angiotensinogen gene. Hypertension 28(5): 907-911

Monteith MS, Wang T, Brown MJ (1995) Differences in transcription and translation of long and short Gsa, the stimulatory G-protein, in human atrium. Clin Sci 89: 487-495

Stephens NG, Parsons A, Schofield P, Kelly F, Cheeseman K, Mitchinson MJ, Brown MJ (1996) Randomised controlled trial of vitamin E in patients with coronary disease: Cambridge Heart Antioxidant Study (CHAOS). Lancet 347: 781-786, 23 March

Stevens PA, Brown MJ (1995) Genetic variability of the ET- 1 and ETA receptor genes in essential hypertension. J Cardiovasc Pharmacol 36 (Supplement) 33: S9-S12

Cardiff

The Therapeutics and Toxicology Group, led by Professor PA Routledge, is part of the Department of Pharmacology, Therapeutics and Toxicology at the University of Wales College of Medicine (UWCM) in Cardiff, Wales. The group is committed to education in clinical pharmacology and therapeutics and in addition to MSc, MD and PhD student opportunities, there is a distance learning University Diploma in Therapeutics. A Diploma/Masters in Medical Toxicology by distance-learning is planned to start in September 1998.

The group is responsible for clinical pharmacology and therapeutics training in Wales and has three specialist registrar posts in the speciality. Specific interest within the group are pharmacovigilance, drug metabolism and toxicology, factors affecting drug response and cardiovascular pharmacology.

Clinical facilities for the group are in Llandough Hospital, including general medical beds, coronary care facilities and a dedicated poisons treatment unit for the Cardiff district. The NHS and academic link is reflected in the activities of the UWCM Therapeutics and Toxicology Centre on the Llandough site. The Centre was recently recognised by the Welsh Development Agency and European Union as a Centre Expertise in the University Sector. Its role is to provide authoritative advice on the acute and chronic toxicity of drugs, chemicals and naturally occurring agents to health professionals, government agencies and industries. It offers bioanalytical services for the measurement of drugs and chemicals and undertakes training in the safe use of such substances for health care professionals and other interested groups. The Unit also provides clinical services for the diagnosis and treatment of individuals with suspected toxicity due to drugs or chemicals.

The Centre has 30 staff, including physicians, scientists, nurses, technical and other support personnel. Six information scientists provide a 24-hour toxicology advisory service for healthcare professionals (Welsh National Poisons Unit). A clinical investigations facility is available for clinical trials and other research. Centre staff also direct the Welsh Adverse Drug Reactions scheme to encourage the spontaneous reporting by health-care professionals of suspected adverse drug reactions to the Committee on Safety of Medicines ('yellow card scheme').

Academic staff: Professor PA Routledge, Drs HG Rees, AD Hutchings, MC Bialas, Senior Clinical Lecturer (to be appointed), HGM Shetty, RW Marchall, RA Bracchi.

Application procedures/enquiries: all enquiries should, in the first instance, be made to Professor PA Routledge.

References

Al-Shareef A, Buss DC, Shetty HGM, Ali N, Routledge PA (1997) The effect of repeated-dose activated charcoal on the pharmacokinetics of sodium valproate in healthy volunteers. Br J Clin Pharmacol 43: 109-11

Bialas MC, Reid P, Beck P, Lazarus JH, Smith PM, Scorer RC, Routledge PA (1996) Changing patterns of poisoning in a UK Health District between 1978-1988 and 1992-1993. Quarterly J Med 89: 893-901

Bialas MC, Shetty HGM, Houghton J, Woods F, Routledge PA (1997a) Nitrofurantoin rechallenge and recurrent toxicity. Postgrad Med J 73: 519-520

Bialas MC, Varley H, Shetty HGM, Routledge PA (1997b) Low grade fever after prosthetic valve insertion and captopril therapy: an iatrogenic cause. Postgrad Med J 73: 764-5

Bialas MC, Evans RJ, Hutchings AD, Alldridge G, Routledge PA (1998) The impact of nationally distributed guidelines on the management of paracetamol poisoning in accident and emergency departments. J Accident Emerg Med 15: 13-17

Buss DC, Marshall RW, Milligan N, McQueen I, Compston DAS, Routledge PA (1997) The effect of intravenous aminophylline on essential tremor. Br J Clin Pharmacol 43: 119-121

Cassidy SL, Hale A, Buss DC, Routledge PA (1997) In-vitro drug adsorption to charcoal, silicas, acrylate copolymer and silicone oil with charcoal and with acrylate copolymer. Hum Exp Toxicol 16: 25-27

Houghton J, Woods F, Richens A, Routledge PA (1996) The Welsh Adverse Drug Reactions Scheme: ten years experience of a regional monitoring centre. Adv React Acute Pois Rev 15: 93-107

Hutchings A, Routledge PA (1996) A single sample saliva test to measure acetylator phenotype using isoniazid. Br J Clin Pharmacol 42: 635-637

Rees HG (1996) Exposure to sheep dip and the incidence of acute symptoms in a group of Welsh farmers. Occup Environ Med 53: 258-263

Cork

The Clinical Pharmacology Unit at University College Cork was established in 1992 by Professor Michael Murphy. The unit is a section of the Department of Pharmacology and Therapeutics.

The unit provides a broad range of research experience. On the one hand it participates in the Irish Centre for Evidence Based Therapy which conducts large scale clinical trials. Professor Murphy is Principal Investigator of the PROSPER trial, evaluating the efficacy of Pravastatin in prevention of coronary heart disease and stroke in elderly patients in a cohort of 5500 individuals. Almost 50 research staff participate in primary care based clinical research. On the other hand, smaller phase II and phase III studies are conducted in a dedicated unit at the Mercy Hospital, Cork. Clinical Pharmacology also has an association with a commercial clinical trials unit, the Shandon Clinic which conducts phase I, phase II and generic bio-equivalence studies. Trainees in clinical pharmacology gain experience through participation in study design, and in regulatory and ethical matters through participation in the Clinical Research Ethics Committee of the Cork Teaching Hospitals. Since the unit provides acute medical care at the Mercy Hospital a broad experience of general medicine as well as specialist clinic experience in the management of hypertension, hyperlipidaemia and heart failure, is available.

A part of the larger Department of Pharmacology and Therapeutics, the Clinical Pharmacology Unit encourages integration of clinical and basic research. Clinical Pharmacology trainees may complement their clinical studies with basic research on mode of action of drugs, in the laboratories of the toxicology and molecular pharmacology faculty. All trainees in the department are encouraged to read for a higher degree, e.g. MD or PhD in the course of their training in the unit.
Academic staff: Professor MB Murphy, Dr BM Buckley, Dr Damian O'Connell, Dr Ashley Allshire, Dr Frank van Pelt, Professor P Leary. Applicants for position should contact Professor Michael Murphy in the first instance.

References

Cronin CC, Higgins TM, Murphy MB, Ferriss JB (1997) Supervised drug administration in patients with hypertension unmasking non-compliance. Postgrad Med J 73: 239-240

Foss JF, O'Connor MF, Yuan CS, Murphy MB, Moss J, Roizen MF (1997) Safety and tolerance of methylnaltrexone in healthy humans: a randomised, placebocontrolled, intravenous, ascending dose, pharmacokinetic study. J Clin Pharmacol 37: 25-30

Murphy DB, Murphy MB (1997) A comparison of effects of tramadol and morphine on gastric emptying in man. Anaesthesia 52: 1212-1229

Murphy DB, Sutton JA, Prescott LF, Murphy MB (1997) Opioid induced delay in gastric emptying: a peripheral mechanism in man. Anesthesiology 87: 765-770

Vaughan CJ, Murphy MB, Buckley BM (1996a) Statins do more than just lower cholesterol. Lancet 348: 1079-1082

Vaughan CJ, Aherne AM, Murphy MB, O'Connell DP (1996b) Immunohistochemical mapping of the dopamine D1B receptor in the kidney. Br J Pharmacol 117: 125P

Vaughan CJ, Gallagher M, Murphy MB (1997a) Left ventricular myxoma presenting with constitutional symptoms and raised serum interleukin-6, both suppressed by naproxen. Eur Heart J 18: 703

Vaughan CJ, Delanty N, Harrington H, Murphy MB (1997b) Treatment of spastic dystonia with transdermal nicotine. Lancet 1997: 350-565

Dublin

The Department has an active research programme in Clinical Pharmacology and Neuropharmacology (Ph.D/MD Degrees by Thesis). The Department participates in the General Internal Medicine service of the major university Teaching Hospital, St James's Hospital, where there are dedicated laboratory facilities and an In-patient Clinical Investigation Area. The Hypertension and Lipid Clinics, Alzheimer's Research Unit, The National Medicines Information Centre and Centre for Pharmacoeconomics are all associated with the Department.

Trinity College is the oldest University in Ireland (1592), and has a full range of faculties including Health Sciences.

The staff of the department consists of 14 full and part-time employees including two clinical pharmacologists, one toxicologist and two senior lecturers.

Application procedures: Letter to Head of Department (J. Feely)

References

Adebayo GI, Gaffney P, Buggy D, Feely J (1994) Acute inhibitory effect of alcohol on sodium-lithium countertransport. Alcohol 11(5): 367-370

Chambers PL (1995) Mechanisms of toxicity and biomarkers to assess adverse effects of chemicals, eds. Mutti A, Chambers PL, Chambers CM, Amsterdam, Elsevier Science Publishers 397 pp

Chan R, Hemeryck L, O'Regan M, Clancy L, Feely J (1995) Oral versus intravenous antibiotics for community acquired lower respiratory tract infection in a general hospital: open, randomised controlled trial. Br Med J 310: 1360-1362

Deegan P, Feely J (1996) Making sensible choices – horses for courses in: Lipids – current Perspectives. Ed J Betteridge. Martin Dunitz, London pp 227-243

Feely J (1994) New Drugs, Third Edition. British Medical Association pp 448

Hall M, McCormack P, Arthurs N, Feely J (1995) The spontaneous reporting of adverse drug reactions by nurses. Br Clin Pharmacol 40: 173-175

McGettigan P, Golden J, Conroy RM, Arthur N, Feely J (1997) Reporting of adverse drug reactions by hospital doctors and the response to intervention. Br J Clin Pharmacol 44: 98-100

O'Connor JJ, Rowan MJ, Anwyl R (1994) Long-lasting enhancement of NMDA activation. Nature 367: 557-559

O'Mahony D, Rowan MJ, Feely J, Walsh JB, Coakley D (1994) Primary auditory pathway and reticular activating system dysfunction in Alzheimer's disease. Neurology 44: 2089-2094

Xu L, Anwyl R, Rowan MJ (1997) Behavioural stress facilitates the induction of long-term depression in the hippocampus. Nature 387: 497-500

Dundee

The department is situated in Ninewells Hospital and Medical School. There are five senior staff (two professors, two readers and one senior clinical lecturer), three clinical lecturers and three technicians. In addition, there are more than 40 research staff, including a number of clinical research fellows. The main research interests of the department are cardiovascular and respiratory clinical pharmacology (including major themes related to heart failure, hypertension and obstructive airways disease), but there is also a large grant funded pharmacoepidemiology unit (the Medicines Monitoring Unit) which is committed to drug safety, pharmacoeconomics and outcomes research. The department has a number of clinical and biochemical research laboratories which are well equipped and are supported by grants from MRC, Wellcome Trust, other medical charities and the pharmaceutical industry. There is a 54-bedded Professorial Medical Unit in the hospital which is responsible for general and cardiovascular medicine. Training is available either through one of the clinical lecturer/specialist registrar posts, which are approved for general medicine/clinical pharmacology training by the JCHMT, or by 2-year clinical research fellowships which would normally lead to a higher degree. Application should be made in response to advertised vacancies.

Inquiries or expressions of interest should be directed to the Head of Department, Professor DG McDevitt.

Edinburgh

Edinburgh is the capital city of Scotland, a thriving business centre, holds many international festivals and has close links to Europe. The University of Edinburgh has a longstanding reputation in Medicine and the Faculty of Medicine was recently given the highest rating nationally for its clinical research activities. The University of Edinburgh's Clinical Pharmacology Unit (CPU) and Clinical Research Centre (CRC) are based at the Western General Hospital, a major teaching hospital in the city of Edinburgh. The CPU has a suite of offices and research laboratories for analytical research, in vitro pharmacology and molecular techniques. The substantial facilities of the Molecular Medicine Centre are immediately adjacent. The CRC is a 22-bedded purposedesigned unit housing ward areas and a suite of offices for clinical research in healthy volunteers and patients. The emphasis is on cardiovascular research, particularly related to the vascular endothelium. The approach involves research 'from molecules to man'. There are around 50 members of staff, including a professor, a senior lecturer and three lecturers. There are close links with cardiology in the University, and with the pharmaceutical industry. Applications (to the Head of Department) for research fellowships are welcomed from high quality overseas trainees, particularly those who are selffunding or are likely to compete successfully for external grant support.

Enquiries to Professor DJ Webb.

References

Haynes WG, Webb DJ (1994) Contribution of endogenous generation of endothelin1 to basal vascular tone in man. Lancet 344: 852-854

Haynes WG, Hand MF, Johnstone HA, Padfield PL, Webb DJ (1994) Direct and sympathetically mediated venoconstriction in essential hypertension: enhanced responses to endothelin. J Clin Invest 94: 1359-1364

Haynes WG, Hand MH, Dockrell MEC, Eadington DW, Lee MR, Benjamin N, Webb DJ (1997) Physiological role of nitric oxide in regulation of renal function in humans. Am J Physiol 272: 364-371

Love MP, Haynes WG, Gray GA, Webb DJ, McMurray JJV (1996) Vasodilator effects of endothelinconverting enzyme inhibition and endothelin ETA receptor blockade in chronic heart failure patients treated with ACE inhibitors. Circulation 94: 2131-2137

Noon JP, Haynes WG, Webb DJ, Shore AC (1996) Local inhibition of nitric oxide generation in man reduces blood flow in the finger pulp but not in the dorsum of the hand. J Physiol 490: 501-508

Noon JP, Walker BR, Shore AC, Holton DW, Edwards HV, Webb DJ, Watt GCM (1997) Capillary rarefaction and impaired microvascular dilatation in young adults with a familial predisposition to hypertension. J Clin Invest 99: 1873-1879

Petrie JR, Ueda S, Webb DJ, Elliott HL, Connell JMC (1996) Endothelial nitric oxide production and insulin sensitivity: a physiological link with implications for pathogenesis of cardiovascular disease? Circulation 93: 1331-1333

Webb DJ (1995) The pharmacology of human blood vessels in vivo. J Vasc Res 32: 215

Webb DJ (1996) Careers in pharmacology: life as an academic clinical pharmacologist. TiPS 17: 557

Webb DG, Vallance PJT (1997) The Endothelium in Hypertension. SpringerVerlag, Berlin 1997 pp 220 [book].

Glasgow

In 1989, a separate Department for Clinical Pharmacology and the Department of Medicine merged to form a Department of Medicine and Therapeutics.

There are approved specialist training posts in clinical pharmacology for up to four trainees at any one time. There are also approved posts for training in Internal Medicine both at a General Professional and Specialist level. Trainees in clinical pharmacology are expected to participate in the MSc Clinical Pharmacology Course, co-ordinated in the department either 1 year full-time or 2 year part-time study. This MSc is open to other biomedical graduates wishing to train in Clinical Pharmacology.

The Clinical Pharmacology Division has access to 46 General Medical beds and a seven-bed Programmed Investigation Unit as well as an eight-bed Clinical Pharmacology Research Centre for study of patients and healthy volunteers. There is close back up from the Cell and Molecular Biology laboratories, Biochemical Pharmacology and Biometrics and Statistics.

The University of Glasgow is one of the oldest in Europe (founded 1451) and one of the largest Medical Schools (1700 undergraduates and 620 postgraduates in 1996/97)

In the Division of Clinical Pharmacology, there are three Professors, two Readers and two Senior Lecturers supported by non-clinical Academic staff, Biochemical Pharmacology, Pharmacy and Biometrics. As of August 1997, the chairman of the division is Dr Martin J Brodie whose address is Epilepsy Unit, Department of Medicine and Therapeutics, Western Infirmary, Glasgow G11 6NT, phone: +44 141 211 2572

Application procedures: Application for the BSc Med Sci (starts October each year) should be made to Nan Scott, Postgraduate Secretary, Department of Medicine, Western Infirmary, Glasgow. Clinical Training posts are advertised nationally but informal enquiries are welcome.

Enquiries to the Head of Department, Professor John Reid.

References

Banerjee S. Ardill JES, Beattie AD, McColl KEL (1996) Effect of omeprazole and feeding on plasma gastrin in patients with achlorhydria. Aliment Pharmacol and Ther 9: 507-512

Brodie MJ, Dichter MA (1996) Drug therapy-antiepileptic drugs. N Engl J Med 334: 168-175

Doig JK, MacFadyen RJ, Sweet CS, Reid JL (1995) Haemodynamic and renal responses to oral losartan potassium during salt depletion or salt repletion in normal human volunteers. J Card Pharmacol 25: 511-517

Dyker AG, Lees KR (1996) The rationale for new therapies in acute ischaemic stroke. J Clin Pharmacol and Ther 21: 377-391

Leach JP, Sills GJ, Butler E, Forrest G Thompson GH, Brodie MJ (1997) Neurochemical actions of the desglycinyl metabolite of remacemide hydrochloride (ARL12495AA) in mouse brain. Br J Pharmacol 121: 923-926

McLeod HL, Murray LS, Wanders J, Setanoians A, Graham MA, Pavlidis N et al (1996) Multicentre phase II pharmacological evaluation of rhizoxin. Br J Cancer 74: 1944-1948

Meredith PA (1996) Generic drugs: therapeutic equivalence. Drug Safety 4: 233-242

Reid JL (1997) Clinical Pharmacology and therapeutics – past, present and future. Br J Clin Pharmacol 44: 101-103

Reid JL, Rubin PC, Whiting B (eds) (1996) Lecture Notes on Clin Pharmacol, 5th ed. (Oxford: Blackwell)

Thomson AH, Kerr S, Wright S (1996) Population pharmacokinetics of caffeine in neonates and young infants. Ther D Monit 18: 245-253

Greenford

Glaxo Wellcome Research & Development has a global Clinical Pharmacology function, with its major activities in the UK, USA and Italy. It employs about 130 staff, including 20 physicians and has two clinical pharmacology units of 12 and 24 beds.

Clinical Pharmacology is responsible for the early evaluation of all potential new drugs in man from GW Research. It has close ties with the research part of the company, as well as important academic links especially with the University of Cambridge, Oxford and London.

Apart from physicians, the department employs pharmacokinetics, research scientists and nurses. Training is provided through guidance and mentoring whilst 'on the job' and by external courses where needed. An important part of training for new physicians is provided by the industrial-academic training posts organized under the auspices of the ABPI.

Vacancies for physicians arise from time to time and are usually advertised in the BMJ and Lancet.

Harlow

SmithKline Beecham Pharmaceuticals (SB) has a 30-bed Clinical Pharmacology Research Unit in Harlow, Essex, and is constructing a further Research Unit within Addenbrooke's Hospital in Cambridge. When the new Unit is open, it is planned that there will be approximately 50 permanent staff members.

The department has a large programme of work to evaluate the clinical pharmacology of the company's extensive portfolio of potential new therapeutic agents.

SB is an active supporter of the ABPI (The Association of the British Pharmaceutical Industry) initiative for the training of Clinical Pharmacologists jointly between the Pharmaceutical Industry and The National Health Service (NHS). SB has a number of partners, in Academic Centres within the NHS, including the University of Oxford and the University of Cambridge, with whom training programmes have been developed which cover the published curriculum. The posts are advertised in the national press.

The training programmes, which will enable the trainees to obtain the CCST, include a year spent within the Clinical Pharmacology Department at SB. The trainee has the opportunity, during the time at SB, to gain experience of the Scientific and Medical challenges related to developing new medicines and the application of Clinical Pharmacology to bringing them to resolution. They are also able to spend time in other departments including Drug Metabolism and Pharmacokinetics, Discovery, Pharmacology and Toxicology.

Inveresk

Inveresk Research has over 20 years of experience in drug development activities. Inveresk performs a range of volunteer and patient clinical studies. Phase I studies are done in a clinical unit with 52 beds supported by laboratories, examination rooms and monitoring equipment. Phase I studies performed include single dose tolerability, multiple dose tolerability, radiolabelled studies, pharmacodynamic studies and pharmacokinetic studies. These volunteer study capabilities are applied to many speciality medical areas, including CNS, respiratory, gastrointestinal, cardiovascular and haematopoietic system. Early phase II patient studies involve dose response, dose finding, efficacy, safety and drug interactions. Phase II studies are carried out with single centre, multi-centre or international designs, and Inveresk has experienced clinical research staff in the UK and selected countries in Europe. In these studies, Inveresk features (1) a computerized trial management system (CTMS) which incorporates data on investigators, monitoring visits, recruited patients, adverse events and clinical trial supplies and tracks case report forms as they are processed, and (2) a clinical trials pharmacy which manages clinical trials supplies. The company has a contract research subsidiary in North America. Other services offered by Inveresk include data review, project design, project management, data management, reporting, regulatory affairs, drug analysis, clinical pathology, statistics and data management and quality assurance.

Leeds
Leeds General Infirmary
The Clinical Pharmacology Unit, led by Dr MP Feely, is part of the University Department of Clinical Medicine and is based a the Division of Medicine, Leeds General Infirmary.

Clinical facilities are based on the beds of the Division of Medicine and include beds for medical cardiology, diabetes and epilepsy as well as general medical beds.

The research interests of the Unit are centred around epilepsy, compliance with drug therapy and respiratory (molecular) pharmacology/asthma. It is a small Unit and much of its work is carried out in collaboration with other clinical and research groups and there has also been a long-standing collaboration with the Pharmacology Department of Leeds General Infirmary in relation to both drug utilisation and compliance research.

Academic staff: Dr M Feely, Dr J Morrison. NHS staff: Dr S Chadha.

References
Feely M (1996) Generic Prescribing. In: Prescribing in General Practice. Ed Harris C. Radcliffe Medical Press, Oxford & New York.
Gelder CM, Thomas PS, Yates DH, Adcock IM, Morrison JF, Barnes PJ (1995) Cytokine expression in normal, atopic and asthmatic subjects using the combination of sputum induction and the polymerase chain reaction. Thorax 50: 1033-1037
Harun RB, Markham AF, Morrison JF (1996) Identification of differentially expressed genes in CD19+veB lymphocytes in allergic asthma. Adv Exp Med Biol 409: 75-380

Harun RB, Smith KK, Leek JP, Markham AF, Norris A, Morrison JF (1997) Characterisation of human SHC p66 cDNA and its processed pseudogene mapping to Xq12-q13.1 Genomics 42: 349-352

Hathaway TJ, Higenbottam TW, Morrison JF, Clelland CA, Wallwork J (1993) Effects of inhaled capsaicin in heart-lung transplant patients and asthmatic subjects. Am Rev Resp Dis 148: 1233-1237

Hatton M, Allen M, Vathenen S, Feely M, Cooke N (1996) Compliance with oral corticosteroids during steroid trials in chronic airways obstruction. Thorax 51: 523-524

Mansur AH, Gelder CM, Holland D, Campbell DA, Griffin A, Cunliffe W, Markham AF, Morrison JF (1996) Non-random usage of T cell receptor alpha gene expression in atopy using anchored PCR. Adv Exp Med Biol 409: 381-389

Newton-Syms FAO, Dawson PH, Cooke J, Feely M, Booth TG, Jerwood D, Calvert RT (1992) A study to evaluate the influence of an academic representative on prescribing by general practitioners. Br J Clin Pharmacol 33: 69-73

Osbaldeston NJ, Lee DM, Cox VM, Hesketh JE, Morrison JF, Blair GE, Goldspink DF (1995) The temporal and cellular expression of c-fos and c-jun in mechanically stimulated rabbit latissimus dorsi muscle. Biochem J 308: 465-471

Sowter BJ, Feely M, Kay EA (1997) An audit of warfarin anticoagulation in teaching hospital patients. Pharm J 259: 612-3

Wolff K, Hay AWM, Raistrick G, Feely M (1993) Use of very low doses of phenobarbitone to investigate compliance in patients on reducing doses of methadone. J Subst Abuse Treat 10: 453-8

Wolff K, Rostami-Hodjegan A, Shires S, Hay AWM, Feely M, Calvert R, Raistrick D, Tucker GT (1997) The pharmacokinetics of methadone in healthy subjects and opiate users. Br J Clin Pharmacol 44: 325-334

University of Leeds – Chapel Allerton Hospital

The group concentrates on pharmacology related rheumatology and the development of drugs for the treatment of rheumatic diseases though this is interpreted brief widely.

We have in the past done work with antibiotics and hypnotics (particularly applied to rheumatology) though our main interest is in desease-modifying drugs for rheumatoid arthritis and a lesser interest is in non-steroidal anti-inflammatory drugs and particularly analgesics. Research interests vary from early phase I pharmacokinetic studies to an interest in economic aspects of the sale of drugs already marketed. We have also held research grants for the study of bowel flora in relation to rheumatoid arthritis and pharmacogenetics.

Wearing a clinical rheumatology hat, we have researach interests in joint hyperlaxity as a model of accelerated osteoarthritis and in performing arts medicine which implies the integration of biomechanics with pharmacology. We have excellent clinical consulting rooms and a large clinical pharmacology laboratory.

Inquiries to professor Howard A Bird.

References

Beyeler C, Daly AK, Armstrong M, Bird HA, Idle JR (1994) Phenotype/genotype relationships for the cytochrome P450 enzyme CYP2D6 in rheumatoid arthritis: influence of drug therapy and disease activity. J Rheumatol 21: 1034

Jamieson AH, Alford CA, Bird HA, Hindmarch I, Wright V (1995) The effect of sleep and nocturnal movement on stiffness, pain and psychomotor performance in ankylosing spondylitis. Clin Exp Rheumatol 13: 73-8

Beyeler C, Banks R, Thompson D, Forbes MA, Cooper EH, Bird H (1995) Bone alkaline phosphatase in rheumatic diseaases. Ann Clin Biochem 32: 379-84.

Astbury C, Beyeler C, Bird HA (1995) Polymorphic acetylation: lack of influence of rheumatic disease activity and concomitant drug administration. Rheumatol Int 14: 257-60

Beyeler C, Armstrong M, Bird HA, Idle JR, Daly AK (1996) Relationship between genotype for the cytochrome P450 CYP2D6 and susceptibility to ankylosing spondylitis and rheumatoid arthritis. Ann Rheum dis 55: 66-8

Taggert A, Gardiner P, McEvoy F, Hopkins R, Bird H (1996) Which is the active moiety of sulfasalazine in ankylosing spondylitis? Arthritis Rheum 39: 1400-5

Bird HA (1996) Modern drug delivery systems. Musculoskeletal Med 3: 6-8

Troughton PR, Platt R, Bird H, El-Manzalawi E, Bassiouni M, Wright V (1996) Synovial fluid interleukin-8 and neutrophil function in rheumatoid arthritis and seronegative polyarth-ritis. Br J Rheumatol 35: 1244-51

Beyeler C, Frey BM, Bird HA (1997) Urinary 6 -hydroxycortisol excretion in rheumatoid artheritis. Br J Rheumatol 36: 54-8

Bradley SM, Le Gallez P, Troughton PR, Gooi HC, Astbury C, Bird Ha (1997) The effect of sulphasalazine on neutropil superoxide generation in rheumatoid arthritis. Br J Rheumatol; 36: 530-4

Leicester

The academic unit of Clinical Pharmacology at the University of Leicester is a division in the Department of Medicine and Therapeutics. The division has facilities for training in clinical and laboratory based clinical pharmacology with a special interest in cardiovascular disease. There are five full time academic members of staff, as well as technical and secretarial support. In addition, the division is associated with the Leicester Royal Infirmary, a major acute teaching hospital and staff of the division have specific responsibilities for General (Internal) Medicine with a special interest in cardiovascular disease. The group is also responsible for the training of junior medical staff with special interests in both Clinical Pharmacology, General (Internal) Medicine and Cardiology. Research interests include early intervention and secondary prevention of myocardial infarction, early diagnosis and therapeutic management of heart failure, intracellular signalling mechanisms in cardiovascular and renal tissue with particular emphasis on hypertension and diabetic complications.

References

Cullen J, Trant J, Moody A, Woods KL, Hudson N, Jivan A, Keal R, Barnett DB, Cherryman G (1996) Detection of posterior extension in inferior myocardial infarction using magnetic resonance imaging, comparison with thallium perfusion imaging. Eur Heart J 17: 24.

Maxwell S, Thorpe G (1996) Tea flavonoids have little short term impact on serum antioxidant activity. Br Med J 313: p229

Rajman I, Lip GG, Cramb R, Maxwell S, Zafaris J, Beevers DG, Kendall MJ (1996) Adverse changes in low-density lipoprotein subfraction profile with oestrogen-only hormone replacement therapy. Q J Med 89: 771-778

Siczkowski M, Ng LL (1996) Glucose-induced changes in activity and phosphorylation of the Na^+/H^+ exchanger NHE-1 vascular myocytes from Wistar-Kyoto and spontaneously hypertensive rats. Metabolism 45 (1): 114-119

Squire IB, MacFadyen RJ, Reid JL, Devlin A, Lees KR (1996) Differing early blood pressure and renin-angiotensin system responses to the first dose of angiotensin converting enzyme inhibitors in congestive heart failure. J Cardiovasc Pharmacol 27: 657-666

Woods KL (1996) Review of research methodology used in clinical trials of magnesium and myocardial infarction – why does controversy persist despite ISIS-4. Coron Art Dis 7: 348-351.

Woods KL, Ketley D, Agusti A, Hagan C, Kala R (1996) Translation of clinical trials into practice: A European population-based study of the use of thrombolysis for acute myocardinal infarction. Lancet 347: 1203-1207

Leics

Astra Charnwood is the UK Research and Development site within the Swedish pharmaceutical company, Astra AB. Over 900 scientific and support staff are engaged in the discovery and development of new medicines. Research at Astra Charnwood is largely focused on novel approaches to inflammatory and immunological mechanisms in the disease areas of respiratory, rheumatology and dermatology. In Development, projects are focused on the following therapeutic areas: respiratory diseases, cardiovascular diseases such as thrombosis and diseases of the central nervous system such as epilepsy. Clinical Pharmacology is part of the Department of Experimental Medicine within the Clinical R&D group. The Department of Experimental Medicine (staff of 25) forms the bridge between the preclinical departments and full scale development and is responsible for first administration to man studies through to concept testing in patients. The Department employs medical and science graduates. Training is directed to developing knowledge and skills in pharmaceutical medicine and especially in the early clinical phases of drug development. Clinical Pharmacology has a 12-bedded unit on site for the performance of healthy volunteer studies.

Specific vacancies are advertised in medical and scientific publications. General enquiries should be directed to the Human Resources Department at Astra Charnwood.

Liverpool

The Department of Pharmacology and Therapeutics, led by Professor Alasdair Breckenridge who holds the chair of clinical pharmacology, has a long tradition of research in the field. It continues to be one of the most highly rated departments of pharmacology in the country. The department has three professors in clinical pharmacology and two in basic pharmacology and prides itself on the collaborative approach to the two disciplines. The clinical side of the department also has two senior lecturers and three recognized posts for training in clinical pharmacology and general (internal) medicine.

The department has an active teaching programme for undergraduates and postgraduates and its clinical facilities are centred on a 24 bedded general medical ward in the adjacent Royal Liverpool Hospital. There are also good investigative facilities for cardiovascular disease and the department runs a hypertension clinic although its range of interests (see references) are much wider than this.

Application procedures/enquiries: all enquiries should, in the first instance, be made to Professor A Breckenridge.

References

Barnes CS, Coker S (1995) Failure of nitric oxide to alter arrhythmias induced by acute myocardial ischaemia or reperfusion in anaesthetised rats. Br J Pharmacol 114: 349-456

Barry MG, Back DJ, Breckenridge AM (1995) Zidovudine therapy in HIV infection – which patients should be treated and when. Br J Clin Pharmacol 40: 107-110

Coleman JW (1996) Keeping up with drug allergy. Clin Exp Allerg 26: 1341-1342

Fishwick J, Mclean WG, Edwards G, Ward SA (1995) The toxicity of Artemisinin and related compounds on neuronal and glial cells in culture. Chem Biol Interact 96: 263-271

Green VJ, Pirmohamed M, Kitteringham N, Knapp MJ, Park BK (1995) Glutathione-S-transferase u genotype (GSTM1*O) in Alzheimer's patients with tacrine transaminitis. Br J Clin Pharmacol 39: 411-415

Haycox A, Barton S, Walley T (1996) Cost effectiveness of lowering cholesterol. Br Med J 313: 1142-1143

Ismail S, Na Banchang K, Na Barwan J, Back DJ, Edwards G (1996) Paracetamol disposition in Thai patients during and after treatment of falciparum malaria. Eur J Clin Pharmacol 48: 65-70

Lloyd Jones G, Walley T, Bligh J (1996) Integrating clinical pharmacology in a new problem based medical undergraduate curriculum. Br J Clin Pharmacol 43: 15-19

Park BK, Pirmohamed M, Kitteringham N (1995) The role of cytochrome P-450 enzymes in hepatic and extrahepatic human drug toxicity. Pharm Ther 68: 385-424

Winstanley PA, Khoo S, Szwandt IS, Edwards G, Wilkins E, Tjia J, Coker S, McKane W, Beeching N, Watkins S, Breckenridge AM (1995) Marked variation in pyrimethamine disposition in AIDS patients treated for cerebral toxoplasmosis. J Antimicrob Chemother 36: 435-439

London
Imperial College School of Medicine

The National Heart and Lung Institute (NHLI) is a Division of the newly formed Imperial College School of Medicine, which includes Hammersmith, St Mary's and Charing Cross Hospitals. The Department of Respiratory Medicine which covers all these hospitals is the largest such department in Europe and covers the whole range of respiratory medicine with research opportunities in many areas, including clinical pharmacology. The Department of Thoracic Medicine at NHLI has a particular interest in respiratory pharmacology, and in particular the therapy of asthma and other obstructive lung diseases. There is a wide range of expertise in molecular and cell biology, animal models of asthma and in clinical studies of asthma. There is an active Clinical Studies Unit that undertakes phase I-III studies with novel asthma drugs. In addition, there is a very active programme of clinical studies in asthma, based at the Royal Brompton Hospital, using sophisticated tests of lung function, airway responsiveness and markers of airway inflammation. Details of the research undertaken in the department may be obtained at the internet address, see address list.

The Professorial group within the Department of Thoracic Medicine has approximately 50 full time researchers, of whom one third are clinical. This group publishes approximately 60 papers per annum in peer-reviewed journals.

The NHLI is a postgraduate research institution with a strong focus on research in heart and lung diseases. It was one of only three clinical institutions in the UK rated as the highest grade (5*) in the recent Research Assessment Exercise and has one of the highest impact of journal citations of any department in the UK.

Enquiries: Professor PJ Barnes.

References

Barnes PJ, Karin M (1997) Nuclear factor-B: a pivotal transcription factor in chronic inflammatory diseases. N Engl J Med 336:1066-1071

Evans DJ, Barnes PJ, Coulby LJ, Spaethe SM, van Alstyne EC, Pechous PA, Mitchell MI, O'Connor BJ (1996) The effect of a leukotriene B4 antagonist LY293111 on allergen-induced responses in asthma. Thorax 51:1178-1184

Fox AJ, Lalloo UG, Belvisi MG, Bernareggi M, Chung KF, Barnes PJ (1996) Bradykinin-evoked sensitization of airway sensory nerves: a mechanism for ACE-inhibitor cough. Nature Med 2: 814-817

Fox AJ, Barnes PJ, Venkatesan P, Belvisi MG (1997) Activation of large conductance potassium channels inhibits the afferent and efferent function of airway sensory nerves. J Clin Invest 99:513-519

Haddad E-B, Rousell J, Lindsay MA, Barnes PJ (1996) Synergy between TNF-a and IL-1b in inducing down-regulation of muscarinic M2 receptor gene expression. J Biol Chem 271:32586-32592

John M, Hirst SJ, Jose P, Robichaud A, Witt C, Twort C, Berkman N, Barnes PJ, Chung KF (1997) Human airway smooth muscle cells express and release RANTES in response to Th1 cytokines: regulation by Th2 cytokines. J Immunol 158: 1841-1847

Keatings VM, Jatakanon A, Worsdell YM, Barnes PJ (1997) Effects of inhaled and oral glucocorticoids on inflammatory indices in asthma and COPD. Am J Respir Crit Care Med 155: 542-548

Kharitonov SA, Yates DH, Barnes PJ (1996) Regular inhaled budesonide decreases nitric oxide concentration in the exhaled air of asthmatic patients. Am J Resp Crit Care Med 153: 454-457

O'Connor BJ, Towse LJ, Barnes PJ (1996) Prolonged effect of tiotropium bromide on methacholine-induced bronchoconstriction in asthma. Am J Respir Crit Care Med 154: 876-880

Yates DH, Kharitonov SA, Barnes PJ (1996) An inhaled glucocorticoid does not prevent tolerance to salmeterol in mild asthma. Am J Respir Crit Care Med 154: 1603-1607

United Medical and Dental School of Guy's and St. Thomas's Hospitals (UMDS)

The department is involved in research in human vascular pharmacology, particularly into the relationship of endothelial function to atherosclerotic risk factors including hypertension, dyslipidaemia and diabetes mellitus. There are two specialist registrars, both of whom are training jointly in general internal medicine as well as clinical pharmacology. In addition, there are currently three PhD students and there is the opportunity for both clinical and non-clinical research fellowships provided applications are made with sufficient notice to seek outside funding.

There are clinical facilities for training in GIM with an inpatient as well as an outpatient service. The department has approximately 122 m^2 of laboratory space including tissue culture and general laboratory facilities, in addition to a blood flow laboratory and general clinical laboratories. There is also a superbly equipped phase I unit (Guy's Drug Research Unit) and the option of training in human toxicology (National Poisons Centre).

UMDS is part of London University, and is currently undergoing merger with King's College.

Staff: Professor JM Ritter (Head of Department & Honorary Consultant), Dr PJ Chowienczyk (Senior Lecturer/Honorary Consultant), Dr A Ferro (Senior Lecturer/Honorary Consultant), Dr M Dawes (Lecturer/Specialist Registrar), Dr R Kelly (Lecturer/Specialist Registrar), Dr TGK Mant (Director, Guy's Drug Research Unit/Honorary Senior Lecturer), Dr G Volans (Poisons Unit/Honorary Senior Lecturer), Dr J Warren (Honorary Senior Lecturer), Dr D Amin (Honorary Lecturer), Dr I Rajman (Honorary Lecturer)

Application Procedures: Specialist Registrar training vacancies are advertised in the Lancet and/or British Medical Journal which specify the application procedure. Informal enquiries should be made regarding other training/fellowship opportunities.

Enquiries: informal enquiries should be made in the first instance to the Head of Department or to one of the Senior Lecturers.

References

Adatia I et al. (1993)Thromboxane A2 and prostacyclin biosynthesis in children and adolescents with pulmonary vascular disease. Circulation 88: 2117-2122

Chowienczyk PJ et al. (1993) Differential inhibition by NG-monomethyl-L-arginine of vasodilator effects of acetylcholine and methacholine in human forearm vasculature. Br J Pharmacol 110: 736-738

Chowienczyk PJ et al. (1994) Sex differences in endothelial function in normal and hypercholesterolaemic subjects. Lancet 344: 305-306

Chowienczyk PJ et al. (1995) Inhibition of acetylcholinesterase selectively potentiates NGmonomethyl-L-arginine-resistant actions of acetylcholine in human forearm vasculature. Clin Sci 88: 111-117

Chowienczyk PJ et al. (1997) Preserved endothelial function in patients with severe hypertriglyceridemia and low functional lipoprotein lipase activity. J Am Coll Cardiol 29: 964-968

Cockcroft JR et al. (1994) Preserved endothelium-dependent vasodilatation in patients with essential hypertension. N Engl J Med 330: 1036-1040

Dawes M et al. (1997) Effects of inhibition of the L-arginine/nitric oxide pathway on vasodilation caused by β-adrenergic agonists in human forearm. Circulation 95: 2293-2297

Edwards JS, Ritter JM (1994) Effects of cytoplasmic pH on Ca2+-stimulated eicosanoid biosynthesis in human platelets. Br J Pharmacol 113: 926-930

Elliott TG et al. (1993) Inhibition of nitric oxide synthesis in forearm vasculature of insulindependent diabetic patients: blunted vasoconstriction in patients with microalbuminuria. Clin Sci 85: 687-693

Ritter JM et al. (1993) Thromboxane A: receptor antagonism and synthase inhibition in essential hypertension. Hypertension 22: 197-203

University College London
Centre for Clinical Pharmacology, Therapeutics & Toxicology

University College of London has been a centre for excellence in pharmacology and physiology for over 100 years, since the days of Sidney Ringer.

Within Clinical Pharmacology, there is a major research interest in vascular reactivity, inflammation, atherogenesis and the role of the endothelium and nitric oxide. The human pharmacology research spans molecular biology, in vitro pharmacology and studies in healthy volunteers and patient groups. The approach is to integrate basic and clinical investigation to ensure rapid progress in areas relevant to human disease. Drugs are used to probe mechanisms and identify novel therapeutic targets.

A number of different groups in medical and basic sciences are interested in problems of cell injury and cell death. The Centre for Clinical Pharmacology, Therapeutics and Toxicology is now working to bring these varied groups into contact so that biologists and geneticists interested in the role of the Bcl2 gene are brought into contact with clinical groups interested in renal injury following transplantation, and toxicologists interested in cell death after paracetamol overdose. The underlying genetic and biochemical mechanisms are so similar in different cell injury models that bringing these groups together to form a joint cytotoxicity group is likely to prove intensely fruitful.

The Centre is also active in Drug Policy and Usage because there is a general interest in the rational and safe use of medicines. This ranges from specific research projects exploring drug utilisation and adverse events, to implementation of local guidelines and providing advice to national and international bodies.

The Centre is involved in teaching human pharmacology, toxicology and therapeutics to medical students. In addition, BSc units in Clinical Pharmacology, Human Vascular Pharmacology and Toxicology are underway or planned. The Centre has a number of PhD students and actively promotes interaction between groups and individuals. Students are expected and encouraged to take a broad view of Clinical Pharmacology, Toxicology and Therapeutics outside the direct area of interest of the research project. There is a seminar programme designed to cover a wide range of pharmacological and toxicological subjects. Students are expected to present their own research and are taught the skills of presentation and communication.

The Centre runs a general medical team and has a specific clinical interest in cardiovascular disorders. There are close links and shared appointments with Clinical Cardiology. Besides, members of the Centre for Clinical Pharmacology, Therapeutics and Toxicology have acted as consultants to government departments and industrial firms concerned with safety and efficacy of chemicals and drugs. This activity continues with the proviso that it must not interfere with the fundamental teaching and research activities of the group.

The total number of researchers exceeds 30 and we are in the process of appointing two new Senior Lecturers and a Lecturer. The research is funded by grants from The Wellcome Trust, British Heart Foundation and MRC.

References

Beales D and McLean AEM (1996) Protection in the late stage of paracetamol induced liver cell injury with fructose, cyclosporin A and trifluoperazine. Toxicology (in press)

Bhagat K, Collier J, Vallance P (1995) Vasodilatation to arachidonic acid in humans: an insight into endogenous prostanoids and effects of aspirin. Circulation 92: 2113-2118

Bhagat K, Collier J, Vallance P (1996) Local venous responses to endotoxin in humans. Circulation 94: 490-497

Bogle R, Vallance P (1996) Functional effects of econazole on inducible nitric oxide synthase: production of a calmodulin-dependent enzyme. Br J Pharmacol 117: 1053-1058

Bogle RG, MacAllister RJ, Whitley GSJ, Vallance P (1995) Induction of NG-monomethyl-L-arginine (LNMMA) uptake by human endothelial cells and murine macrophages: A possible mechanism for differential inhibition of nitric oxide biosynthesis. Am J Physiol 269: C750-756

Cruickshank JM, Prichard BNC (1994) Beta Blockers in Clinical Practice, Churchill Livingstone, Edinburgh

Petros A, Bennett D, Vallance P (1991) Effect of nitric oxide synthase inhibitors on hypotension in patients with septic shock. Lancet 338: 1557-1558

Smith CCT, Prichard BNC, Betteridge DJ (1992) Plasma and platelet free catecholamines in patients with familial hypercholesterolaemia. Clin Sci 82:113-116

Vallance P, Collier J, Moncada S (1989) Effects of endothelium-derived nitric oxide on peripheral arterial tone in man. Lancet (ii): 997-1000

Vallance P, Leone A, Calver A, Collier J, Moncada S (1992) Accumulation of an endogenous inhibitor of nitric oxide synthesis in chronic renal failure. Lancet 339: 572-576

Nottingham

The Division of Therapeutics is part of the Section of Medicine within the School of Medical and Surgical Sciences at the University of Nottingham. The current Head of Division is Dr IP Hall.

The Division of Therapeutics has two main roles, namely research and training in Clinical Pharmacology. Major research interests within the Division include (1) regulation of receptor expression and coupling (particularly in airway tissues), (2) regulation of intracellular second messenger pathways and (3) the genetics of complex disease, (particularly the pharmacogenetics of asthma). Professor Rubin, the previous Head of Department, has maintained links with the Division in his new role as Dean of the Medical School in Nottingham and has interests in the medical disorders of pregnancy. The Division of Therapeutics co-ordinates training in clinical pharmacology both at the postgraduate and undergraduate level.

Facilities within the division include a dedicated phase I-III clinical unit, and fully equipped laboratories including human tissue culture facilities and fully equipped molecular biology laboratories.

Academic staff: one professor, four doctors.

Inquiries: should all be addressed in the first instance to Dr IP Hall.

References

Dewar JC, Wilkinson J, Wheatley A. Thomas S, Doull I, Morton N, Lio P, Harvey J, Liggett SB, Holgate ST, Hall IP (1997) The glutamine 27 β_2 adrenoceptor polymorphism is associated with elevated IgE levels in asthmatic families. J Allerg Clin Immunol 100: 261-265

Green SA, Turki J, Bejarna P, Hall IP, Liggett SB (1995) Influence of β_2-adrenergic receptor genotypes on signal transduction in human airway smooth muscle cells. Am J Respir Cell and Mol Biol 13: 25-33

Hall IP, Wheatley A, Wilding P, Liggett SB (1995) Association of the Glu 27 β_2 adrenoreceptor polymorphism with lower airway reactivity in asthmatic subjects.

Jobson TM, Billington C, Hall IP (in press) Regulation of proliferation of human colonic subepithelial myofibroblasts by mediators important in inflammatory bowel disease. J Clin Invest

Kume H, Hall IP, Washabau RJ, Tagaki K, Kotlikoff MI (1994) β_2-Adrenergic agonists regulate Kca channels in airway smooth muscle by cAMP dependent and independent mechanisms. J Clin Invest 93: 371-379

McCreath G, Hall IP, Hill SJ (1994) Agonist induced desensitization of histamine H1-receptor mediated inositol phospholipid hydrolysis in human umbilical vein endothelial cells. Br J Pharmacol 113: 823-830

Panettieri RA, Hall IP, Murray RK (1995) Thrombin increases cytosolic calcium and induces human airway smooth muscle cell proliferation. Am J Respir Cell Mol Biol 13: 205-213

Tan S, Hall IP, Dewar J, Dow E, Lipworth B (1997) Association between β_2 adrenoceptor polymorphism and susceptibility to bronchodilator desensitisation in moderately severe asthmatics. Lancet 350: 995-1000

Sandwich

Pfizer Inc. is a research-based health-care company with global operations. In 1997, Pfizer anticipates investing approximately $2 billion on research and development.

The European Early Clinical Research Group is located on three sites. Sandwich is the European headquarters for Pfizer Central Research and is where the majority of staff within the department are based. There is also a 18-bed Clinical Research Unit in Canterbury (UK) and a 30-bed unit in Brussels. The department provides clinical advice to all Sandwich-based drug discovery teams and is responsible for clinical methodology development, phase I and early phase II studies. The clinical trials are conducted at the Pfizer units, at Contract Research Organisations or at academic centres. Training is thus provided in clinical pharmacology and pharmaceutical medicine. The department also co-funds training registrar positions within the UK scheme set up by the ABPI and the Royal College of Physicians.

The Early Clinical Research Group employs approximately 65 people; a mixture of physicians, post-doctorate scientists, life science graduates, nurses, administrative and technical staff.

Interested physicians and/or scientists should write to Dr M J Allen, including a copy of their CV.

Sheffield

The two Sections have an integrated programme with interests spanning from the molecular biology of cytochromes P450, drug metabolism, PK/PD modelling including population approaches, pharmacogenetics, clinical trials design, risk assessment and management, evidence-based therapy. Special areas of therapeutic interest include hypertension, hyperlipidaemia, cancer, diabetes and drugs of abuse. The Section of CP & T has care of patients in 30 acute medical beds and runs general medical and hypertension outpatient clinics.

The Section is involved in teaching of Medical/Dental undergraduate and postgraduates and non-clinical Honours BSc Pharmacology students.

Within the two Sections, there are five clinical and eight non-clinical academic staff, a clinical trial research physician, three research fellows, a research nurse, six research technicians, two teaching technicians, 15 postgraduate students, a research administrator and two secretaries.

References

Chadwick IG et al. (1996) No relation between angiotensin-converting enzyme gene polymorphism and dermal responses to bradykinin in healthy subjects. Br J Clin Pharmacol 91: 617

Ellis SW et al. (1996) Evidence that aspartic acid 301 is a critical substrate-contact residue in the active site of cytochrome P450 2D6. J Biol Chem 270: 29055

Ghahramani P et al. (1997) Cytochromes P450 mediating the N-demethylation of amitriptyline. Br J Clin Pharmacol 43: 137

Haq IU et al. (1996) Lipid-lowering for prevention of coronary heart disease: what policy now? Clin Sci 91: 399

Lennard L et al. (1997) Thiopurine methyltransferase deficiency in childhood lymphoblastic leukaemia: 6-mercaptopurine dosage strategies. Med Pediat Oncology 29: 252

Ramsay LE et al. (1996) The Sheffield table for primary prevention of coronary heart disease: corrected. Lancet 348: 1251

Rostami-Hodjegan A et al. (1996) Caffeine urinary metabolite ratios as markers of enzyme activity: a theoretical assessment. Pharmacogenetics 6: 121

Tucker GT (1994) Clinical implications of genetic polymorphism in drug metabolism. J Pharm Pharmacol 46:417

Williams ML et al. (1994) Interindividual variation in the isomerization of 4-hydroxytamoxifen by human liver microsomes: involvement of cytochromes P450. Carcinogenesis 15: 2733

Yeo WW et al. (1995) Resolution of ACE inhibitor cough after stopping enalapril: Changes in subjective symptoms, capsaicin dose-response and skin response to bradykinin. Br J Clin Pharmacol 40: 423

Southampton

Clinical Pharmacology in Southampton has laboratory space in both the Biomedical Sciences Building and in the Southampton University Hospitals where the Group delivers its clinical responsibilities. Besides teaching medical undergraduates, there is a strong postgraduate research training programme.

Research interests are focused on cardiovascular clinical pharmacology; drugs in the elderly; compliance with drug therapy; drug metabolism and toxicokinetics and the immunopharmacology of asthma and cutaneous diseases. Links have been established with the Drug Safety Research Unit at Bursledon for pharmacovigilance studies. The group provides a back-up to the Regional Drug Information Centre and members serve also on national committees concerned with drug regulation and formulary committees.

The group comprises Professor CF George (clinical pharmacology), Professor MK Church (immunopharmacology), Professor AG Renwick (biochemical pharmacology; Head), two senior lecturers and a lecturer.

Applications/enquiries should be directed to Professor AG Renwick.

Welwyn Garden City

The Department of Clinical Pharmacology Operations of Roche is headquartered in the UK, where 25 medical and scientific staff manage all Roche clinical pharmacology studies throughout the world. These staff become involved with, and have published on, new medicines being developed for a wide range of therapeutic indications on many aspects of clinical pharmacology.

The department operates a Clinical Pharmacology Unit on the Roche campus, employing a further 15 medical and nursing staff conducting studies ranging from entry-into-man through to studies on over-the-counter medication, with expertise in cardiovascular and central nervous system techniques and methodologies. For specialized investigations, several links have been made with external academic groups.

Roche has five research sites, with Welwyn Garden City concentrating on research in virology (the others in Basle, Switzerland; New Jersey and California, USA; and Japan).

New employees receive training 'on-the-job', by specific short courses with invited trainers, and by externally organized courses. Staff have the opportunity to study for academic qualifications such as the Diploma in Clinical Pharmacology or the Diploma and MSc in Pharmaceutical Medicine.

In addition, the Department collaborates with the Department of Medicine, Western General Hospital, Edinburgh, in a joint Clinical Pharmacology training programme.

Inquiries should be addressed to Dr McClelland.

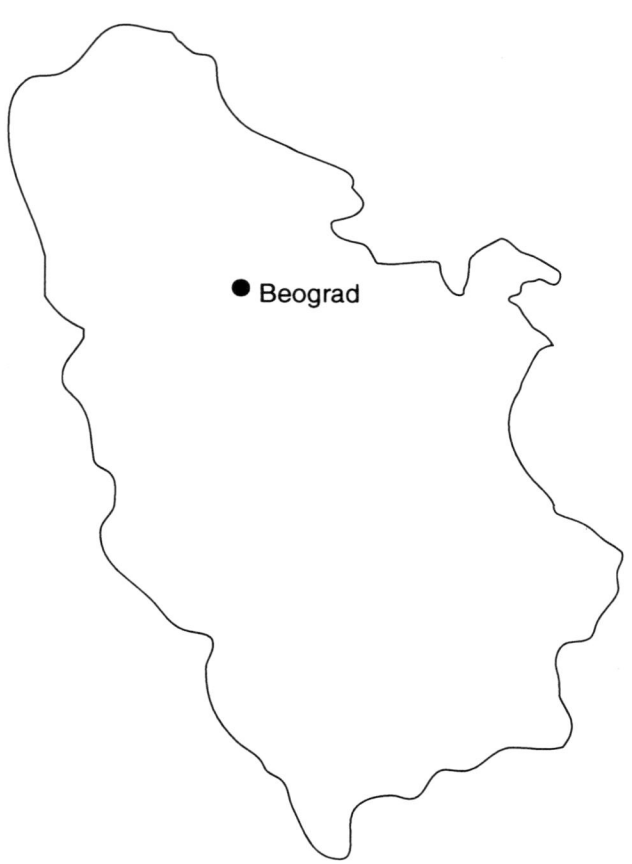

Yugoslavia

Clinical pharmacology has been an independent medical speciality since 1981. The training lasts 3 years after graduation as MD. Of the 36 months, 13 are spent in experimental pharmacology, nine with formal lectures and 14 with clinical training. At present there are 34 trainees enrolled in the programme. A shorter training programme only lasting 18 months also exists for specialists in internal medicine, anaesthesiology, paediatrics, infectious diseases and psychiatry. At present, another 107 trainees are enrolled in this programme.

The Section of Clinical Pharmacology is part of the Society of Pharmacology in Yugoslavia and it has about 100 members at the moment. The section was established in 1994. Four times a year, the section organizes scientific meetings in collaboration with the Yugoslavian Society of Pharmacology. Joint meetings are also organized in collaboration with the section of Pharmacotherapy which is part of the Serbian Medical Association. The section has several goals for the future. It will work for improving the quality of all types of drug trials. It will also participate in the activities at the National Centre for Drug Adverse Effects located at the University Clinical Centre of Serbia in Belgrade. The section will also seek to improve teaching in clinical pharmacology at all levels. The section has introduced the area of pharmacoepidemiology in Yugoslavia as well as the areas of pharmacoeconomy, drug information and drug utilization. Finally, it is responsible for 'Pharmacy' which is the official publication of the Section of Clinical Pharmacology.

There are five medical schools in Yugoslavia: Belgrade, Novi Sad, Kragujevac, Nis, and Pristina. At the universities in Belgrade, Kragujevac and Novi Sad, there are joint departments of pharmacology, clinical pharmacology and toxicology. There is an increasing understanding of the need for teaching clinical pharmacology to medical students. The most recent proposal says 30 lectures given during the last year in medical school. The departments of pharmacology, clinical pharmacology and toxicology will be responsible for the course.

There are three smaller units of clinical pharmacology at the departments of neurology, infectious diseases and the Institute of Oncology and Radiology in Serbia. There are no separate departments or institutes of Clinical Pharmacology in Yugoslavia.

Addresses

Belgrade
Professor T Kažić
Section of Clinical Pharmacology
Institute of Clinical Pharmacology, Pharmacology and Toxicology
Belgrade University Medical School
POB 662
11000 Belgrade
Phone: +381 11 688 348
Fax: +381 11 686 025

Dr Radulovš Siniša
Department of Clinical Pharmacology
Institute for Oncology and Radiology of Serbia
Pasterova 14
11000 Belgrade
Phone: +381 11 235 2358
Fax: +381 11 685 300